A PRACTICAL GUIDE TO FETAL ECHOCARDIOGRAPHY

NORMAL AND ABNORMAL HEARTS *Second Edition*

Alfred Abuhamad, MD

Professor of Obstetrics & Gynecology
Professor of Radiology
Chairman, Department of Obstetrics & Gynecology
Eastern Virginia Medical School
Norfolk, Virginia

Rabih Chaoui, MD

Professor of Obstetrics & Gynecology
Prenatal Diagnosis and Human Genetics Center
Berlin, Germany

🟤 Wolters Kluwer | Lippincott Williams & Wilkins
Health

Philadelphia • Baltimore • New York • London
Buenos Aires • Hong Kong • Sydney • Tokyo

Acquisitions Editor: Brian Brown
Product Manager: Ryan Shaw
Vendor Manager: Alicia Jackson
Senior Manufacturing Manager: Benjamin Rivera
Senior Marketing Manager: Angela Panetta
Design Coordinator: Holly McLaughlin
Production Service: Cadmus Communications

Printed in China

Library of Congress Cataloging-in-Publication Data
ISBN-13: 978-0-7817-9757-3
ISBN-10: 0-7817-9757-8
Abuhamad, Alfred.
  A practical guide to fetal echocardiography : normal and abnormal hearts / Alfred Abuhamad, Rabih Chaoui. – 2nd ed.
      p. ; cm.
  Includes bibliographical references and index.
  ISBN 978-0-7817-9757-3
    1. Fetal heart–Ultrasonic imaging. I. Chaoui, Rabih. II. Title.
  [DNLM: 1. Fetal Heart–ultrasonography. 2. Heart Defects, Congenital–ultrasonography. 3. Ultrasonography, Prenatal–methods. WQ 210.5 A1651p 2010]
    RG628.3.E34A28 2010
    618.3'26107543–dc22

                                                                    2009031203

Care has been taken to confirm the accuracy of the information presented and to describe generally accepted practices. However, the authors, editors, and publisher are not responsible for errors or omissions or for any consequences from application of the information in this book and make no warranty, expressed or implied, with respect to the currency, completeness, or accuracy of the contents of the publication. Application of the information in a particular situation remains the professional responsibility of the practitioner.

The authors, editors, and publisher have exerted every effort to ensure that drug selection and dosage set forth in this text are in accordance with current recommendations and practice at the time of publication. However, in view of ongoing research, changes in government regulations, and the constant flow of information relating to drug therapy and drug reactions, the reader is urged to check the package insert for each drug for any change in indications and dosage and for added warnings and precautions. This is particularly important when the recommended agent is a new or infrequently employed drug.

Some drugs and medical devices presented in the publication have Food and Drug Administration (FDA) clearance for limited use in restricted research settings. It is the responsibility of the health care provider to ascertain the FDA status of each drug or device planned for use in their clinical practice.

To purchase additional copies of this book, call our customer service department at (800) 638-3030 or fax orders to (301) 223-2320. International customers should call (301) 223-2300.

Visit Lippincott Williams & Wilkins on the Internet: at LWW.com. Lippincott Williams & Wilkins customer service representatives are available from 8:30 am to 6:00 pm, EST.

RRS1308

*To our parents for their unwavering support and commitment
to excellence throughout the years, and to*

*Sami and Nicole
Kathleen, Amin and Ella,*

With love and admiration.

$\mathcal{F}$or a variety of reasons, when I was invited to write a brief foreword to this book, I could not say no. However, only after I received the chapter drafts did I realize what a bonus it was to have an advance copy in my hands, months before the book comes out. I often groan when I hear people say, when describing a novel, "I couldn't put the book down," because the phrase is so over used. Well, this book messed up my whole weekend because I could not put it down.

Why? Because it encompasses not only what anyone in the field needs to know about various abnormalities of the fetal heart, but, most importantly, it tells the reader how to tweak the utmost information out of today's available equipment in order to screen for cardiac abnormalities and to pinpoint the exact problem if an anomaly is suspected. Each chapter is replete with helpful hints on how to optimize one's image, and how to utilize selectively M mode, pulse wave Doppler, color Doppler, 3-D technology (TUI, STIC, inversion mode, enhanced color flow, etc) in route to solving many diagnostic puzzles. To keep the reader on track, key points are summarized at the end of each chapter.

The book is laid out in a logical sequence, starting with general information on the epidemiology of cardiac defects and how to screen for them. Then there are two "how-to" and "what to look for" chapters on the four chamber view and outflow tracts, followed by chapters each on color Doppler, pulse Doppler, 3-D with its bells and whistles, and another on the use of fetal echocardiography in early gestation (to satisfy a new trend in prenatal diagnosis). The last chapters cover comprehensively virtually every cardiac abnormality a fetus can have, including cardiomyopathies and arrhythmias.

The authors form a formidable team of two of the best-known clinician/investigators who are recognized internationally for their work in fetal echocardiography and also in various other aspects of prenatal diagnosis. Dr. Chaoui trained in Europe, and Dr. Abuhamad spent his formative years in the United States. For years I have been impressed with the quality and depth of Dr. Chaoui's contributions. My contact with Dr. Abuhamad has been first hand, starting from the first day he set foot in Yale as a fellow. On the second day, everyone in the division knew he would be one of the brightest stars in the field.

Fetal echocardiographers generally come into the field via one of two pathways: pediatric cardiology or perinatology (a few such as Benaceraff and Jeanty, who have roots in Radiology, are exceptions). Those pursuing the first pathway are immersed in all aspects of cardiac dynamics from the start—training that is put into play daily in the care of children and, often, fetuses with cardiac abnormalities. Doctors Abuhamad and Chaoui arrived by the second route—one that requires self-education, rather than a formalized program. This is evident in the way we, the readers, are methodically taught in each chapter.

From my standpoint, this will become the ultimate text on the fetal heart. Actually, and I am reluctant to say this as an author of books that have had modest sales, this may be one of the very best ultrasound- related books around—period!

— *John C. Hobbins, MD.*

*I*t is with great pleasure that we introduce this second edition of *A Practical Guide to Fetal Echocardiography: Normal and Abnormal Hearts*, a product of intense work and collaboration on this important and rapidly progressing field of fetal cardiology. As we decided to embark on this project, we strived to ensure that this book provides the most up-to-date and comprehensive reference on this subject written in an easy to read style and illustrated with the most informative figures. In keeping with progress in fetal imaging, we also included detailed information on the use of color Doppler and three-dimensional ultrasound in fetal echocardiography and an in-depth discussion on the evolving topic of cardiac imaging in the first trimester. In order to maintain the systematic and methodical approach of this book, the authors chose the difficult path of writing the book in its entirety without outside collaboration.

The book is divided into two parts, part one covers the normal heart with a focus on detailed normal anatomy as seen from multiple imaging planes, screening and prevention of congenital heart disease, genetic aspects of cardiac anomalies and the role of color, pulsed Doppler, three dimensional ultrasound and early gestation scanning in fetal echocardiography. Detailed discussion on fetal cardiac malformations is presented in the second part of the book in a uniform format that includes the definition, spectrum of disease and incidence, the use of gray scale, color Doppler, three-dimensional and early gestation ultrasound in the diagnosis of each cardiac abnormality followed by the differential diagnosis, prognosis and outcome. Schematics and drawings illustrate cardiac anomalies and the book relies on the liberal use of tables outlining common and differentiating features of various cardiac malformations.

Congenital heart disease is the most common congenital malformation with a significant impact on neonatal morbidity and mortality. Prenatal diagnosis of congenital heart disease has been suboptimal over the years owing in large part to the complexity of cardiac anatomy and the inherent difficulty of the ultrasound examination of the fetal heart. We feel that this book provides a comprehensive reference to the practitioners involved in prenatal diagnosis and we sincerely hope that this book enhances the detection rate of congenital heart disease which should translate into improved outcome for our smallest of patients.

This book would not have been a reality without the support of several people, first and foremost, our families and friends who unselfishly allowed us to spend long hours away from them in completing this task, the artistic talents of Ms. Patricia Gast who performed all the superb drawings in this book in an efficient and accurate manner, Dr. Elena Sinkovskaya, pediatric cardiologist, for her assistance in reviewing several chapters and providing valuable input, Ms. Kerry Jones for her professionalism and outstanding administrative support, Dr. Cornelia Tennstedt for her superb expertise in cardiac pathology and who generously provided the anatomic figures in the book, Dr. Kai-Sven Heling, Dr. Chaoui's clinical partner, for his cooperation throughout the years in the field of fetal echocardiography and the professional editorial team at Lippincott Williams and Wilkins. Finally, we would like to thank Skype, the internet software, for the ease with which we (the authors) communicated several times per week across 2 continents.

In closing, we owe a great debt of gratitude to two giants in the field of ultrasound, Dr. John Hobbins (for Dr. Abuhamad) and Dr. Rainer Bollmann (for Dr. Chaoui) who gave us our ultrasound roots and provided mentorship and guidance.

We sincerely hope that this book contributes to your academic and clinical success.

Alfred Abuhamad, MD—Norfolk, Virginia

Rabih Chaoui, MD—Berlin, Germany

CONTENTS

INCIDENCE OF CONGENITAL HEART DISEASE

Congenital heart disease (CHD) is the most common severe congenital abnormality (1). Half of the cases of CHD are minor and are easily corrected by surgery, with the remainder accounting for over half of the deaths from congenital abnormalities in childhood (1). Moreover, CHD results in the most costly hospital admissions for birth defects in the United States (2). The incidence of CHD is dependent on the age at which the population is initially screened and the definition of CHD used. Inclusion of a large number of premature neonates in a study may increase the incidence of CHD. Both patent ductus arteriosus and ventricular septal defects are common in premature infants. An incidence of 8 to 9 per 1000 live births has been reported in large population studies (1). Of all cases of CHD, 46% are diagnosed by the first week of life, 88% by the first year of life, and 98% by the fourth year of life (1). The incidence of CHD is also influenced by the inclusion of bicuspid aortic valve, the incidence of which is estimated at 10 to 20 per 1000 live births (3,4). Bicuspid aortic valve may be associated with considerable morbidity and mortality in affected individuals (3). Furthermore, accounting for subtle anomalies such as persistent superior vena cava (5 to 10 per 1000 live births) and isolated aneurysm of the atrial septum (5 to 10 per 1000 live births) results in an overall incidence of CHD approaching 50 per 1000 live births (5). CHD remains the most common severe abnormality in the newborn; its prenatal diagnosis allows for better pregnancy counseling and improved neonatal outcome. Table 1-1 lists incidence by specific type of CHD (6).

RISK FACTORS FOR CONGENITAL HEART DISEASE

The majority of fetuses with CHD have no known risk factors (7). In spite of this, fetal echocardiography has been traditionally performed on pregnancies with identifiable risk factors for CHD. Risk factors for CHD can be grouped into two main categories: fetal factors and maternal factors (Table 1-2). The association of CHD with a prior family history of such, or in the presence of fetal chromosomal abnormalities, will be discussed in the following chapter.

Fetal Risk Factors

Extracardiac Anatomic Abnormalities
The presence of extracardiac abnormalities in a fetus is frequently associated with CHD and is thus an indication for fetal echocardiography. The risk of CHD is dependent on the specific type of fetal malformation. Abnormalities detected in more than one organ system increase the risk of CHD and also of concomitant chromosomal abnormalities. Nonimmune hydrops in the fetus is frequently associated with CHD. Incidence of abnormal cardiac anatomy is reported in about 10% to 20% of fetuses with nonimmune hydrops (8,9). Table 1-3 lists extracardiac fetal abnormalities and the incidence of associated CHD (10–24).

Fetal Cardiac Arrhythmia
The presence of fetal cardiac rhythm disturbances may be associated with an underlying structural heart disease. Isolated extrasystoles account for more than 90% of fetal cardiac arrhythmias (25). Overall, about 1% of fetal cardiac arrhythmias are associated with CHD (8). Complete heart block, on the other hand, is associated with structural cardiac abnormalities in about 50% of fetuses, with the remaining pregnancies associated with the presence of maternal Sjögren antibodies (26). Diagnosis and management of fetal cardiac rhythm disturbances is discussed in detail in Chapter 25.

Suspected Cardiac Anomaly on Routine Ultrasound
A risk factor with one of the highest yields for CHD is the suspicion for the presence of a cardiac abnormality during routine ultrasound scanning. CHD is confirmed in about 40% to

TABLE 1-1	Types and Incidence of Human Congenital Heart Disease

Defect	Incidence per 1000 live births
VSD	3.570
PDA	0.799
ASD	0.941
AVSD	0.348
PS	0.729
AS	0.401
CoA	0.409
TOF	0.421
D-TGA	0.315
HRH	0.222
Tricuspid atresia	0.079
Ebstein anomaly	0.114
Pulmonary atresia	0.132
HLH	0.266
Truncus	0.107
DORV	0.157
SV	0.106
TAPVC	0.094

VSD, ventricular septal defect; PDA, patent ductus arteriosus; ASD, atrial septal defect; AVSD, atrioventricular septal defect; PS, pulmonary stenosis; AS, aortic stenosis; CoA, coarctation of the aorta; TOF, tetralogy of Fallot; D-TGA, complete transposition of the great arteries; HRH, hypoplastic right heart; HLH, hypoplastic left heart; DORV, double outlet right ventricle; SV, single ventricle; TAPVC, total anomalous pulmonary venous connection.
(Modified from Hoffman JI, Kaplan S. The incidence of congenital heart disease. *Circ Res* 2004;94:1890–1900, with permission.)

50% of pregnancies referred with this finding (8,9). In view of this, and the fact that most infants born with CHD are born to pregnancies without risk factors, systemic ultrasound examination of the fetal heart should not be limited to pregnant mothers with known risk factors. The value of routine ultrasound in the screening for CHD is discussed in Chapter 3.

Thickened Nuchal Translucency
Measurement of fetal nuchal translucency (NT) thickness in the late first and early second trimesters of pregnancy is currently established as an effective method for individual risk

TABLE 1-2	Risk Factors for Congenital Heart Disease

Fetal
Chromosomal abnormalities
Extracardiac anatomic abnormalities
Fetal cardiac arrhythmia
Suspected cardiac anomaly on routine ultrasound
Thickened nuchal translucency
Monochorionic placentation

Maternal
Family history of congenital heart disease
Maternal metabolic disorders (diabetes, phenylketonuria)
Maternal teratogen exposure (drug related)
Pregnancy of assisted reproduction
Maternal obesity

TABLE 1-3	Incidence of Associated Congenital Heart Disease (CHD) with Extracardiac Malformation

Extracardiac malformation	% CHD
Nonimmune hydrops (8,9)	10–20
Single umbilical artery (10)	9.1
Ureteral obstruction (11)	2.1
Bilateral renal agenesis (11)	42.8
Unilateral renal agenesis (11)	16.9
Horseshoe kidney (11)	38.8
Renal dysplasia (11)	5.4
Isolated hydrocephalus (12)	4.4
Agenesis of corpus callosum (13)	14.8
Tracheoesophageal fistula (14)	14.7
Duodenal atresia (15)	17.1
Jejunal/ileal atresia (16)	5.2
Imperforate anus (17)	11.7
Omphalocele (18)	19.5
Pentalogy of Cantrell (19)	77.8
Beckwith-Wiedemann syndrome (20)	92.3
Diaphragmatic hernia (21)	9.6
Meckel-Gruber syndrome (22)	13.8
Dandy-Walker syndrome (23)	4.3

(Modified from Copel JA, Pilu G, Kleinman CS. Congenital heart disease and extracardiac anomalies: associations and indications for fetal echocardiography. *Am J Obstet Gynecol* 1986;154:1121–1132, with permission.)

assessment for fetal chromosomal abnormalities. Several reports have noted an association between increased NT and genetic syndromes and major fetal malformations including cardiac defects (27,28). The prevalence of major cardiac defects increases exponentially with fetal NT thickness, without an obvious predilection to a specific type of CHD (29). An NT thickness of greater than or equal to 3.5 mm in a chromosomally normal fetus has been correlated with a prevalence of CHD of 23 per 1000 pregnancies, a rate that is higher than pregnancies with a family history of CHD (29,30). In this setting of an NT that is greater than or equal to 3.5 mm, referral for fetal echocardiography is thus warranted. Finding an NT thickness of greater than or equal to 3.5 mm may lead to an earlier diagnosis of all major types of CHD (31). Table 1-4 lists the prevalence of CHD with NT thickness in chromosomally normal fetuses (30).

Monochorionic Placentation

The incidence of CHD in fetuses of monochorionic placentation is increased (32,33). This increased risk of CHD is noted even after excluding cardiac effects of twin–twin transfusion syndrome (TTTS) (32). In a cohort study of 165 sets of monochorionic twins, the overall risk of at least one of a twin pair having a structural CHD was 9.1% (32). This risk was 7% for monochorionic–diamniotic twins and 57.1% for at least one twin member of monochorionic–monoamniotic twins (32). If one twin member is affected, the risk that the other twin member is also affected is 26.7% (32). A systemic literature review of 830 fetuses from monochorionic–diamniotic twin pregnancies confirms an increased risk for CHD independent of TTTS (33). Ventricular septal defects were the most common type of CHD in non-TTTS fetuses, and pulmonary stenosis and atrial septal defects were significantly more prevalent in fetuses of pregnancies complicated with TTTS (33).

Maternal Risk Factors

Maternal Metabolic Disease

Maternal metabolic disorders, mainly diabetes mellitus, have a significant effect on the incidence of CHD. The incidence of CHD is fivefold higher in infants of diabetic mothers when

TABLE 1-4	Prevalence of Congenital Heart Disease (CHD) with Nuchal Translucency Thickness in Chromosomally Normal Fetus

Nuchal translucency	Prevalence CHD[a]
<2.0 mm	1.9/1000[b]
2.0–2.4 mm	4.8/1000[b]
2.5–3.4 mm	6.0/1000[b]
≥3.5 mm	23/1000[b]

[a] Prevalence in study population 2.6/1000.
[b] Per 1000 pregnancies.
(From Bahado-Singh RO, Wapner R, Thom E, et al. Elevated first-trimester nuchal translucency increases the risk of congenital heart defects. *Am J Obstet Gynecol* 2005;19:1357–1361, with permission.)

compared to controls (34). Ventricular septal defects and transposition of the great arteries are common cardiac defects in fetuses of diabetic pregnancies (34). Poor glycemic control in the first trimester of gestation, as evidenced by an elevated glycohemoglobin level (HgA1c), has been strongly correlated with an increased risk of structural defects in infants of diabetic mothers (35,36). Although some studies have identified a level of glycohemoglobin above which the risk for fetal structural abnormalities is increased (35), other studies have failed to identify a critical level of glycohemoglobin providing an optimal predictive power for CHD screening (37). Fetal echocardiography should therefore be offered to all pregnancies with initial glycohemoglobin levels above the upper limits of normal (37).

Another metabolic disorder that is associated with CHD is phenylketonuria. Women with phenylketonuria should be aware of the association of fetal CHD with elevated maternal phenylalanine levels (38). This is particularly important as phenylketonurics usually follow unrestricted dietary regimens in adulthood. Fetal exposure during organogenesis to maternal phenylalanine levels exceeding 15 mg/dL is associated with a 10- to 15-fold increase in congenital heart disease (39). Other fetal abnormalities in phenylketonurics include microcephaly and growth restriction (38). In the presence of maternal metabolic disease, preconception counseling and tight metabolic control immediately prior to and during organogenesis is required in order to reduce the incidence of fetal CHD.

Maternal Teratogen Exposure (Drug-related Congenital Heart Disease)

The effects of maternal exposure to drugs during cardiogenesis has been widely studied. Numerous drugs have been implicated as cardiac teratogens. Evidence suggests that the overall contribution of teratogens to CHD is small (40). Available literature suggests that maternal use of lithium, anticonvulsants, ethanol, isotretinoin, indomethacin, angiotensin-converting enzyme (ACE) inhibitors, and selective serotonin reuptake inhibitors may increase the risk of cardiovascular abnormalities in the newborn (Table 1-5).

Initial retrospective reports regarding the teratogenic risk of lithium treatment in pregnancy showed a strong association between lithium use and Ebstein anomaly in the fetus (41). More recent controlled studies, however, have consistently reported a lower risk for CHD in exposed fetuses. Four case-control studies of Ebstein anomaly involving a total of 208 affected children found no association with maternal lithium intake in pregnancy (42–45). A cohort study on the effect of lithium exposure in pregnancy showed no significant risk to the fetus (46). These findings suggest that the teratogenic risk of lithium exposure is lower than previously reported, and that the risk/benefit ratio of prescribing lithium in pregnancy should be evaluated in light of this modified risk estimate.

Anticonvulsants, a class of drugs that includes phenytoin and sodium valproate, are commonly used in the treatment of epilepsy or pain management in pregnancy. An incidence of congenital defects varying from 2.2% to 26.1% has been noted in pregnancies exposed to phenytoin (47). Some evidence suggests that the teratogenic effect of phenytoin is related to elevated amniotic fluid levels of oxidative metabolites secondary to low activity of the clearing enzyme epoxide hydrolase (48). A fetal hydantoin syndrome consisting of variable degrees of

TABLE 1-5	Drug-related Congenital Heart Disease	

Drug	Frequency of association	Common cardiac abnormalities
Lithium	Rare	Ebstein abnormality
Hydantoin	Moderate	Mixed abnormalities
Trimethadione	High	Septal defects
Valproic acid	Rare	Mixed abnormalities
Ethanol	High	Septal defects
Isotretinoin	Moderate	Conotruncal abnormalities
Indomethacin	Moderate	Premature constriction of ductus arteriosus
ACE inhibitors (1st trimester)	Moderate	Septal defects
ACE inhibitors (2nd and 3rd trimesters)	High	ACE inhibitor fetopathy
SSRIs (1st trimester)	Rare	Septal defects
SSRIs (2nd and 3rd trimesters)	Moderate	PPHN

ACE, angiotensin-converting enzyme; SSRIs, selective serotonin reuptake inhibitors; PPHN, persistent pulmonary hypertension of the newborn.

hypoplasia and ossification of distal phalanges and craniofacial abnormalities has been described (49). CHD is often observed in conjunction with this syndrome (50). Trimethadione, an anticonvulsant primarily used in the treatment of petit mal seizures, is associated with a high incidence of congenital defects. Defects include craniofacial deformities, growth abnormalities, mental retardation, limb abnormalities, and genitourinary abnormalities (51). Cardiac abnormalities are common, with septal defects occurring in about 20% of exposed fetuses (51). Valproic acid has also been associated with congenital defects, with the most serious abnormality being neural tube defects (1% to 2%) (52). Although some reports have suggested an increased risk of CHD in fetuses exposed to valproic acid (53), others could not establish a causal relationship (52,54).

The fetal alcohol syndrome, consisting of facial abnormalities, growth restriction, mental retardation, and cardiac abnormalities, has been well described in women consuming heavy amounts of alcohol in pregnancy (55). Cardioteratogenic effects of ethanol in the chick embryo have been confirmed in concentrations comparable to human blood alcohol levels (56). CHD has been identified in 25% to 30% of infants with fetal alcohol syndrome, with septal defects representing the most common lesions (55,57).

Isotretinoin is a vitamin A derivative prescribed for the treatment of severe cystic acne. Since its introduction, several reports have appeared in the literature describing the teratogenic effect of this medication. A characteristic pattern of malformations is observed, which includes central nervous system, craniofacial, branchial arch, and cardiovascular abnormalities (58). Cardiac abnormalities are usually conotruncal in origin (59,60). The mechanism of teratogenicity is probably related to free radical generation by metabolism with prostaglandin synthase (61).

Indomethacin, a nonsteroidal anti-inflammatory drug, is used in the treatment of preterm labor. In the fetus, indomethacin therapy may lead to premature constriction of the ductus arterior (see Chapter 13 for details). Several neonatal complications, which appear to be limited to indomethacin exposure beyond 32 weeks of gestation, include oliguria, necrotizing enterocolitis, and intracranial hemorrhage (62). Cardiovascular complications include a higher risk for patent ductus arteriosus requiring surgical ligation in indomethacin-exposed infants (62).

ACE inhibitors are commonly used antihypertensive medications. Fetal exposure to ACE inhibitors in the first trimester of pregnancy has been associated with an increased risk of major congenital malformation that was 2.7 times greater than the background risk or the risk of fetuses exposed to other antihypertensive medications (63). The increase in major malformations primarily affects the cardiovascular (risk ratio, 3.72) and central nervous systems (risk ratio, 4.39) (63). Atrial and ventricular septal defects represent the most common cardiac abnormalities (63). Fetal exposure to ACE inhibitors in the second and third trimesters of pregnancy is associated with "ACE inhibitor fetopathy," which includes oligohydramnios, intrauterine growth restriction, hypocalvaria, renal failure, and death (64).

Selective serotonin reuptake inhibitors (SSRIs) represent a new class of antidepressants that has gained wide acceptance for the treatment of depression and anxiety during pregnancy (65). Specific SSRI medications include citalopram (Celexa), fluoxetine (Prozac), paroxetine (Paxil), and sertraline (Zoloft). Pregnancies exposed to SSRIs in the first trimester have shown an increased risk of congenital heart defects (66–68). Paroxetine has been singled out as the SSRI with the greatest association with congenital heart malformations, primarily atrial and ventricular septal defects (68). A meta-analysis of seven studies noted a significant overall increased risk of 74% for cardiac malformations in women exposed to paroxetine in the first trimester of pregnancy (69). The U.S. Food and Drug Administration, Health Canada, and the drug manufacturer issued a warning in 2005 to health care professionals regarding the potential risk to infants born to mothers receiving paroxetine during the first trimester of pregnancy (70). Two recent large controlled studies, however, do not support the association of overall SSRI exposure in the first trimester of pregnancy with an increased risk of congenital heart defects or of most other categories of birth defects (71,72). Individual SSRIs may confer increased risks for some specific defects, but it should be recognized that the specific defects implicated are rare and the absolute risks are small (71,72).

SSRI exposure after the 20th week of gestation has been associated with an increased risk of persistent pulmonary hypertension of the newborn (PPHN) (73). PPHN occurs in 1 to 2 per 1000 live births and is associated with increased morbidity and mortality. SSRI exposure increases this risk to about 6 to 12 per 1000 neonates, a sixfold increase over the background risk (73). Possible mechanisms of action include an accumulation of serotonin in the lung in exposed fetuses (74). Serotonin has vasoconstrictor properties and a mitogenic effect on pulmonary smooth muscle cells, which may result in the proliferation of smooth muscle cells, the characteristic histologic pattern in PPHN (75,76).

Pending further studies, SSRI use during pregnancy should be individualized. Health care workers and their patients must weigh both the benefits and the potential risks of SSRI treatment in the context of the risk of recurrence of depression if maintenance therapy is discontinued.

Pregnancies of Assisted Reproductive Technology

Infants born to pregnancies of assisted reproductive technology are more likely to be born preterm, of low birth weight, and small for gestational age (77). This increased neonatal morbidity applies to multiple and singleton births (78). The evidence relating to the risk of birth defects is somewhat less clear. A report of systematically reviewed and pooled epidemiologic data assessing the risk of birth defects suggests a 30% to 40 % increase following assisted reproductive technologies (in vitro fertilization [IVF] and/or intracytoplasmic sperm injection [ICSI]) (79). Another population-based study on congenital malformations in children born after IVF with matched controls noted a fourfold increase in CHD in the IVF population, with the majority of cardiac anomalies representing atrial and ventricular septal defects (80). This same rate of fourfold increase in CHD was also noted in pregnancies conceived through ICSI (81).

Maternal Obesity

The prevalence of obesity, which is defined as a body mass index (BMI) greater than or equal to 30 kg/m^2, is increasing at an exponential rate. An established association between neural tube defects and prepregnancy maternal obesity exists (82). Several studies have noted an increased risk of congenital heart defects in obese pregnant mothers when compared to average-weight mothers (83,84). This increased risk is relatively small: 1.18-fold for the obese mother and 1.40-fold for the morbidly obese mother (BMI >35 kg/m^2). Atrial and ventricular septal defects contribute to the majority of this increased risk (84).

PREVENTION OF CONGENITAL HEART DISEASE

Current evidence suggests that folic acid supplementation taken preconceptionally significantly reduces the risk of CHD (85–88). Analysis of a randomized, controlled trial evaluating the efficacy of 0.8 mg of folic acid showed a 50% reduction in risk for a range of cardiac malformations (85). Other studies have shown a significant reduction in conotruncal abnormalities in newborns of pregnant women who took folic acid prenatally (86,87).

The mechanism of action of the effect of folic acid on the reduction in the risk of cardiac malformations has not been elucidated. Methylenetetrahydrofolate reductase (MTHFR) enzyme activity may be involved in this process (89). An association exists between homocysteine elevations, methylenetetrahydrofolate reductase gene variants, and CHD (89–91). In a controlled study, fasting homocysteine levels have been shown to be higher in mothers of infants affected by CHD (90). Current data support folic acid as the active ingredient involved in fetal cardiac embryogenesis and that periconceptional folic acid use may reduce the risk for congenital cardiac malformations (92).

▓ KEY POINTS: CONGENITAL HEART DISEASE: INCIDENCE, RISK FACTORS, AND PREVENTION

- The incidence of CHD is around 8 to 9 per 1000 live births.
- The overall incidence of CHD may be in the order of 50 per 1000 live births if all subtle cardiac anomalies are counted including bicuspid aortic valve, aneurysm of the atrial septum, and persistent superior vena cava.
- The incidence of CHD is reported in 10% to 20% of fetuses with nonimmune hydrops.
- Complete heart block in a fetus is associated with CHD in about 50% of cases.
- The suspicion for CHD during a routine ultrasound is a risk factor with the highest yield for CHD (40% to 50%).
- Most infants born with CHD are born to pregnancies without risk factors.
- A nuchal translucency thickness that is greater than or equal to 3.5 mm warrants referral for fetal echocardiography.
- Fetuses of monochorionic pregnancies are at an increased risk for CHD.
- The incidence of CHD is fivefold higher in infants of diabetic mothers, with ventricular septal defects and transposition of the great arteries accounting for the majority of cardiac malformations.
- Fetal exposure in the first trimester to maternal phenylalanine levels exceeding 15 mg/dL is associated with a 10- to 15-fold increase in CHD.
- The risk of lithium exposure to the fetus is lower than previously reported.
- Anticonvulsant exposure during the first trimester of pregnancy confers significant risk to the fetus.
- CHD has been identified in 25% to 30% of infants with fetal alcohol syndrome.
- ACE inhibitor exposure to the fetus in the first trimester results in an increased risk of CHD. Exposure in the second and third trimesters results in "ACE inhibitor fetopathy."
- SSRI exposure in the first trimester may be associated with increased CHD. Exposure beyond the 20th week of gestation is associated with a sixfold increase in persistent pulmonary hypertension of newborn.
- A fourfold increase in CHD is noted in fetuses of IVF pregnancies.
- Fetuses of obese mothers have a small increased risk for CHD.
- Folic acid supplementation taken preconceptionally reduces the risk for CHD.

References

1. Hoffman JIE, Christianson R. Congenital heart disease in a cohort of 19,502 births with long-term follow-up. *Am J Cardiol* 1978;42:641–647.
2. Yoon PW, Olney RS, Khoury MJ, et al. Contribution of birth defects and genetic diseases to pediatric hospitalizations. A population-based study. *Arch Pediatr Adolesc Med* 1997;151:1096–1103.
3. Ward C. Clinical significance of the bicuspid aortic valve. *Heart* 2000;83:81–85.
4. Keith JD. Bicuspid aortic valve. In: Keith JD, Rowe RD, Vlad P, eds. *Heart disease in infancy and childhood.* New York: Macmillan, 1978;728–735.
5. Woodrow Benson D. The genetics of congenital heart disease: a point of revolution. *Cardiol Clin* 2002;20:385–394.
6. Hoffman JI, Kaplan S. The incidence of congenital heart disease. *Circ Res* 2004;94:1890–1900.
7. Allan LD. Echocardiographic detection of congenital heart disease in the fetus: present and future. *Br Heart J* 1995;74:103–106.
8. Friedman AH, Copel JA, Kleinman CS. Fetal echocardiography and fetal cardiology: indications, diagnosis and management. *Semin Perinatol* 1993;17(2):76–88.
9. Crawford DC, Chita SK, Allan LD. Prenatal detection of congenital heart disease: factors affecting obstetric management and survival. *Am J Obstet Gynecol* 1988;159:352–356.

10. Abuhamad AZ, Shaffer W, Mari G, et al. Single umbilical artery: does it matter which artery is missing? *Am J Obstet Gynecol* 1995;173:728–732.
11. Greenwood RD, Rosenthal A, Nadas AS. Cardiovascular malformations associated with congenital anomalies of the urinary system. *Clin Pediatr* 1976;15:1101.
12. Burton BK. Recurrence risks for congenital hydrocephalus. *Clin Genet* 1979;16:47.
13. Parrish ML, Roessmann U, Levinsohn MW. Agenesis of the corpus callosum: a study of the frequency of associated malformations. *Ann Neurol* 1979;6:349.
14. Greenwood RD, Rosenthal A. Cardiovascular malformations associated with tracheoesophageal fistula and esophageal atresia. *Pediatrics* 1976;57:87.
15. Fonkalsrud EW, DeLorimier AA, Hays DM. Congenital atresia and stenosis of the duodenum. A review compiled from the members of the Surgical Section of the American Academy of Pediatrics. *Pediatrics* 1969;43:79.
16. DeLorimier AA, Fonkalsrud EW, Hays DM. Congenital atresia and stenosis of the jejunum and ileum. *Surgery* 1969;65:819.
17. Greenwood RD, Rosenthal A, Nadas AS. Cardiovascular malformations associated with imperforate anus. *J Pediatr* 1975;86:576.
18. Greenwood RD, Rosenthal A, Nadas AS. Cardiovascular malformations associated with omphalocele. *J Pediatr* 1974;85:818.
19. Toyama WM. Combined congenital defects of the anterior abdominal wall, sternum, diaphragm pericardium and heart: a case report and review of the syndrome. *Pediatrics* 1972;50:778.
20. Greenwood R, Sommer A, Rosenthal A, et al. Cardiovascular abnormalities in the Beckwith-Wiedemann syndrome. *Am J Dis Child* 1977;131:293.
21. Greenwood RD, Rosenthal A, Nadas AS. Cardiovascular abnormalities associated with congenital diaphragmatic hernia. *Pediatrics* 1976;57:92.
22. Opitz JM, Howe JJ. The Meckel syndrome (dysencephalia splanchnocystica, the Gruber syndrome). *Birth Defects* 1969;5(2):167.
23. Sawaya R, McLaurin RL. Dandy-Walker syndrome: clinical analysis of 23 cases. *J Neurosurg* 1981;55:89.
24. Copel JA, Pilu G, Kleinman CS. Congenital heart disease and extracardiac anomalies: associations and indications for fetal echocardiography. *Am J Obstet Gynecol* 1986;154:1121–1132.
25. Creasy RK, Resnik R. *Maternal fetal medicine. Principles and practice,* 3rd ed. Philadelphia: WB Saunders, 1994;326.
26. Crawford D, Chapman M, Allan LD. The assessment of persistent bradycardia in prenatal life. *Br J Obstet Gynecol* 1985;92:941–944.
27. Souka AP, Krampl E, Bakalis S, et al. Outcome of pregnancy in chromosomally normal fetuses with increased nuchal translucency in the first trimester. *Ultrasound Obstet Gynecol* 2001;18:9–17.
28. Nicolaides KH. Nuchal translucency and other first-trimester sonographic markers of chromosomal abnormalities. *Am J Obstet Gynecol* 2004;191:45–67.
29. Atzei A, Gajewska K, Huggon IC, et al. Relationship between nuchal translucency thickness and prevalence of major cardiac defects in fetuses with normal karyotype. *Ultrasound Obstet Gynecol* 2005;26:154–157.
30. Bahado-Singh RO, Wapner R, Thom E, et al. Elevated first-trimester nuchal translucency increases the risk of congenital heart defects. *Am J Obstet Gynecol* 2005;19:1357–1361.
31. Makrydimas G, Sotiriadis A, Huggon IC, et al. Nuchal translucency and fetal cardiac defects: a pooled analysis of major fetal echocardiography centers. *Am J Obstet Gynecol* 2005;192(1):89–95.
32. Manning N, Archer N. A study to determine the incidence of structural congenital heart disease in monochorionic twins. *Prenat Diagn* 2006;11:1062–1064.
33. Bahtiyar MO, Dulay AT, Weeks BP, et al. Prevalence of congenital heart defects in monochorionic/diamniotic twin gestations: a systematic literature review. *J Ultrasound Med* 2007;11:1491–1498.
34. Rowland TW, Hubbell JP Jr, Nadas AS. Congenital heart disease in infants of diabetic mothers. *J Pediatr* 1973;83:815–820.
35. Miller E, Hare JW, Cloherty JP, et al. Elevated maternal hemoglobin A1c in early pregnancy and major congenital anomalies in infants of diabetic mothers. *N Engl J Med* 1981;304:1331–1334.
36. Yinen K, Aula P, Stenman U, et al. Risk of minor and major fetal malformations in diabetics with high haemoglobin A1c values in early pregnancy. *Br Med J* 1984;289:345–346.
37. Shields LE, Gan EA, Murphy HF, et al. The prognostic value of hemoglobin A1c in predicting fetal heart disease in diabetic pregnancies. *Obstet Gynecol* 1993;81:954–957.
38. Levy HL, Waisbren SE. Effects of untreated maternal phenylketonuria and hyperphenylalaninemia on the fetus. *N Engl J Med* 1983;309:1269.
39. Lenke RL, Levy HL. Maternal phenylketonuria and hyperphenylalaninemia: an international survey of the outcome of untreated and treated pregnancies. *N Engl J Med* 1980;303:1202.
40. Tikkanen J, Heinonen OP. Maternal exposure to chemical and physical factors during pregnancy and cardiovascular malformations in the offspring. *Teratology* 1991;43:591–600.
41. Schou M, Godfield MD, Weinstein MR, et al. Lithium and pregnancy. I: report from the Register of Lithium Babies. *BMJ* 1973;2:135–136.
42. Kallen B. Comments on teratogen update: lithium. *Teratology* 1988;38:597.
43. Edmonds LD, Oakley GP. Ebstein's anomaly and maternal lithium exposure during pregnancy. *Teratology* 1990;41:551–552.
44. Zalstein E, Xoren G, Einarson T, et al. A case-control study on the association between first trimester exposure to lithium and Ebstein's anomaly. *Am J Cardiol* 1990;65:817–818.
45. Sipek A. Lithium and Ebstein's anomaly. *Cor Vasa* 1989;31:149–156.
46. Jacobson SJ, Jones K, Johnson X, et al. Prospective multicenter study of pregnancy outcome after lithium exposure during first trimester. *Lancet* 1992;339:530–533.

47. Hanson JW, Buehler BA. Fetal hydantoin syndrome: current status. *J Pediatr* 1982;101:816–818.
48. Buehler BA, Delimont D, Van Waes M, et al. Prenatal prediction of risk of the fetal hydantoin syndrome. *N Engl J Med* 1990;322:1567–1572.
49. Meadow SR. Anticonvulsant drugs and congenital abnormalities. *Lancet* 1968;2:1296.
50. Nora JJ, Nora AH. The environmental contribution to congenital heart diseases. In: Nora JJ, Takao A, eds. *Congenital heart disease: causes and processes.* Mount Kisco, NY: Futura, 1984;15–27.
51. Briggs GG, Freeman RK, Yaffe SJ. *Drugs in pregnancy and lactation,* 4th ed. Philadelphia: Lippincott, Williams & Wilkins, 1994;845.
52. Centers for Disease Control, U.S. Department of Health and Human Services. Valproate: a new cause of birth defects-report from Italy and follow-up from France. *MMWR Morb Mortal Wkly Rep* 1983;32:438–439.
53. Thisted E, Ebbesen F. Malformations, withdrawal manifestations, and hypoglycaemia after exposure to valproate in utero. *Arch Dis Child* 1993;69(3 Spec No):288–291.
54. Lindhout D, Meinardi H. Spina bifida and in-utero exposure to valproate. *Lancet* 1984;2:396.
55. Jones KL, Smith DW, Ulleland CN, et al. Pattern of malformation in offspring of alcoholic mothers. *Lancet* 1973;1:7815.
56. Bruyere HJ Jr, Kapil RP. Cardioteratogenic dose of ethanol in the chick embryo results in egg white. *J Appl Toxicol* 1990;10(1):69–71.
57. Clarren SK, Smith DW. The fetal alcohol syndrome. *N Engl J Med* 1978;298:1063.
58. Lammer EJ, Chen DR, Hoar RM, et al. Retinoic acid embryopathy. *N Engl J Med* 1985;313:837–841.
59. Anonymous. Birth defects caused by isotretinoin-New Jersey. *MMWR Morb Mortal Wkly Rep* 1988;37: 171–172, 177.
60. Rosa FW. Retinoic acid embryopathy. *N Engl J Med* 1986;315:262.
61. Kubow S. Inhibition of isotretinoin teratogenicity by acetylsalicylic acid pretreatment in mice. *Teratology* 1992;45:55–63.
62. Norton ME, Merrill J, Cooper BAB, et al. Neonatal complications after the administration of indomethacin for preterm labor. *N Engl J Med* 1993;329:1602.
63. Cooper WO, Hernandez-Diaz S, Arbogast PG, et al. Major congenital malformations after first-trimester exposure to ACE inhibitors. *N Engl J Med* 2006;354:2443–2451.
64. Tabacova S, Little R, Tsong Y, et al. Adverse pregnancy outcomes associated with maternal enalapril antihypertensive treatment. *Pharmacoepidemiol Drug Saf* 2003;8:633–646.
65. Mann JJ. The medical management of depression. *N Engl J Med* 2005;353:1819–1834.
66. Cole JA, Ng EW, Wphross SA, et al. Paroxetine in the first trimester of pregnancy and the prevalence of congenital malformations [Abstract]. *Pharmacoepidemiol Drug Saf* 2006;15:S6.
67. Kallen B, Otterblad Olausson P. Antidepressant drugs during pregnancy and infant congenital heart defect [Letter]. *Reprod Toxicol* 2006;21:221–222.
68. SSRI antidepressant and birth defects. *Prescurie Int* 2006;15:222–223.
69. Bar-Oz B, Einarson T, Einarson A, et al. Paroxetine and congenital malformations: meta-analysis and consideration of potential confounding factors. *Clin Ther* 2007;5:918–926.
70. U.S. Food and Drug Administration. FDA public health advisory, paroxetine. Available at: http://www.fda.gov/cder/drug/advisory/paroxetine200512.htm. 2007.
71. Louik C, Lin AE, Werler MM, et al. First-trimester use of selective serotonin-reuptake inhibitors and the risk of birth defects. *N Engl J Med* 2007;26:2675–2683.
72. Alwan S, Reefhuis J, Rasmussen SA, et al. Use of selective serotonin-reuptake inhibitors in pregnancy and the risk of birth defects. *N Engl J Med* 2007;356:2684–2692.
73. Chambers CD, Hernandez-Diaz S, Van Marter LJ, et al. Selective serotonin-reuptake inhibitors and risk of persistent pulmonary hypertension of the newborn. *N Engl J Med* 2006;6:579–587.
74. Suhara T, Sudo Y, Yoshida K, et al. Lung as reservoir for antidepressants in pharmacokinetic drug interactions. *Lancet* 1998;9099:332–335.
75. McMahon TJ, Hood JS, Nossaman BD, et al. Analysis of responses to serotonin in the pulmonary vascular bed of the cat. *J Appl Physiol* 1993;1:93–102.
76. Runo JR, Loyd JE. Primary pulmonary hypertension. *Lancet* 2003;361:1533–1544.
77. Jackson RA, Gibson KA, Wu YW, et al. Perinatal outcomes in singletons following in vitro fertilization: a meta-analysis. *Obstet Gynecol* 2004;103:551–563.
78. Helmerhorst FM, Perquin DAM, Donker D, et al. Perinatal outcome of singletons and twins after assisted conception: a systematic review of controlled studies. *Br Med J* 2004;328:261.
79. Hansen M, Bower C, Milne E, et al. Assisted reproductive technologies and the risk of birth defects—a systematic review. *Hum Reprod* 2005;20:328–338.
80. Koivurova S, Hartikainen AL, Gissler M, et al. Neonatal outcome and congenital malformations in children born after in-vitro fertilization. *Hum Reprod* 2002;5:1391–1398.
81. Kurinczuk JJ, Bower C. Birth defects in infants conceived by intracytoplasmic sperm injection: an alternative interpretation. *Br Med J* 1997;315:1260–1266.
82. Kallen K. Maternal smoking, body mass index, and neural tube defects. *Am J Epidemiol* 1998;147: 1103–1111.
83. Watkins ML, Rasmussen SA, Honein MA, et al. Maternal obesity and risk for birth defects. *Pediatrics* 2003;111:1152–1158.
84. Cedegren MI, Kallen AJ. Maternal obesity and infant heart defects. *Obes Res* 2003;11:1065–1071.
85. Czeizel AE. Periconceptional folic acid containing multivitamin supplementation. *Eur J Obstet Gynecol Reprod Biol* 1998;78:151–161.
86. Shaw GM, O'Malley CD, Wasserman CR, et al. Maternal periconceptional use of multivitamins and reduced risk for conotruncal heart defects and limb deficiencies among offspring. *Am J Med Genet* 1995;59:536–545.

87. Scanlon KS, Ferencz C, Loffredo CA, et al. Preconceptional folate intake and malformations of the cardiac outflow tract. Baltimore–Washington Infant Study Group. *Epidemiology* 1998;9:95–98.
88. Botto LD, Mulinare J, Erickson JD. Occurrence of congenital heart defects in relation to maternal multivitamin use. *Am J Epidemiol* 2000;151:878–884.
89. Junker R, Kotthoff S, Vielhaber H, et al. Infant methylenetetrahydrofolate reductase 677TT genotype is a risk factor for congenital heart disease. *Cardiovasc Res* 2001;51:251–254.
90. Kapusta L, Haagman MLM, Steegers EAP, et al. Congenital heart defects and maternal derangement of homocysteine metabolism. *J Pediatr* 1999;135:773–774.
91. Westrom KD, Johanning GL, Johnston KE, et al. Association of the C677T methylenetetrahydrofolate reductase mutation and elevated homocysteine levels with congenital cardiac malformations. *Am J Obstet Gynecol* 2001;184:806–817.
92. Bailey LB, Berry RJ. Folic acid supplementation and the occurrence of congenital heart defects, orofacial clefts, multiple births, and miscarriage. *Am J Clin Nutr* 2005;81(suppl):1213S–1217S.

INTRODUCTION

The fetal heart undergoes complex developmental changes in the first few weeks of gestation and is anatomically fully developed by the eighth week of embryonic life (1). The presence of congenital heart defects in the fetus is a result of abnormal cardiac development during its embryogenesis. Current knowledge suggests that the genetic contribution to congenital heart defects has been significantly underestimated in the past. Recent advances in microscopic techniques have added significantly to the knowledge of early cardiac development and how congenital heart defects originate (2). Human cardiovascular genetics is a field that is progressing at a rapid pace, and clinically available genetic tests for various forms of cardiac abnormalities are made available at variable speed (3). Online resources listed at the end of this chapter will provide an updated list of available genetic testing. Table 2-1 displays, in chronologic order, important milestones in fetal cardiac development, and Table 2-2 lists associated cardiac defects with the corresponding stage of cardiac development.

CONGENITAL HEART DEFECTS AND NUMERICAL CHROMOSOMAL ABNORMALITIES

The frequency of chromosomal abnormalities in infants with congenital heart defects has been estimated as 5% to 15% from postnatal data (4–6). In a population-based case-control study of 2102 live-born infants, ascertained by their cardiovascular malformations, chromosomal abnormalities were found in 13% (5). In this study, Down syndrome occurred in 10.4% of infants with cardiovascular malformations, with the other trisomies each occurring in less than 1% of cases (5). Similar data were reported from three large registries of congenital malformations, involving 1.27 million births (6). The frequency of abnormal karyotype in fetuses with cardiac defects is higher and has been reported in the range of 30% to 40% by several studies (7–9). This higher rate of chromosomal abnormalities in fetuses with cardiac defects, when compared to their live-born counterparts, is mainly due to an increased prenatal mortality in fetuses with aneuploidy, which has been estimated at 30% for trisomy 21, 42% for trisomy 13, 68% for trisomy 18, and 75% for Turner syndrome (10). Not only is the association of congenital cardiac defects and chromosomal abnormalities lower in live-born infants when compared to fetuses, but also the distribution of chromosomal abnormalities is more skewed toward Down syndrome in the neonatal population (5,6), again probably due to the high prenatal mortality of trisomy 18, trisomy 13, and monosomy X.

Certain specific cardiac diagnoses are more commonly associated with chromosomal abnormalities than others. Prenatal and postnatal studies are concordant with regard to the specific cardiac diagnoses that are more likely to be associated with chromosomal abnormalities. In general, malformations of the right side of the heart are less commonly associated with karyotypic abnormalities. Specific cardiac diagnoses like transposition of the great vessels and heterotaxy syndromes are not usually associated with chromosomal abnormalities. Endocardial cushion defect, ventricular (perimembranous) and atrial septal defects, tetralogy of Fallot, double outlet right ventricle, and hypoplastic left heart syndrome, on the other hand, are more commonly associated with chromosomal abnormalities in the fetus and newborn. Table 2-3 lists specific cardiac diagnoses in infants with noncomplex cardiovascular defects from three large registries (6) and the corresponding incidence of associated numerical chromosomal abnormalities.

The majority of fetuses with cardiac defects and chromosomal abnormalities have other associated extracardiac abnormalities, in the order of 50% to 70% (7,9). The distribution of extracardiac abnormalities usually follows the typical pattern noted within each chromosomal syndrome with no predominance of any specific abnormality. In the fetus with an apparently

TABLE 2-1	Chronology of Cardiac Development

Feature	Weeks of development (from fertilization)
Angiogenetic clusters	Early 3
Formation of heart tubes	Early 3
Cardiac pumping	Early 3
Fusion of heart tubes	Early 3
Looping of heart tube	Mid 3
Appearance of intraventricular septum	Mid 3/late 3
Septum primum	End 3/early 4
Appearance of endocardial cushions	End 4
Conotruncal ridges	Late 4/early 5
Conotruncal septum	Early 5/mid 5
Septum secundum	Late 5/early 6
Fusion of endocardial cushions	Early 6
Obliteration of membranous septum	Mid 7/end 7

(Adapted from O'Rahilly R, Müller F. *Human embryology and teratology*. New York: Wiley-Liss, 1992;107–117, with permission.)

isolated cardiac abnormality, the incidence of chromosomal abnormalities is still significantly increased (15% to 30%), and thus appropriate genetic counseling is warranted (7,9,11).

When the diagnosis of a chromosomal abnormality is made in a fetus, an echocardiogram is indicated in view of the common association of cardiac malformations with karyotypic abnormalities. Data obtained from postnatal studies suggest that the incidence of cardiac defects is 40% to 50% in trisomy 21, 25% to 35% in Turner syndrome, and more than 80% in trisomy 13 and 18 (12,13). Cardiac defects tend to be specific to the type of chromosomal abnormality. Table 2-4 lists the most common numerical chromosomal abnormalities and their associated congenital cardiac defects.

CONGENITAL HEART DEFECTS AND CHROMOSOMAL DELETION SYNDROMES

DiGeorge and Velocardiofacial Syndromes

DiGeorge and velocardiofacial syndromes represent the two most common syndromes of a heterogeneous group of disorders that share a monosomic deletion of chromosome 22q11 The prevalence of this deletion has been estimated at 1 in 4000 live births (14). Phenotypic abnormalities of chromosome 22q11 deletion syndrome include thymus hypoplasia or aplasia, cardiac outflow tract abnormalities, cleft palate, velopharyngeal insufficiency, and dysmorphic facial features (15). The clinical feature of the 22q11 deletion is highly variable. Cardiovascular anomalies, which can be present in up to 85% of cases; immunodeficiency; and speech delay appear to be the most frequent phenotypic manifestations (15,16). Other abnormalities include neonatal hypocalcemia due to parathyroid hypoplasia, feeding and behavioral disorders, learning disabilities, and cleft anomalies (3). When a fetus or a child is diagnosed with the 22q11 deletion, karyotypic evaluation of the parents is critical as approximately 6% to 28% of parents will be found to carry the deletion with a 50% transmission to future offspring (16). Risk of recurrence is small (1%) if neither parent carries the deletion. Fluorescence in situ hybridization (FISH) for 22q11 deletion must be specifically requested in addition to routine karyotyping when looking for this deletion, as shown in Figure 2-1. The specific type of congenital heart disease is more commonly associated with the 22q11 deletion. Interrupted aortic arch, pulmonary atresia with ventricular septal defect (VSD), common arterial trunk, and conoventricular septal defects are most commonly associated with the 22q11 deletion. Table 2-5 estimates the 22q11 deletion with types of congenital heart disease. Once a cardiac anomaly is diagnosed prenatally, the additional demonstration of a hypoplastic or absent fetal thymus on an ultrasound examination increases the risk of an association with a

TABLE 2-2	Stages of Cardiac Development and Congenital Cardiac Defects
Stage	**Associated cardiac defect**
Primitive heart tube	Lethal defects
Looping	Dextrocardia Situs inversus totalis Ventricular inversion Corrected TGA Heterotaxy syndrome
Wedging/ventricular development	Double outlet RV Double inlet LV Single ventricle (R or L) Hypoplastic ventricle (R or L) Ventricular septal defects
Atrial septation	Common atrium Atrial septal defects (primum, secundum, sinus venosus)
Systemic and pulmonary veins	Left SVC to coronary sinus Bilateral SVCs Interruption of IVC with azygous continuation Total anomalous pulmonary venous connection Partial anomalous pulmonary venous connection Cor triatriatum
Atrioventricular valves	Ebstein anomaly Atrioventricular septal defect Atresia of AV valve Hypoplasia of valve annulus
Aortic and pulmonary outflow tracts	Common arterial trunk Double outlet RV Double inlet LV Probably transposition/malposition Tricuspid atresia TOF VSDs IAA Straddling tricuspid valve Absent ductus arteriosus
Aortic arch	Interrupted aortic arch Right aortic arch Aberrant subclavian arteries TOF PDA Hypoplastic pulmonary trunk

TGA, transposition of the great arteries; RV, right ventricle; LV, left ventricle; R, right; L, left; SVC, superior vena cava; IVC, inferior vena cava; AV, atrioventricular; TOF, tetralogy of Fallot; VSDs, ventricular septal defects; IAA, interrupted aortic arch; PDA, persistent ductus arteriosus.
(Adapted from Collins-Nakai R, McLaughlin P. How congenital heart disease originates in fetal life. *Cardiol Clin* 2002;20:367–383, with permission.)

deletion 22q11 The thymus is demonstrated in a transverse plane of the chest at the level of the upper sternum (three-vessel-trachea view) anterior to the three vessels (Fig. 2-2A). Thymic aplasia or hypoplasia may be suspected at this plane level (Fig. 2-2B). Note that the presence of a thymus on ultrasound does not rule out a 22q11 deletion (17).

TABLE 2-3	Number of Infants with Identified Chromosomal Anomalies According to Cardiac Defect Type (Noncomplex Cardiovascular Defects Only)

	Chromosomal anomaly		
Cardiovascular defect	No	Yes	Percentage
Corrected transposition	16	0	0.0
D-TGA	969	9	0.9
Pulmonary atresia without VSD	195	4	2.0
TAPVC	287	6	2.0
ASD + pulmonary valve stenosis	117	5	4.1
HLHS	799	35	4.2
Tricuspid valve atresia	132	6	4.3
Pulmonary valve stenosis	374	17	4.3
Common arterial trunk	217	10	4.4
Aortic valve stenosis	235	11	4.5
Interrupted aortic arch	179	11	5.8
Ebstein anomaly	110	8	6.8
Coarctation of aorta	403	32	7.4
Single ventricle	91	9	9.0
VSD + coarctation of aorta	207	21	9.2
Tetralogy of Fallot	1077	123	10.3
DORV	174	25	12.6
VSD	2134	474	18.2
ASD	868	319	26.9
VSD + ASD	447	207	31.7
AVSD	317	687	68.4

D-TGA, D-transposition of great arteries; VSD, ventricular septal defect; TAPVR, total anomalous pulmonary venous connection; ASD, atrial septal defect; HLHS, hypoplastic left heart syndrome; DORV, double outlet right ventricle; AVSD, atrioventricular septal defect.
(Modified from Harris JA, Francannet C, Pradat P. The epidemiology of cardiovascular defects, part 2: a study based on data from three large registries of congenital malformations. *Pediatr Cardiol* 2003;24:222–235, with permission.)

Williams-Beuren Syndrome

Williams-Beuren syndrome, also known as Williams syndrome, is associated with a microdeletion at chromosome 7q11.23. The prevalence of this deletion has been estimated at 1 in 10,000 live births (18). Phenotypic abnormalities are variable but include characteristic facies, personality and cognitive abnormalities, infantile hypercalcemia, and skeletal, renal, and cardiac anomalies (18). Cardiovascular anomalies are present in 80% to 90% of cases and typically include supravalvular aortic stenosis, often in conjunction with supravalvular pulmonary stenosis and peripheral pulmonary stenosis. These cardiac abnormalities probably result from the deletion of the elastin gene (19). The supravalvular and peripheral pulmonary stenosis regress with time, whereas the supravalvular aortic stenosis progresses in many cases (19). The prenatal diagnosis of supravalvular aortic or pulmonary stenosis warrants specific testing of the fetus by FISH for this deletion. Although most cases occur de novo, autosomal dominant transmission from a carrier parent is possible. Recurrence risk is small (<5%) if neither parent is a carrier (18,19).

CONGENITAL HEART DEFECTS AND SINGLE GENE DISORDERS

Noonan Syndrome

Noonan syndrome is an autosomal dominant disorder with a prevalence of 1 in 1000 to 2500 live births (20). The syndrome, which affects both sexes equally, is characterized by dysmorphic facies, short stature, webbed neck, skeletal deformities, cryptorchidism, bleeding diatheses, and cardiac anomalies (20). Cardiac involvement is observed in 80% to 90% of affected fetuses, with valvular pulmonary stenosis (70%) and hypertrophic cardiomyopathy

TABLE 2-4 Representative Numerical Chromosomal Disorders and Their Association with Congenital Heart Defects

Chromosomal disorder	Main features	Percent with CHD	Heart anomaly
Trisomy 9	Severe prenatal and postnatal growth retardation, marked microcephaly, deep-set eyes, low-set ears, severe mental retardation; two thirds die in infancy	65–80	PDA, LSVC, VSD, TOF/PA, DORV
Trisomy 13 (Patau syndrome)	Polydactyly, cleft lip and palate, scalp defects, hypotelorism, microphthalmia or anophthalmia, colobomata of irides, holoprosencephaly, microcephaly, deafness, profound mental retardation, rib abnormalities, omphalocele, renal abnormalities, hypospadias, cryptorchidism, uterine abnormalities; 80% die in the first year	80	ASD, VSD, PDA, HLHS, CoA, laterality defects
Trisomy 18 (Edwards syndrome)	IUGR, polyhydramnios, micrognathia, short sternum, hypertonia, rocker-bottom feet, overlapping fingers and toes, TEF, CDH, omphalocele, renal anomalies, biliary atresia, profound mental retardation; 90% die in first year	90–100	ASD, VSD, PDA, TOF, DORV, CoA, BAV, BPV, polyvalvular nodular dysplasia
Trisomy 21 (Down syndrome)	Hypotonia, hyperextensibility, epicanthal fold, simian crease, clinodactyly of fifth finger, brachydactyly, variable mental retardation, premature aging	40–50	AVSD, VSD, ASD, TOF
Monosomy X (Turner syndrome, 45, X)	Lymphedema of hands and feet, widely spaced hypoplastic nipples, webbed neck, primary amenorrhea, short stature, normal intelligence	25–35	CoA, BAV, valvar AS, HLHS, aortic dissection
Klinefelter syndrome (47,XXY)	Usually normal appearing, tall stature, small testes, delayed puberty, emotional and behavioral problems common, variable mental retardation	50	MVP, venous thromboembolic disease, PDA, ASD
Trisomy 8 mosaicism	Skeletal/vertebral anomalies, widely spaced eyes, broad nasal bridge, small jaw, high arched palate, cryptorchidism, renal anomalies (50%), long survival	25	VSD, PDA, CoA, TAPVC, common arterial trunk

CHD, congenital heart disease; PDA, patent ductus arteriosus; LSVC, left superior vena cava; VSD, ventricular septal defect; TOF/PA, tetralogy of Fallot with pulmonary atresia; DORV, double outlet right ventricle; ASD, atrial septal defect; HLHS, hypoplastic left heart syndrome; CoA, coarctation of the aorta; IUGR, intrauterine growth restriction; TEF, tracheoesophageal fistula; CDH, congenital diaphragmatic hernia; BAV, bicuspid aortic valve; BPV, bicuspid pulmonary valve; AS, aortic stenosis; AVSD, atrioventricular septal defect; MVP, mitral valve prolapse; PS pulmonary stenosis; TAPVC, total anomalous pulmonary venous connection.
(Source: Pierpont ME, Basson C, Woodrow Benson D, et al. Genetic basis for congenital heart defects: current knowledge. *Circulation* 2007;115:3015–3038.)

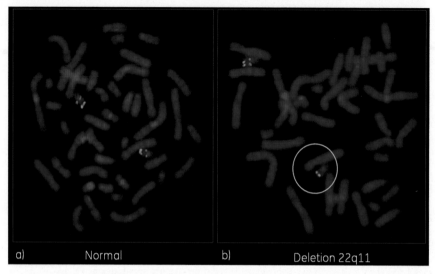

Figure 2-1. A: Normal fetal karyotype; chromosomes 22 are tagged by green color and the DiGeorge critical region is identified by a specific marker (red). **B:** Fetus with a 22q11 deletion. One of the two 22 chromosomes (*white circle*) is missing the DiGeorge critical region consistent with the 22q11 deletion. (Courtesy of Professor Gundula Thiel.)

TABLE 2-5	Estimated 22q11 Deletion Frequency in Congenital Heart Defects

Cardiac defect	Estimated deletion frequency (%)
Interrupted aortic arch	50–89
VSDs	10
with normal aortic arch[a]	3
with aortic arch anomaly[b]	45
Common arterial trunk	34–41
Tetralogy of Fallot (including pulmonary atresia with VSD and absent pulmonary valve syndrome)	10–40
Isolated aortic arch anomalies	24
Double outlet right ventricle	<5
Transposition of the great arteries	<1

VSD, ventricular septal defect.
[a]Left-sided aortic arch with normal branching pattern.
[b]Includes right aortic arch and/or abnormal branching pattern, cervical location, and/or discontinuous branch pulmonary arteries.
(Adapted from Pierpont ME, Basson C, Woodrow Benson D, et al. Genetic basis for congenital heart defects: current knowledge. *Circulation* 2007;115:3015–3038; and Chaoui R, Kalache KD, Heling KS, et al. Absent or hypoplastic thymus on ultrasound: a marker for deletion 22q11 in fetal cardiac defects. *Ultrasound Obstet Gynecol* 2002;20:546–552, with permission.)

(20%) accounting for the majority of cardiac lesions. The pulmonary stenosis is typically due to dysplastic leaflets rather than fused commissures, which is a type of valve stenosis that is rarely seen in non-Noonan individuals (18). Other heart anomalies observed in Noonan syndrome include atrioventricular septal defect, atrial septal defect, tetralogy of Fallot, mitral valve abnormalities, and aortic coarctation.

Mutations in the gene *PTPN11* on the chromosome locus 12q24.1 have been identified in almost half the cases. Other identified genes include *SOS1* and *KRAS*. Prenatal testing is available when the mutation is previously identified in a family member. Noonan syndrome should be clinically suspected in a fetus with increased nuchal translucency or cystic hygroma,

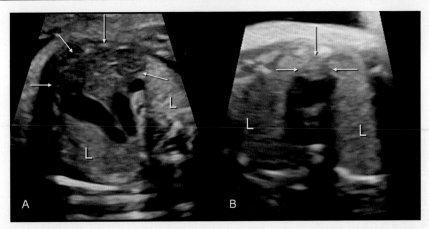

Figure 2-2. A: Normal fetus at 32 weeks' gestation: The thymus (*white arrows*) is visualized anterior to the three vessels in a transverse view at the upper chest level. **B:** Fetus at 30 weeks' gestation with 22q11 deletion: The thymus is hypoplastic (*white arrows*). L, right and left lungs.

thickened nuchal fold, unilateral or bilateral pleural effusion, and hydrops in the setting of a normal fetal karyotype. Cardiac anomalies may be progressive and are only detected in 27% of cases prenatally (21).

The absence of a mutation in the *PTPN11, KRAS,* and *SOS1* genes does not rule out Noonan syndrome given its genetic heterogeneity.

Alagille Syndrome

Alagille syndrome is an autosomal dominant disorder with a prevalence of 1 in 70,000 to 100,000 live births (22). The syndrome is characterized by cholestasis, dysmorphic facies, and skeletal, ocular, and cardiac anomalies (22). Originally, the diagnosis required the presence of paucity of bile ducts on liver biopsy in addition to three of the aforementioned characteristics. Cardiac involvement is observed in 90% of affected fetuses, with pulmonary artery branch stenosis accounting for the majority of cardiac lesions. Other cardiac lesions include tetralogy of Fallot, pulmonary stenosis, and coarctation of the aorta.

Mutations or deletions in the gene *JAG1* on the chromosome locus 20p11.2 have been identified in cases with Alagille syndrome. De novo mutations occur in 50% to 60% of cases. Prenatal testing is available when the mutation is previously identified in a family member. Given the variable expressivity of this syndrome, the severity of the phenotype in an identified fetus is difficult to predict (23).

Holt-Oram Syndrome

Holt-Oram syndrome, also known as heart-hand syndrome, is an autosomal dominant disorder, with complete penetrance and very variable expression, and a prevalence of 1 in 100,000 live births (24). The syndrome is characterized by cardiac anomalies in fetuses with upper limb deformities. Preaxial radial ray malformations occur in all affected fetuses and is required for the diagnosis. Cardiac anomalies are present in 85% to 95% of cases. Secundum atrial septal defects and muscular ventricular septal defects are the most common cardiac lesions (25). Conduction defects occur in 40% of cases.

Mutations in the gene *TBX5* on the chromosome locus 12q24.1 have been identified in cases with Holt-Oram syndrome (24). De novo mutations occur in 30% to 40% of cases. The absence of a detected *TBX5* mutation does not preclude the diagnosis.

Table 2-6 is a comprehensive list of nonnumerical chromosomal disorders and their association with congenital heart defects, and Table 2-7 is a list of genes known to be associated with congenital heart defects.

TABLE 2-6   Representative Nonnumerical Chromosomal Disorders and Their Association with Congenital Heart Defects

Chromosomal disorder	Main features	Percent with CHD	Heart anomaly
Deletion 4p (Wolf-Hirschhorn syndrome)	Pronounced microcephaly, widely spaced eyes, broad nasal bridge (Greek helmet appearance), downturned mouth, micrognathia, preauricular skin tags, elongated trunk and fingers, severe mental restriction and seizures; one third die in infancy	50–65	ASD, VSD, PDA, aortic atresia, dextrocardia, TOF, tricuspid atresia
Deletion 5p (cri-du-chat)	Catlike cry, prenatal and postnatal growth retardation, round face, widely spaced eyes, epicanthal fold, simian crease, severe mental restriction, long survival	30–60	VSD, ASD, PDA
Deletion 7q11.23 (Williams-Beuren syndrome)	Infantile hypercalcemia, skeletal and renal anomalies, cognitive deficits, "social" personality, elfin facies	53–85	Supravalvar AS and PS, PPS
Deletion 8p syndrome	Microcephaly, growth retardation, mental retardation, deep-set eyes, malformed ears, small chin, genital anomalies in males, long survival	50–75	AVSD, PS, VSD, TOF
Deletion 10p	Frontal bossing, short down-slanting palpebral fissures, small low-set ears, micrognathia, cleft palate, short neck, urinary/genital and upper limb anomalies	50	BAV, ASD, VSD, PDA, PS, CoA, common arterial trunk
Deletion 11q (Jacobsen syndrome)	Growth restriction, developmental delay, mental retardation, thrombocytopenia, platelet dysfunction, widely spaced eyes, strabismus, broad nasal bridge, thin upper lip, prominent forehead	56	HLHS, valvar AS, VSD, CoA, Shone complex
Deletion 20p12 (Alagille syndrome)	Bile duct paucity, cholestasis, skeletal or ocular anomalies, broad forehead, widely spaced eyes, underdeveloped mandible	85–94	Peripheral PA hypoplasia, TOF, PS
Deletion 22q11 (DiGeorge, velocardiofacial, and conotruncal anomaly face syndrome)	Hypertelorism, micrognathia, low-set posteriorly rotated ears, "fish mouth," thymic and parathyroid hypoplasia, hypocalcemia, feeding/speech/learning and behavioral disorders, immunodeficiency, palate/skeletal/renal anomalies	75	IAA-B, truncus arteriosus, isolated aortic arch anomalies, TOF, conoventricular VSD

CHD, congenital heart defects; ASD, atrial septal defect; VSD, ventricular septal defect; PDA, patent ductus arteriosus; TOF, tetralogy of Fallot; AS, aortic stenosis; PS, pulmonic stenosis; PPS, peripheral pulmonary stenosis; AVSD, atrioventricular septal defect; BAV, bicuspid aortic valve; CoA, coarctation of the aorta; HLHS, hypoplastic left heart syndrome; PA, pulmonary artery; IAA-B, interrupted aortic arch type B.
(Modified from Pierpont ME, Basson C, Woodrow Benson D, et al. Genetic basis for congenital heart defects: current knowledge. *Circulation* 2007;115:3015–3038, with permission.)

TABLE 2-7	Genes Associated with Congenital Heart Defects	

Condition	Gene(s)	Chromosome location
Nonsyndromic CHD		
Familial congenital heart disease (ASD, atrioventricular block)	NKX2.5 (CSX)	5q34-q35
D-TGA, DORV	CFC1	2q21
D-TGA	PROSIT240	12q24
Tetralogy of Fallot	ZFPM2/FOG2	8q23
	NKX2.5	5q34-35
	JAG1	20p12
Atrioventricular septal defect	CRELD1	3p21
ASD/VSD	GATA4	8p23
Heterotaxy	ZIC3	Xq26
	CFC1	2q21
	ACVR2B	3p21.3-p22
	LEFTA	1q42.1
Supravalvar aortic stenosis	ELN	7q11
Syndromes		
Holt-Oram syndrome	TBX5	12q24
Alagille syndrome (PPS)	JAG1	20p12
Char syndrome (PDA)	TFAP2B	6p12
Noonan syndrome	PTPN11	12q24
	KRAS	12p1.21
	SOS1	2p21
CHARGE association	CHD7	8q12
Ellis-van Creveld syndrome	EVC, EVC2	4p16
Marfan syndrome	FBN1	15q21.1
Marfan-like syndrome	TGFBR2	3p22
Cardiofaciocutaneous syndrome	KRAS	12p12.1
	BRAF	7q34
	MEK1	15q21
	MEK2	7q32
Costello syndrome	HRAS	11p15.5

CHD, congenital heart defect; ASD, atrial septal defect; D-TGA, D-transposition of great arteries; DORV, double outlet right ventricle; VSD, ventricular septal defect; PPS, peripheral pulmonary stenosis; PDA, patent ductus arteriosus; CHARGE, coloboma, heart anomaly, choanal atresia, retardation, genital, and ear anomalies.
(Source: Pierpont ME, Basson C, Woodrow Benson D, et al. Genetic basis for congenital heart defects: current knowledge. *Circulation* 2007;115:3015–3038.)

 FAMILIAL RECURRENCE OF CONGENITAL HEART DEFECTS

Although the factors that regulate fetal cardiac development are not well understood, traditionally the etiology of most congenital heart defects has been ascribed to multifactorial causation with interaction between genetic and environmental factors. Analyzing a large cohort of children with congenital heart defects, the Baltimore Washington Infants Study revealed that about 30% of congenital heart defects presented an association with genetic disorders, while about 70% are apparently isolated, nonsyndromic in type (26). In this group of isolated congenital heart defects, only about 3% to 5% presented familial recurrence (26). Based on this multifactorial model, recurrence risk for an isolated congenital cardiovascular malformation is modified for each family based on the number of affected relatives and the severity of the abnormality in the proband. Large population studies estimate a recurrence risk of 3% for two healthy nonconsanguineous parents with one affected child (27). The risk of recurrence increases to 10% with two affected siblings (27,28). Table 2-8 lists recurrence risk estimates in nonsyndromic congenital heart defects based on the multifactorial model of inheritance.

TABLE 2-8	Recurrence Risks in Nonsyndromic Congenital Heart Defects (Normal Parents and One Affected Offspring)

Anomaly	Recurrence risk (%)
Ventricular septal defect	4.2
Atrial septal defect	3
Tetralogy of Fallot	2.5–3
Pulmonary stenosis	2.7
Coarctation of the aorta	1.8
Aortic stenosis	2.2
Transposition of great arteries	1–1.8
Corrected transposition of great arteries	5.8
Atrioventricular septal defect	3–4
Hypoplastic left heart	2.2
Tricuspid atresia	1.0
Ebstein's anomaly	1.0

(From Nora JJ, Berg K, Nora AH. Cardiovascular diseases: genetics, epidemiology and prevention. New York: Oxford University Press, 1991;53–80, and Calcagni G, Digilio CM, Sarkozy A, et al. Familial recurrence of congenital heart disease: an overview and review of the literature. *Eur J Pediatr* 2007;166:111–116, with permission.)

TABLE 2-9	Congenital Cardiac Lesions and Their Associations with Syndromes

Pulmonary artery valve stenosis	• Noonan syndrome • Alagille syndrome • Costello syndrome • Leopard syndrome • Trisomy 8
Pulmonary artery branch stenosis	• Alagille syndrome • Williams-Beuren syndrome
Aortic artery valve stenosis	• Jacobsen syndrome (del 11q) • Autosomal trisomies 13, 18 • Noonan syndrome • Turner syndrome
Supravalvular aortic stenosis	• Williams-Beuren syndrome
Coarctation of the aorta	• Turner syndrome
Secundum atrial septal defect	• Holt-Oram syndrome • Ellis-van Creveld syndrome
Ventricular septal defect	• Holt-Oram syndrome • Autosomal trisomies 21, 18, 13 • 22q11 deletion syndrome
Atrioventricular septal defect	• Autosomal trisomies 21, 18, 13
Tetralogy of Fallot	• 22q11 deletion syndrome • Alagille syndrome • Cat-eye syndrome • Autosomal trisomies 21, 18, 13 • Other
Common arterial trunk/interruption of aortic arch	• 22q11 deletion syndrome • Trisomy 8 • Deletion 10p
Double outlet right ventricle	• Autosomal trisomies 9, 13, 18 • Duplication 2p, 12p
Tricuspid atresia	• Most are sporadic
Ebstein anomaly	• Most are sporadic
Total anomalous venous connection	• Most are sporadic

(Source: Pierpont ME, Basson C, Woodrow Benson D, et al. Genetic basis for congenital heart defects: current knowledge. *Circulation* 2007;115:3015–3038.)

The contribution of genetic factors increases in significance when congenital heart defects are grouped by pathogenic developmental mechanism rather than by anatomic phenotype (29,30). In a population-based epidemiologic study, the sibling recurrence risk for hypoplastic left heart syndrome was 13.5%, significantly different from what is expected from a multifactorial pattern (31). These studies and others suggest that variability in risk among the lesions may be greater than previously estimated, and that genetic factors may play a more prominent role in some forms of isolated congenital heart abnormalities than previously expected.

 ## SUMMARY

This chapter reviews some of the known associations between congenital heart defects, chromosome abnormalities, and single gene disorders. An attempt was made to present an association between genetic and cardiac malformations that are clinically relevant with an emphasis on the most prevalent of the syndromes. Table 2-9 lists various congenital cardiac lesions and their known association with genetic syndromes. Additional resources that present more comprehensive information on this topic are available at the end of this chapter.

Significant progress has been made in our understanding of the genetic basis of congenital heart disease in the past decade. Despite these significant advances, the direct cause of congenital heart disease remains poorly understood. It is highly likely that new genetic techniques will continue to expand the knowledge in this field, which will lead to the development of novel approaches to diagnosis, prevention, and therapy.

■ KEY POINTS: GENETIC ASPECTS OF CONGENITAL HEART DEFECTS

- Chromosomal abnormalities in infants with congenital heart defects are estimated at around 5% to 15%.
- Chromosomal abnormalities in fetuses with congenital heart defects are estimated at around 30% to 40%.
- Specific cardiac diagnoses most likely to be associated with chromosomal abnormalities include atrioventricular septal defect, ventricular and atrial septal defects, and tetralogy of Fallot.
- Specific cardiac diagnoses least likely to be associated with chromosomal abnormalities include transposition of great arteries and heterotaxy syndromes.
- The incidence of congenital heart defects is 40% to 50% in trisomy 21, 25% to 35% in Turner syndrome, and more than 80% in trisomies 13 and 18.
- Cardiovascular anomalies are noted in up to 85% of fetuses with the 22q11 deletion (DiGeorge syndrome).
- The most common cardiac abnormalities associated with the 22q11 deletion include tetralogy of Fallot, common arterial trunk, and aortic arch abnormalities (interrupted aortic arch).
- Cardiovascular anomalies are noted in up to 90% of fetuses with the 7q11.23 deletion (Williams-Beuren syndrome).
- The most common cardiac abnormalities associated with the 7q11.23 deletion include supravalvular aortic stenosis and supravalvular pulmonary stenosis.
- Cardiac involvement is observed in 80% to 90% of fetuses with Noonan syndrome, with valvular pulmonary stenosis and hypertrophic cardiomyopathy accounting for the majority of cardiac lesions.
- Cardiac involvement is observed in 90% of fetuses with Alagille syndrome, with pulmonary branch stenosis accounting for the majority of cardiac lesions.
- Preaxial radial ray malformations are required for the diagnosis of Holt-Oram syndrome (heart-hand).
- Cardiac involvement is observed in 85% to 95% of fetuses with Holt-Oram syndrome, with secundum atrial septal defects and muscular ventricular septal defects accounting for the majority of cardiac lesions.
- Of all congenital heart defects, 70% are isolated, nonsyndromic in type and 30% are associated with a genetic disorder.
- In general, recurrence risks in nonsyndromic congenital heart defects are in the order of 1% to 5%.

■ ADDITIONAL RESOURCES

■ Online Mendelian Inheritance in Man (http://www.ncbi.nlm.nih.gov/omim/):
Reviews for genetic disorders and the ability to search based on dysmorphic features
■ GeneTests (http://www.genetests.org/):
Reviews for genetic disorders for which a gene has been identified and details on availability of clinical testing
■ Genetic Alliance (http://www.geneticalliance.org/):
Support groups and information for families on various genetic disorders

References

1. O'Rahilly R, Müller F. *Human embryology and teratology.* New York: Wiley-Liss, 1992;107–117.
2. Collins-Nakai R, McLaughlin P. How congenital heart disease originates in fetal life. *Cardiol Clin* 2002;20:367–383.
3. Pierpont ME, Basson C, Woodrow Benson D, et al. Genetic basis for congenital heart defects: current knowledge. *Circulation* 2007;115:3015–3038.
4. Hook EB. Contribution of chromosome abnormalities to human morbidity and mortality. *Cytogenet Cell Genet* 1982;33:101–106.
5. Ferencz C, Neill CA, Boughman JA, et al. Congenital cardiovascular malformations associated with chromosome abnormalities: an epidemiologic study. *J Pediatr* 1989;114:79–86.
6. Harris JA, Francannet C, Pradat P. The epidemiology of cardiovascular defects, part 2: a study based on data from three large registries of congenital malformations. *Pediatr Cardiol* 2003;24:222–235.
7. Copel JA, Cullen M, Green JJ, et al. The frequency of aneuploidy in prenatally diagnosed congenital heart disease: an indication for fetal karyotyping. *Am J Obstet Gynecol* 1988;158:409–413.
8. Schwanitz G, Zerres K, Gembruch U, et al. Prenatal detection of heart defects as an indication for chromosome analysis. *Ann Genet* 1990;33:78–83.
9. Eydoux P, Choiset A, Le Porrier N, et al. Chromosomal prenatal diagnosis: study of 936 cases of intrauterine abnormalities after ultrasound assessment. *Prenat Diagn* 1989;9:255–268.
10. Hook EB. Chromosome abnormalities and spontaneous fetal death following amniocentesis: further data and associations with maternal age. *Am J Hum Genet* 1983;35:110–116.
11. Berg KA, Clark EB, Astemborski JA, et al. Prenatal detection of cardiovascular malformations by echocardiography: an indication for cytogenetic evaluation. *Am J Obstet Gynecol* 1988;159:477–481.
12. Pierpont MEM, Moller JH. Chromosomal abnormalities. In: Pierpont MEM, Moller JH, eds. *The genetics of cardiovascular disease.* Boston: Nijhoff, 1987;13–24.
13. Wyllie JP, Wright MJ, Burn J, et al. Natural history of trisomy 13. *Arch Dis Child* 1994;71:343–345.
14. Devriendt K, Fryns JP, Mortier G, et al. The annual incidence of DiGeorge/velocardiofacial syndrome. *J Med Genet* 1998;35:789–790.
15. Perez E, Sullivan K. Chromosome 22q11 deletion syndrome: DiGeorge and velocardiofacial syndromes. *Curr Opin Pediatr* 2002;14:678–683.
16. Digilio MC, Angioni A, De Saints M, et al. Spectrum of clinical variability in familial deletion 22q11: from full manifestation to extremely mild clinical anomalies. *Clin Genet* 2003;63:308–313.
17. Chaoui R, Kalache KD, Heling KS, et al. Absent or hypoplastic thymus on ultrasound: a marker for deletion 22q11 in fetal cardiac defects. *Ultrasound Obstet Gynecol* 2002;20:546–552.
18. Manning N, Kaufman L, Roberts P. Genetics of cardiological disorders. *Semin Fetal Neonatal Med* 2005;10:259–269.
19. Ewart AK, Morris CA, Atkinson D, et al. Hemizygosity at the elastin locus in a developmental disorder: Williams syndrome. *Nat Genet* 1993;5:11–16.
20. Noonan JA. Noonan syndrome: an update and review for the primary pediatrician. *Clin Pediatr* 1994;33:548–555.
21. Menashe M, Arbel R, Raveh D, et al. Poor prenatal detection rate of cardiac anomalies in Noonan syndrome. *Ultrasound Obstet Gynecol* 2002;19:51–55.
22. Krantz ID, Piccoli DA, Spinner NB. Alagille syndrome. *J Med Genet* 1997;34:152–157.
23. McElhinney DB, Krantz ID, Bason L, et al. Analysis of cardiovascular phenotype and genotype-phenotype correlation in individuals with a JAG1 mutation and/or Alagille syndrome. *Circulation* 2002;106:2567–2574.
24. Basson CT, Cowley GS, Soloman SD, et al. The clinical and genetic spectrum of the Holt-Oram syndrome: heart-hand syndrome. *N Engl J Med* 1994;330:885–891.
25. Bossert T, Walther T, Gummert J, et al. Cardiac malformations associated with the Holt-Oram syndrome: report on family and review of the literature. *Thorac Cardiovasc Surg* 2002;50:312–314.
26. Ferencz C, Rubin JD, Loffredo CA, et al. *Epidemiology of congenital heart disease: the Baltimore-Washington Infant Study.* New York: Futura Publishing Company, 1993;1981–1989.
27. Nora JJ, Berg K, Nora AH. *Cardiovascular diseases: genetics, epidemiology and prevention.* New York: Oxford University Press, 1991;53–80.
28. Calcagni G, Digilio CM, Sarkozy A, et al. Familial recurrence of congenital heart disease: an overview and review of the literature. *Eur J Pediatr* 2007;166:111–116.
29. Maestri NE, Beaty TH, Boughman JA. Etiologic heterogeneity in the familial aggregation of congenital cardiovascular malformations. *Am J Human Genet* 1989;45:556–564.
30. Bulbul ZR, Rosenthal D, Brueckner M. Genetic aspects of heart disease in the newborn. *Semin Perinatol* 1993;17(2):61–75.
31. Boughman JA, Berg KA, Astemborski JA, et al. Familial risks of congenital heart defect assessed in a population-based epidemiologic study. *Am J Med Genet* 1987;26:839–849.

INTRODUCTION

Congenital heart disease (CHD) is the most common congenital abnormality in the human fetus, and it accounts for more than half of the deaths from congenital abnormalities in childhood (1). Several risk factors for CHD, including maternal and fetal factors, have been reported (Chapter 1). Fetal echocardiography has been shown to identify the majority of structural cardiac abnormalities (2), and has traditionally been reserved for pregnancies at increased risk for CHD. Most neonates born with CHD, however, have no preidentified risk factors (2). In fact, of all pregnancies referred for fetal echocardiography, the highest incidence of CHD (50%) occurs in pregnancies with a suspected CHD on a routine ultrasound examination (3). In order to improve the prenatal detection of CHD, a screening test, which can be offered to all pregnancies, is required.

Despite the accuracy of fetal echocardiography, second-trimester detection of CHD occurs infrequently in the population at present (4). In a randomized design study in the United States, the detection rate of CHD in the second trimester of pregnancy was 4 of 22 (18%) and 0 of 17 (0%) in tertiary and nontertiary centers, respectively (5,6). Similar disappointingly low rates (15% at 18 weeks) have been reported in a large randomized controlled trial in Europe (7). A prenatal CHD detection rate of 21% was also reported in a study involving more than 77,000 infants over a period of 5 years (1999 to 2003) (8), and a detection rate of 35% was noted in a large population-based study that included first-trimester risk assessment by nuchal translucency (9). Other studies have shown enhanced prenatal detection of CHD, albeit with significant room for improvement. A nonselected population-based study has recently shown a 57% prenatal detection rate for major CHD, with a 44% detection rate of isolated cardiac lesions (10). Prenatal diagnosis of CHD in cases referred to a pediatric cardiology group has increased from 8% to 50% in the period from 1992 to 2002 in one center in the United States (11). Despite these encouraging studies, prenatal detection rates for isolated CHD have remained significantly below 50% and have lagged behind detection rates of other congenital malformations. Efforts should be directed toward enhancing the detection of CHD in utero in view of evidence suggesting improved neonatal morbidity and mortality in prenatally diagnosed CHD (12,13). Targeted education and training of sonographers and sonologists have been shown to improve detection of CHD in the population (14,15). Recent research directed toward lessening the operator dependency of the ultrasound examination by using automated three-dimensional sonography shows significant promise (16–18). Until the ultrasound technology becomes more standardized and automated, a high level of suspicion for the presence of CHD and attention to anatomic details should be part of every ultrasound examination.

 THE FOUR-CHAMBER VIEW

With the widespread use of routine ultrasound examination in pregnancy, the four-chamber view of the fetal heart has been proposed as a screening test for CHD (19) (Fig. 3-1). The four-chamber view of the heart has several features that make it a good screening test for CHD. It is part of the basic obstetric ultrasound examination (20,21). It does not require specialized ultrasound skills as it is easily imaged in a transverse view of the fetal chest. It is obtainable in all fetal positions and in more than 95% of ultrasound examinations performed after 19 weeks of gestation (22).

Several specific cardiac abnormalities are associated with a normal four-chamber view of the fetal heart. This represents a major limitation for the routine use of the four-chamber view in screening for CHD in pregnancy. Table 3-1 lists cardiac abnormalities that are commonly associated with a normal four-chamber view of the fetal heart, and Table 3-2 lists cardiac

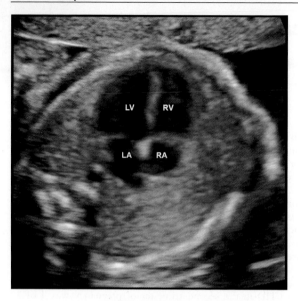

Figure 3-1. Normal four-chamber view of the fetal heart obtained in a transverse view of the chest. LA, left atrium; LV, left ventricle; RA, right atrium; RV, right ventricle.

TABLE 3-1	Cardiac Abnormalities Commonly Associated with a Normal Four-chamber View of the Heart

Tetralogy of Fallot
Transposition of great arteries
Double outlet right ventricle
Small ventricular septal defects
Common arterial trunk
Mild semilunar valves stenosis
Aortic arch abnormalities

abnormalities that are commonly associated with an abnormal four-chamber view of the fetal heart.

A four-chamber view (Fig. 3-1) of the fetal heart should be considered normal only when the following conditions are met:

1. The fetal situs is normal.
2. The size of the heart in relation to the chest is normal.

TABLE 3-2	Cardiac Abnormalities Commonly Associated with an Abnormal Four-chamber View of the Heart

Mitral/aortic atresia
Tricuspid/pulmonary atresia
Ebstein anomaly/tricuspid valve dysplasia
Atrioventricular septal defect
Large ventricular septal defects
Single ventricle (double inlet)
Severe aortic/pulmonary stenosis
Severe coarctation of the aorta
Total anomalous venous connection
Cardiomyopathies/heart tumors

TABLE 3-3	The Four-chamber View of the Heart and Prenatal Screening for Congenital Heart Disease				
Author (ref.)/year	**n**	**Incidence of CHD**	**Risk status**	**Sensitivity (%)**
Copel et al. (3)/1987	1022	72/1000	High risk	92
Sharland and Allan (23)/1992[a]	23,861	2.8/1000	Low risk	77
Vergani et al. (24)/1992	5336	5.9/1000	Low risk	81
Achiron et al. (25)/1992	5347	4.3/1000	Low risk	48
Bromley et al. (26)/1992	—	—	Mixed	63
Wigton et al. (27)/1993	10,004	3.6/1000	Low risk	38
Kirk et al. (28)/1994	5111	10/1000	Low risk	47
Tegnander et al. (29)/1995	7459	12/1000	Low risk	39

[a] Limited to abnormalities commonly detected by four-chamber view.

3. The two atria are equal in size and the flap of the foramen ovale is seen within the left atrium.

4. The two ventricles are equal in size and contractility, with the moderator band imaged in the apex of the right ventricle.

5. The atrial and ventricular septae are normal appearing.

6. The atrioventricular valves are normal appearing where the tricuspid valve appears to insert more apically on the ventricular septum.

Detailed discussion of ultrasonographic fetal cardiac anatomy is presented in the following chapters.

The validity of the four-chamber view in screening for CHD in the fetus has been evaluated by several investigators (3,23–29). Studies differ in the prevalence of CHD in the study population, the risk status of the targeted pregnancies, the operator's expertise, the ascertainment bias, and the study design. These differences undoubtedly contribute to wide variation in the sensitivity of the four-chamber view in screening for CHD in pregnancy. Clinical factors that may affect the ability to obtain a satisfactory four-chamber view include maternal obesity, fetal position within the uterus, gestational age, and prior maternal abdominal surgery (30). In general, studies evaluating the four-chamber view in low-risk populations are associated with a low sensitivity for the detection of CHD (25,27–29). Even within the same ultrasound laboratory, a significant difference in the sensitivity of the four-chamber view is noted between that in low-risk pregnancies and that in high-risk pregnancies (31). Data from studies evaluating the validity of the four-chamber view in screening for CHD are summarized in Table 3-3.

EXTENDED BASIC EXAMINATION

When feasible, views of the outflow tracts should be attempted as part of an "extended basic" screening examination of the fetal heart, because defects of the great vessels are associated with an abnormal four-chamber view in only 30% of cases (32). The extended basic screening examination includes demonstration of the left and right ventricular outflow tracts as they emerge from their respective ventricular chambers. The left ventricular outflow tract view, which illustrates the four chambers of the heart and the aorta as it arises from the left ventricle, is commonly known as the five-chamber view (Fig. 3-2) and is visualized in 90% of pregnant women with adequate training and experience (30). The five-chamber view allows for the visualization of the outflow of the left ventricle and the membranous ventricular septum. Demonstrating continuity of the anterior wall of the aorta with the membranous ventricular septum (Fig. 3-2) is critical in the evaluation of the fetal heart because it rules out an overriding aorta, which is the hallmark of tetralogy of Fallot, truncus arteriosus, and double outlet right ventricle. The right ventricular outflow tract view can be obtained by maintaining the transverse plane of the four-chamber view and sliding the ultrasound transducer toward the fetal head (Fig. 3-3). This view demonstrates the pulmonary artery arising from the right ventricle and coursing to the left. The pulmonary artery divides into right and left branches; the pulmonary valve leaflets should be seen to move freely and the size of the pulmonary artery

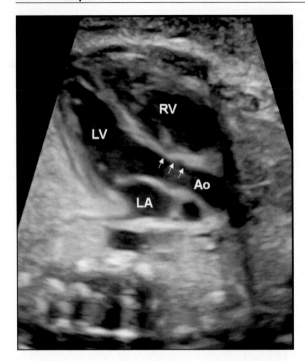

Figure 3-2. Left ventricular outflow tract view (five-chamber view) showing the aorta as it emerges from the left ventricle. Note the continuity of the anterior wall of the aorta with the ventricular septum (*white arrows*). Ao, aorta; LA, left atrium; LV, left ventricle; RV, right ventricle.

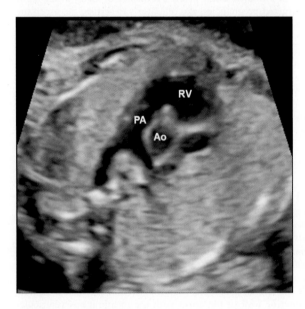

Figure 3-3. Right ventricular outflow tract view showing the pulmonary artery as it emerges from the right ventricle. The pulmonary artery size is slightly larger than the aorta in fetal life. Ao, aorta; PA, pulmonary artery; RV, right ventricle.

should be slightly larger than the aortic root. Detailed discussion of right and left ventricular outflow anatomy is presented in Chapter 6.

In general, studies evaluating the extended basic cardiac examination (outflow tracts) of the fetal heart in screening for CHD have shown a better detection of CHD when compared to the four-chamber view. This is probably related in part to the technical expertise required to obtain these images. Data from various studies on the validity of adding extended views of

TABLE 3-4	Comparison of Studies on Congenital Heart Disease Screening with the Four-chamber View and Visualization of the Great Arteries (Extended Basic Examination)

Author (ref.)/year	Study design	Population	Sensitivity of four-chamber view (%)	Sensitivity of extended examination (%)
Achiron et al. (25)/1992	Prospective	Low risk	48	78
Bromley et al. (26)/1992	Retrospective	High and low risk	63	83
Wigton et al. (27)/1993	Retrospective	Unselected	33.3	38.9
Kirk et al. (28)/1994	Prospective	Low risk	47	78
Rustico et al. (33)/1995	Prospective	Low risk	Unknown	35.4
Stumpflen et al. (34)/1996	Prospective	Unselected	Unknown	88.5
Kirk et al. (35)/1997	Prospective	Unselected	Unknown	66
Stoll et al. (36)/2002	Retrospective, case control	Unselected	Unknown	19.9
Carvalho et al. (37)/2002	Prospective	Unselected	Unknown	76
Tegnander et al. (29)/1995	Prospective	Unselected	Unknown	57
Ogge et al. (38)/2006	Prospective	Low risk	60.3	65.5

(Modified from Oggè G, Gaglioti P, Maccanti S, et al.; and Gruppo Piemontese for Prenatal Screening of Congenital Heart Disease. Prenatal screening for congenital heart disease with four-chamber and outflow-tract views: a multicenter study. *Ultrasound Obstet Gynecol* 2006;28:779–784, with permission.)

the great arteries to the four-chamber view of the heart in screening for CHD in the fetus are presented in Table 3-4 (25–29, 33–38).

SCREENING FOR CONGENITAL HEART DISEASE IN EARLY GESTATION

Several studies have suggested that nuchal translucency, performed in the first and early second trimesters, between 10 and 14 weeks of gestation, may be a good screening test for CHD (39–41). An association exists between increased nuchal translucency thickness and major CHD (9). Early reports noted a 40% sensitivity for major CHD detection for a nuchal translucency measurement at the 99th percentile or greater for a specific crown–rump length measurement (39). Studies performed following the original study reported lower sensitivity, with a range of 13% to 36% (9,40–42). Variation in reported sensitivity may be explained by the risk level of the study population, the inclusion of fetuses with cystic hygroma in the study, the study design, and ascertainment bias. Despite the relatively low sensitivity noted in recent studies, nuchal translucency measurement is expected to enhance detection of CHD as it

TABLE 3-5	Nuchal Translucency (NT) and Prenatal Screening for Congenital Heart Disease (CHD)

Author (ref.)/year	n	Incidence of major CHD	NT threshold (percentile)	Sensitivity (%)	PPV (%)
Hyett et al. (39)/1999	29,154	1.7/1000	99th	40	6.3
Michailidis et al. (41)/2001	6606	1.7/1000	99th	27	4.1
Hafner et al. (40)/2003	12,978	2.1/1000	95th	25.9	1.1
Bahado-Singh et al. (42)/2005	8167	2.1/1000	95th	29.4	0.8
Simpson et al. (9)/2007	34,266	1.5/1000	99th	13.5	3.3

PPV, positive predictive value.
(Modified from Simpson L, Malone F, Bianchi D, et al.; for the First and Second Trimester Evaluation of Risk Research Consortium. Nuchal translucency and the risk of congenital heart disease. *Obset Gynecol* 2007;109:376–383, with permission.)

directs pregnancies with a thickened measurement to targeted evaluation of the fetal heart, preferably by experienced operators. In a meta-analysis assessing the performance of nuchal translucency measurements in screening for CHD that would benefit from prenatal detection, the authors report that, using nuchal translucency measurements, the estimated detection rate of 52% (95% confidence interval [CI] 42–71) was noted, with a false-positive rate of 5% (43). A nuchal translucency measurement, obtained between 10 and 14 weeks of gestation, that is greater than or equal to 3.5 mm is an indication for fetal echocardiography. Table 3-5 compares various studies on this subject. Detailed discussion on the detection of major CHD in the first-trimester ultrasound examination is presented in Chapter 10 and chapters addressing specific cardiac malformations.

■ KEY POINTS: PRENATAL SCREENING FOR CONGENITAL HEART DISEASE

■ Fetal echocardiography has been shown to identify the majority of structural cardiac abnormalities.

■ Most neonates born with CHD have no preidentified risk factors.

■ Prenatal detection rates of isolated CHD have remained below 50% in the general population and have lagged behind detection rates of other congenital malformations.

■ There is wide variation in the sensitivity of the four-chamber view in screening for CHD in pregnancy.

■ Defects of the great vessels are associated with an abnormal four-chamber view in only 30% of cases.

■ Studies evaluating the outflow tracts views of the fetal heart in screening for CHD have shown a better detection of CHD when compared to the four-chamber view.

■ An association exists between increased nuchal translucency thickness and major CHD.

■ A nuchal translucency measurement, obtained between 10 and 14 weeks of gestation, that is greater than or equal to 3.55 mm, is an indication for fetal echocardiography.

References

1. Hoffman JIE, Christianson R. Congenital heart disease in a cohort of 19,502 births with long-term follow-up. *Am J Cardiol* 1978;42:641.
2. Allan LD, Sharland GK, Milburn A, et al. Prospective diagnosis of 1,006 consecutive cases of congenital heart disease in the fetus. *J Am Coll Cardiol* 1994;23:1452.
3. Copel JA, Pilu G, Green J, et al. Fetal echocardiographic screening for congenital heart disease: the importance of the four-chamber view. *Am J Obstet Gynecol* 1987;157:648–655.
4. Garne E, Still C, Clementi M, and the Euroscan Group. Evaluation of prenatal diagnosis of congenital heart diseases by ultrasound: experience from 20 European registries. *Ultrasound Obstet Gynecol* 2001;17:386–391.
5. Ewigman BG, Crane JP, Frigoletto FD, et al. Effect of prenatal ultrasound on perinatal outcome. *N Engl J Med* 1993;329:821–827.
6. Personal Communication, Data from Radius trial, presented at International Perinatal Doppler Society, Toronto, 1994.
7. Westin M, Saltvedt S, Bergman G, et al. Routine ultrasound examination at 12 or 18 gestational weeks for prenatal detection of major congenital heart malformations? A randomized controlled trial comprising 36,299 fetuses. *BJOG* 2006;3:675–682.
8. Nikkila A, Bjorkhem G, Kallen B. Prenatal diagnosis of congenital heart defects: a population based study. *Acta Paediatr* 2006;96:49–52.
9. Simpson L, Malone F, Bianchi D, et al.; for the First and Second Trimester Evaluation of Risk Research Consortium. Nuchal translucency and the risk of congenital heart disease. *Obset Gynecol* 2007;109:376–383.
10. Tegnander E, Williams W, Johanses OJ, et al. Prenatal detection of heart defect in a non-selected population of 30,149 fetuses-detection rates and outcome. *Ultrasound Obstet Gynecol* 2006;27:252–265.
11. Mohan UR, Kleinman CS, Kern JH. Fetal echocardiography and its evolving impact 1992 to 2002. *Am J Cardiol* 2005;96:134–136.
12. Mahle WT, Clancy RR, McGaurn SP, et al. Impact of prenatal diagnosis on survival and early neurological morbidity in neonates with hypoplastic left heart syndrome. *Pediatrics* 2001;107:1277–1282.
13. Bonner D, Coltri A, Butera G, et al. Detection of transposition of the great arteries in fetuses reduces neonatal morbidity and mortality. *Circulation* 1999;99:916–918.
14. Tegnander E, Eik-Nes SH. The examiner's ultrasound experience has a significant impact on the detection rate of congenital heart defects at the second-trimester fetal examination. *Ultrasound Obstet Gynecol* 2006;28:8–14.
15. Hunter S, Heads A, Wyllie J, et al. Prenatal diagnosis of congenital heart disease in the northern region of England: benefits of a training program for obstetric ultrasonographers. *Heart* 2000;84:294–298.
16. Abuhamad A. Automated multiplanar imaging: a novel approach to ultrasonography. *J Ultrasound Med* 2004;23(5):573–576.

17. Abuhamad A, Falkensammer P, Zhao Y. Automated sonography: defining the spatial relationship of standard diagnostic fetal cardiac planes in the second trimester of pregnancy. *J Ultrasound Med* 2007;26:501–507.
18. Abuhamad A, Falkensammer P, Reichartseder F, et al. Automated retrieval of standard diagnostic fetal cardiac ultrasound in the second trimester of pregnancy: a prospective evaluation of the software. *Ultrasound Obstet Gynecol* 2008;31(1):30–36.
19. Allan LD, Crawford DC, Chita SK, et al. Prenatal screening for congenital heart disease. *Br Med J* 1986;292:1717.
20. *American Institute of Ultrasound in Medicine practical guidelines for the performance of obstetric ultrasound examinations.* Laurel, MD: American Institute of Ultrasound in Medicine, 2007.
21. International Society of Ultrasound in Obstetrics and Gynecology. Cardiac screening examination of the fetus: guidelines for performing the 'basic' and 'extended basic' cardiac scan. *Ultrasound Obstet Gynecol* 2006;27:107–113.
22. Shultz SM, Pretorius DH, Budorick NE. Four-chamber view of the fetal heart: demonstration related to menstrual age. *J Ultrasound Med* 1994;13:285–289.
23. Sharland GK, Allan LD. Screening for congenital heart disease prenatally. Results of a 2 1/2-year study in the South East Thames Region. *Br J Obstet Gynecol* 1992;99:220–225.
24. Vergani P, Mariani S, Ghidini A, et al. Screening for congenital heart disease with the four-chamber view of the fetal heart. *Am J Obstet Gynecol* 1992;167:1000–1003.
25. Achiron R, Glaser J, Gelernter, et al. Extended fetal echocardiographic examination for detecting cardiac malformations in low risk pregnancies. *Br Med J* 1992;304:671.
26. Bromley B, Estroff JA, Sanders SP, et al. Fetal echocardiography: Accuracy and limitations in a population at high and low risk for heart defects. *Am J Obstet Gynecol* 1992;166:1473–1481.
27. Wigton TR, Sabbagha RE, Tamura RK, et al. Sonographic diagnosis of congenital heart disease: comparison between the four-chamber view and multiple cardiac views. *Obstet Gynecol* 1993;82:219–224.
28. Kirk JS, Riggs TW, Comstock CH, et al. Prenatal screening for cardiac anomalies: the value of routine addition of the aortic root to the four chamber view. *Obstet Gynecol* 1994;84(3):427–431.
29. Tegnander E, Eik-Nes SH, Johansen OJ, et al. Prenatal detection of heart defects at the routine fetal examination at 18 weeks in a non-selected population. *Ultrasound Obstet Gynecol* 1995;5:372–380.
30. DeVore GR, Medaris AL, Bear MD, et al. Fetal echocardiography: factors that influence imaging of the fetal heart during the second trimester of pregnancy. *J Ultrasound Med* 1993;12:659–663.
31. Ott WJ. The accuracy of antenatal fetal echocardiography screening in high- and low-risk patients. *Am J Obstet Gynecol* 1995;172:1741–1749.
32. Paladini D, Rustico M, Todros T, et al. Conotruncal anomalies in prenatal life. *Ultrasound Obstet Gynecol* 1996;8:241–246.
33. Rustico MA, Benettoni A, D'Ottavio G, et al. Fetal heart screening in low-risk pregnancies. *Ultrasound Obstet Gynecol* 1995;6:313–319.
34. Stumpflen I, Stumpflen A, Wimmer MA, et al. Effect of detailed fetal echocardiography as part of routine prenatal ultrasonographic screening on detection of congenital heart disease. *Lancet* 1996;348:854–857.
35. Kirk JS, Comstock CH, Lee W, et al. Sonographic screening to detect fetal cardiac anomalies: a 5-year experience with 111 abnormal cases. *Obstet Gynecol* 1997;89:227–232.
36. Stoll C, Dott B, Alembick Y, et al. Evaluation and evolution during time of prenatia diagnosis of congenital heart diseases by routine fetal ultrasonographic examination. *Am Genet* 2002;45:21–27.
37. Carvalho JS, Mavrides E, Shinebourne EA, et al. Improving the effectiveness of routine prenatal screening for major congenital heart defects. *Heart* 2002;88:387–391.
38. Oggè G, Gaglioti P, Maccanti S, et al.; and Gruppo Piemontese for Prenatal Screening of Congenital Heart Disease. Prenatal screening for congenital heart disease with four-chamber and outflow-tract views: a multicenter study. *Ultrasound Obstet Gynecol* 2006;28:779–784.
39. Hyett J, Perdu M, Sharland G, et al. Using fetal nuchal translucency to screen for major congenital cardiac defects at 10–14 weeks of gestation: population based cohort study. *BMJ* 1999;318:81–85.
40. Hafner E, Schuller T, Metzenvauer M, et al. Increased nuchal translucency and congenital heart defects in a low-risk population. *Prenat Diagn* 2003;23:985–989.
41. Michailidis GD, Economides DL. Nuchal translucency measurement and pregnancy outcome in karyotypically normal fetuses. *Ultrasound Obstet Gynecol* 2001;17:102–105.
42. Bahado-Singh RO, Wapner R, Thom E, et al. Elevated first-trimester nuchal translucency increases the risk of congenital heart defects. *Am J Obstet Gynecol* 2005;192:1357–1361.
43. Wald NJ, Morris JK, Walker K, et al. Prenatal screening for serious congenital heart defects using nuchal translucency: a meta-analysis. *Prenat Diagn* 2008;28:1094–1104.

GENERAL ANATOMIC LANDMARKS
OF THE FETAL HEART

FETAL VISCERAL SITUS

The first step in the ultrasonographic evaluation of the fetal heart is the assessment of the fetal visceral situs (laterality of fetal organs). Establishing the fetal visceral situs allows for an accurate determination of ventricular and atrial situs and therefore should be part of every fetal ultrasound examination. Three types of visceral situs exist: situs solitus, situs inversus, and situs ambiguous (Table 4-1). Situs solitus refers to the normal arrangement of vessels and organs within the body. Situs inversus, with an incidence of about 0.01% of the population, refers to a mirror-image arrangement of organs and vessels to situs solitus. Situs inversus is associated with a slight increase in the incidence of complex congenital heart disease (CHD), in the order of 0.3% to 5% (1). Furthermore, in about 20% of cases of situs inversus, Kartagener syndrome is noted, which primarily involves ciliary dysfunction with recurrent respiratory infection and reduced fertility (2). Situs ambiguous (heterotaxy), which refers to visceral malpositions and malformations different from situs solitus or inversus, is commonly associated with complex congenital heart disease, abnormalities in venous drainage, bowel malrotations and obstruction, and splenic, biliary, and bronchial tree abnormalities. The incidence of situs ambiguous has been estimated around 1 per 10,000 infants (3). Two types of heterotaxy exist: right isomerism and left isomerism. In right isomerism, also referred to as asplenia, both sides of the body show the right morphology; in left isomerism, also referred to as polysplenia, both sides of the body show the left morphology. Chapter 22 presents a detailed overview of fetal heterotaxy.

Although the current method for the determination of fetal situs relies on the position of the stomach and heart in the abdomen and chest, respectively, careful attention should be paid to the position of the aorta and inferior vena cava below the diaphragm, the presence of bowel dilatation, the presence of a gallbladder, and the presence and location of the spleen (Fig. 4-1). It is generally agreed that the positions of the aorta and inferior vena cava below the diaphragm are more reliable criteria for the determination of right or left isomerism.

Technique

1. Locate the fetal head within the uterus and determine the presenting part (e.g., cephalic, breech).
2. Determine the fetal lie within the uterus by obtaining a sagittal view of the fetal spine. (longitudinal lie: when the fetal spine is parallel to the maternal spine; transverse lie: when

TABLE 4-1	Types of Visceral Situs	
	Findings	
Situs	**Right side**	**Left side**
Solitus (normal)	Morphologic right atrium	Morphologic left atrium
	Major hepatic lobe	Stomach
	Inferior vena cava	Descending aorta
	Trilobed lung	Bilobed lung
	Short eparterial bronchus	Long hyparterial bronchus
Inversus	Morphologic left atrium	Morphologic right atrium
	Stomach	Major hepatic lobe
	Descending aorta	Inferior vena cava
	Bilobed lung	Trilobed lung
	Long hyparterial bronchus	Short eparterial bronchus
Ambiguous (heterotaxy)	Variable	Variable

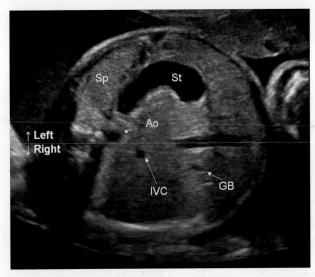

Figure 4-1. Transverse views of the fetal abdomen identifying left-sided and right-sided structures. St, stomach; Ao, descending aorta; Sp, spleen; GB, gallbladder, IVC, inferior vena cava.

the fetal spine is perpendicular to the maternal spine; oblique lie: when the fetal spine is oblique to the maternal spine) (Fig. 4-2).

3. After establishing the exact position of the fetus with steps 1 and 2, determine the location of the fetal left side with regard to the maternal abdomen (fetal left side is anterior [closer to the transducer], posterior [closer to the posterior uterine wall], right lateral [closer to maternal right uterine wall], left lateral [closer to maternal left uterine wall]) (Fig. 4-2).

4. Obtain a transverse view of the fetal abdomen by rotating the transducer 90 degrees from the sagittal view of the lower thoracic spine. The fetal stomach is imaged in the left side of the abdomen, the descending aorta is posterior to the left, and the inferior vena cava is anterior to the right (Fig. 4-2, plane A). By sliding the transducer toward the fetal chest, a four-chamber view of the heart is imaged. Note that the apex of the heart is pointing toward the left side of the fetal chest (Fig. 4-2, plane B). Determining that the stomach, descending aorta, and cardiac apex are located on the fetal left side and the inferior vena cava is located on the right side establishes normal visceral situs.

Other methods for determining fetal situs during the ultrasound examination have been described. Cordes et al. (4) described a technique that involves orienting the transducer in a standardized way so that the fetal head is on the right side of the screen in a fetal sagittal plane as a starting point and then rotating the transducer 90 degrees clockwise to obtain the caudocranial transverse views. Another method reported by Bronshtein et al. (5) is referred to as the right-hand rule for abdominal scanning and the left-hand rule for transvaginal scanning (Fig. 4-3). The palm of the hand corresponds to the face of the fetus, and the examiner holds the hand according to the side of the fetal face; the fetal heart and stomach are shown by the examiner's thumb.

FETAL THORACIC ANATOMY

The thoracic cavity is bound anteriorly by the sternum, posteriorly by the vertebral column, and laterally by the ribs. The clavicles, the first ribs, and the body of the first vertebrae border the thoracic cavity superiorly and the diaphragm inferiorly.

The ribs develop from the mesenchymal costal processes of the thoracic vertebrae during embryogenesis. Chondrification begins at 6.5 weeks, and a well-formed cartilaginous thoracic cage is present toward the end of the embryonic period. Enchondral ossification of the ribs occurs mostly during the first trimester of gestation (6). When development is completed, the

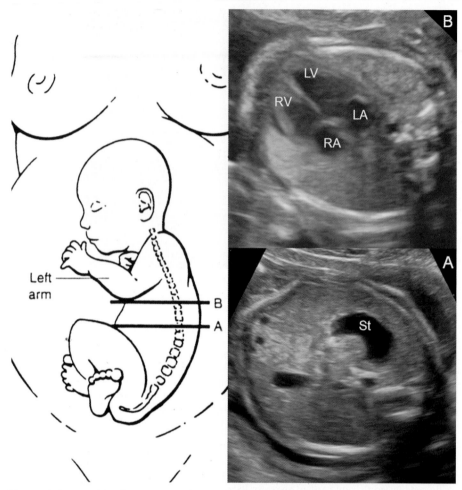

Figure 4-2. Determining the fetal orientation within the uterus; the head is in the uterine fundus and the breech part is presenting. The fetal lie is longitudinal and the spine is located in proximity to the maternal left side. The left side of the fetus is therefore anterior. **Plane A** is obtained by rotating the transducer 90 degrees from a sagittal view of the lower thoracic spine. Note the anterior location of the stomach (St) within the abdomen, thus confirming normal abdominal situs. **Plane B** is obtained by sliding the transducer cephalad from plane A. Note the anterior location of the heart with the cardiac apex pointing toward the fetal left side. RV, right ventricle; LV, left ventricle; RA, right atrium; LA, left atrium.

skeleton of the thorax consists of 12 thoracic vertebrae, 12 pairs of ribs and costal cartilages, and the sternum. Anteriorly, the superior seven costal cartilages articulate with the sternum; the 8th, 9th, and 10th cartilages articulate with the cartilages next above (join with one another but do not reach the sternum); and the 11th and 12th ribs are floating with no anterior articulation (7). Posteriorly, the ribs articulate with the thoracic vertebrae. Although individual ribs incline inferiorly in the adult, in fetal life ribs assume a more horizontal orientation within the thoracic cavity. In view of this rib orientation in the fetus, large segments of individual ribs can be imaged by obtaining transverse views of the abdomen and chest (Figs. 4-1 and 4.2).

The heart occupies the central portion of the thoracic cavity in the middle mediastinum. It is covered anteriorly by the lower two thirds of the sternum and the costal cartilage of the

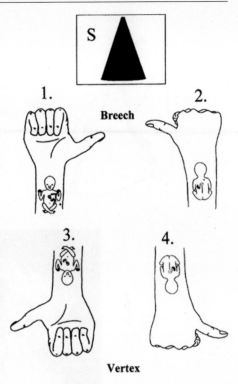

Figure 4-3. A diagram of the fetus is presented in back posterior (1 and 3) and back anterior (2 and 4) positions. In transabdominal scanning the ultrasound beam (S) is directed from top to bottom. The palm of the right hand represents the face of the fetus, and the fetal heart and stomach are on the same side of the examiner's thumb. (Modified from Bronshtein M, Gover A, Zimmer EZ. Sonographic definition of the fetal situs. *Obstet Gynecol* 2002;99(6):1129–1130, with permission.)

second through the sixth ribs. The heart is bordered by the lungs laterally and posteriorly and by the diaphragm inferiorly. The descending thoracic aorta and the esophagus lie posterior to the heart. The thymus is located in the anterior upper mediastinum, between the sternum anteriorly and the great vessels posteriorly. The heart of a fetus lies horizontally in the thorax, and a four-chamber-view plane of the heart is obtained in almost the same plane as a transverse plane of the chest (8). With growth, the cardiac apex swings downward and the postnatal heart is positioned more vertically in the thoracic cavity. The fetal rib corresponding to a four-chamber-view plane of the heart is the fourth rib (9,10). The ultrasonographic technical advantage that the fetal ribs provide when obtaining transverse views of the chest and abdomen is further discussed in Chapter 5.

The external surface of the heart contains several grooves that separate the atria from the ventricles (Fig. 4-4). The atrioventricular or coronary groove (Fig. 4-4A,C) separates the atria from the ventricles. Within this groove lie the coronary sinus and the main trunk of the coronary arteries. The anterior interventricular groove, which contains the anterior interventricular descending branch of the left coronary artery, separates the right from left ventricle anteriorly (Fig. 4-4A,C). The posterior interventricular groove contains the posterior descending coronary artery and the middle cardiac vein (Fig. 4-4B). The atria are separated externally by the interatrial grooves (not shown). These external grooves are filled with fatty tissue in the adult.

The right and left lungs occupy the majority of the thoracic cavity, with the heart occupying the central portion. The right lung is composed of three lobes—superior, middle, and inferior—with a short eparterial main bronchus. The left lung is composed of two lobes—superior and inferior—with a long hyparterial main bronchus. Each lobe, which is further subdivided into lobules, is supplied by a secondary bronchus. Tertiary bronchi supply various segments within each lobe. Individual lung lobes are not seen on ultrasound unless there is a pleural effusion.

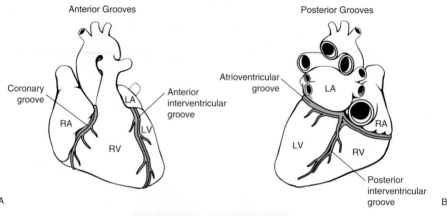

Anterior Grooves

Posterior Grooves

A

B

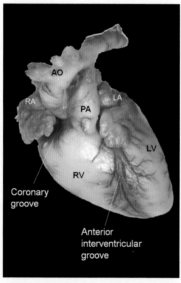

C

Figure 4-4. Anterior **(A)** and posterior **(B)** views of the heart demonstrating the external grooves outlining the divisions of the cardiac chambers. **C:** Cardiac specimen of a 22-week fetus showing the anterior and coronary grooves. LA, left atrium; RA, right atrium; LV, left ventricle; RV, right ventricle; PA, pulmonary artery; AO, aorta.

FETAL CARDIAC AXIS

The fetal cardiac axis can be readily determined by obtaining a transverse view of the chest at the level of the four-chamber-view plane of the heart. A line is drawn from the spine to the anterior chest wall, thus dividing the chest into equal halves. The cardiac axis is the angle that the interventricular septum makes with this line (Fig. 4-5). The normal cardiac axis, which is independent of gestational age, lies at a 45-degree angle to the left of the midline (11) (Figs. 4-5 and 4-6A). Studies have differed slightly with regard to the definition of an abnormal cardiac axis; the authors suggest a cardiac axis of greater than 65 degrees or less than 25 degrees to be abnormal. In a study that defined an abnormal cardiac axis at less than 28 degrees or greater than 59 degrees, the sensitivity in detecting congenital heart disease or intrathoracic anomalies was 79% (12). Cardiac anomalies occurred in fetuses with small and large cardiac axes (12). Defining left axis deviation at greater than 75 degrees, one study noted fetal

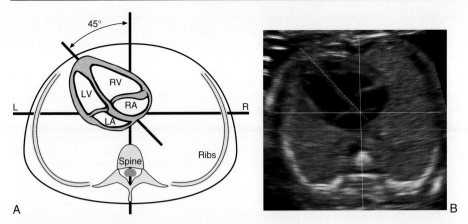

Figure 4-5. Measurement of the cardiac axis from a four-chamber-view plane of the fetal chest with the corresponding plane on ultrasound. LA, left atrium; RA, right atrium; LV, left ventricle; RV, right ventricle; L, left; R, right.

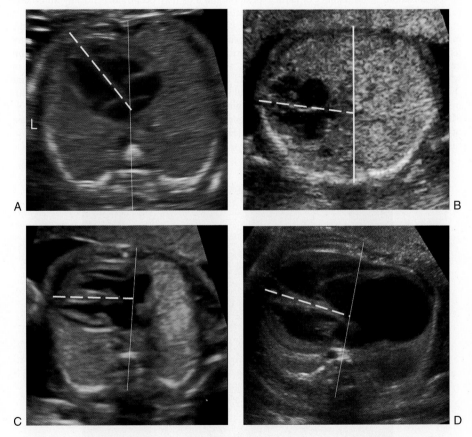

Figure 4-6. **A:** Normal heart with a cardiac axis of 45 degrees. In comparison, three fetuses (B–D) with abnormal cardiac axis (nearly 90 degrees). **B:** Right lung lesion shifting the heart to the left with axis deviation. **C:** Tetralogy of Fallot with a normal four-chamber view but with deviated cardiac axis. **D:** Cardiomegaly in a fetus with Ebstein anomaly. L, left.

anomalies in 76% of fetuses (13). In left cardiac axis deviation, tetralogy of Fallot (Fig. 4-6C), coarctation of the aorta and Ebstein anomaly (Fig. 4-6D) represent the most common cardiac lesions, whereas double outlet right ventricle, atrioventricular septal defect, and common atrium represent the most common cardiac lesions in right axis deviation (12–14). Abnormal cardiac axes are also noted in fetuses with abdominal wall defects such as omphaloceles (59% with cardiac axis deviation) and gastroschisis (14% with abnormal cardiac axis deviation) (15). Figure 4-6B–D shows three fetuses with different abnormal cardiac axes of nearly 90 degrees. The specific embryologic event that results in an abnormal cardiac axis in some fetuses with cardiac abnormalities is not currently known; however, an overrotation of the bulboventricular loop in early embryogenesis has been proposed as the underlying mechanism (11,12,15). In rare occasions involving complex congenital heart disease, the apex of the heart may not be identifiable. Chapter 10 reports on fetal cardiac axis in early gestation.

FETAL CARDIAC POSITION

Fetal cardiac position refers to the position of the heart within the chest and is independent of the fetal cardiac axis. *Dextrocardia* is a term used to describe a heart that is located in the right chest (Figs. 4-7–4-9), *mesocardia* refers to a central position of the heart in the chest (Fig. 4-10), and *levocardia* refers to a left-sided position (Fig. 4-6). These terms describe the position of the heart in the chest and convey no information regarding fetal situs, cardiac axis, cardiac anatomy, or chamber organization. Abnormalities of cardiac position and axis may occur independently and therefore should be reported separately (e.g., dextrocardia with axis to the left).

The incidence of dextrocardia in tertiary referral centers is 0.22% to 0.84%, with the majority of cases associated with congenital heart disease in that setting (16,17). Two other terms have been used in the literature to describe the heart in the right chest: dextroposition and dextroversion. *Dextroposition* of the heart, a form of dextrocardia, refers to a condition in which the heart is located in the right chest and the cardiac apex points medially or to the left (Figs. 4-7 and 4-8). This condition usually results from extrinsic factors, such as a space-occupying lesion in the left thoracic cavity (diaphragmatic hernia [Fig. 4-8A], left lung mass [Fig. 4-8B], or pleural effusion [Fig. 4-7]), or from agenesis of the right lung (Fig. 4-8C) or hypoplasia of the right lung (i.e., with Scimitar syndrome [Fig. 4-8D]). Dextroposition is a transitory position of the heart in the right chest, which is expected to regress when the extracardiac

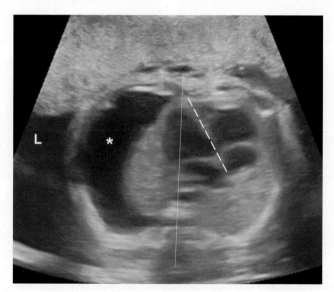

Figure 4-7. Transverse view of the chest in a fetus with a left pleural effusion (*). Note the location of the heart in the right chest with the cardiac apex pointing to the left (L) (dextroposition).

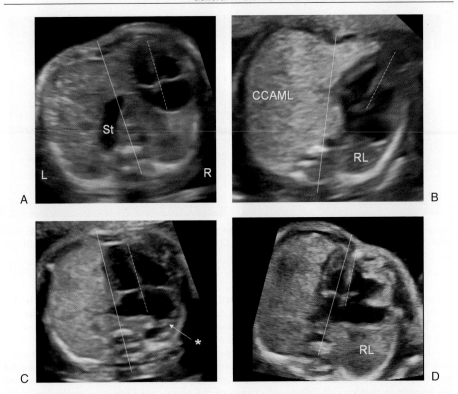

Figure 4-8. Four other conditions with dextroposition. **A:** Left-sided congenital diaphragmatic hernia. **B:** Left-sided congenital cystic adenomatoid malformation of the lung (CCAML). In A and B the heart is shifted to the right hemithorax. **C:** The very rare condition of right lung agenesis (*). **D:** The rare condition of a hypoplastic right lung (RL) in Scimitar syndrome. St, stomach.

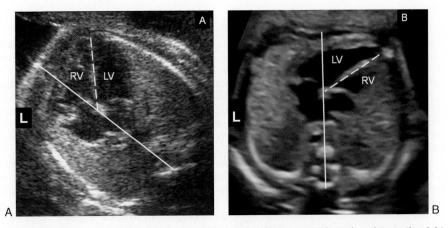

Figure 4-9. Dextroversion: The heart is mainly in the right chest and the axis points to the right. **A:** Fetus with situs inversus with the anterior ventricle being the right ventricle (RV) (mirror-image rotation). **B:** Fetus with a transposition of the great vessels and dextroversion. The heart is rotated to the right side and the left ventricle (LV) is anterior. L, left.

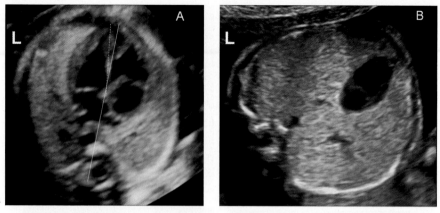

Figure 4-10. Mesocardia in the fetus: The heart is in the central position in the chest. **A:** Isolated mesocardia without cardiac anomaly. **B:** Chest in a fetus with laryngeal atresia with the heart squeezed between dilated lungs. L, left.

malformation is treated. When the heart is located in the right chest with the cardiac axis pointing to the right side, the term *dextroversion* has been used (Fig. 4-9). Dextroversion is found in situs inversus and situs ambiguous and is commonly associated with congenital heart disease, with the majority involving a discordant atrioventricular connection (Fig. 4-9) (18).

Levocardia, a term denoting the normal position of the heart in the left chest, is often used when visceral situs abnormalities are present. Levocardia can be associated with normal situs (normal anatomy), situs inversus, or situs ambiguous. Excessive left cardiac axis rotation can be seen in tetralogy of Fallot, coarctation of the aorta, and Ebstein anomaly (Fig. 4-6). *Levoposition* of the heart refers to the condition where the heart is displaced farther toward the left chest, usually in association with a space-occupying lesion on the right side (Fig. 4-6B).

Mesocardia indicates an atypical location of the heart, in the central chest, with the cardiac apex pointing toward the midline of the chest (Fig. 4-10). Mesocardia is associated with congenital heart disease primarily involving abnormal ventriculoarterial connections such as transposition of great vessels and double outlet right ventricle. Bilateral lung volume enlargement, such as laryngeal atresia, is also associated with mesocardia (Fig. 4-10B).

FETAL CARDIAC DIMENSIONS

The fetal heart occupies approximately one third of the thoracic cavity. Fetal cardiac dimensions can be easily assessed by measuring the ratio of cardiac circumference or area to the chest circumference or area obtained at the level of the four-chamber view (Fig. 4-11). The cardiothoracic (C/T) circumference is fairly constant throughout gestation, with a mean value of 0.45 at 17 weeks and 0.50 at term (19). The mean C/T circumference in the first half of pregnancy increases slightly with gestational age, from 0.38 at 11 weeks to 0.45 at 20 weeks, with all values at less than 0.50 in normal fetuses (20). The C/T area is an alternate method for assessing cardiac dimensions and normal values are fairly constant throughout gestation, with a mean value between 0.25 and 0.35 (21).

Fetal cardiomegaly (Fig. 4-6D), defined as C/T area greater than 2 standard deviations in one series, encompasses heterogeneous etiologies including cardiac and extracardiac abnormalities (21). Holosystolic tricuspid regurgitation with right atrial enlargement is a common pathogenetic feature and is seen in almost 90% of fetal cardiomegaly cases (21). Fetal hydrops is also commonly seen in association with cardiomegaly, up to 50% in some series (21). Table 4-2 lists common causes of fetal cardiomegaly.

An increased C/T circumference can also be observed in the presence of reduced chest volume rather than an enlarged heart, and thus, it is important to compare the measured chest circumference to gestational age nomograms as part of this evaluation. Reduced chest volume

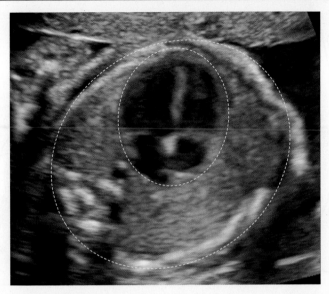

Figure 4-11. Fetal cardiothoracic circumference obtained as a ratio of cardiac to chest circumference at the level of the four-chamber view. The cardiothoracic area is obtained as a ratio of the cardiac area over the chest area.

TABLE 4-2	**Common Causes of Fetal Cardiomegaly**
Etiology	
Cardiac	Ebstein anomaly
	Tricuspid valve dysplasia
	Atrioventricular septal defect
	Sustained fetal arrhythmia (heart block)
	Dilative cardiomyopathy
	Premature constriction of ductus arteriosus
Extracardiac	Arteriovenous malformations as sacrococcygeal teratoma, aneurysm of vein of Galen, and placental chorioangioma
	Recipient in twin–twin transfusion syndrome
	Severe fetal anemia
	Uncontrolled maternal diabetes

can result from some forms of lethal skeletal dysplasias or in the presence of severe pulmonary hypoplasia. Reduced chest circumference is typically associated with a poor outcome.

 SPATIAL RELATIONSHIPS OF CARDIAC CHAMBERS AND OUTFLOW TRACTS

Figure 4-12 represents right anterior (A), anterior (B), left posterior (C), and posterior (D) views of the surface of the fetal heart in the chest. The right atrium occupies a right anterior position within the heart (Fig. 4-12A). The right ventricle is positioned anteriorly and occupies the majority of the anterior surface of the fetal heart (Fig. 4-12B). The left ventricle occupies the left posterior surface of the fetal heart (Fig. 4-12C), and the left atrium is positioned posteriorly (Fig. 4-12D) over the spine. Figure 4-13 is a drawing of three parasternal long-axis anatomic sections through the fetal heart from right to left, showing the spatial relationships of

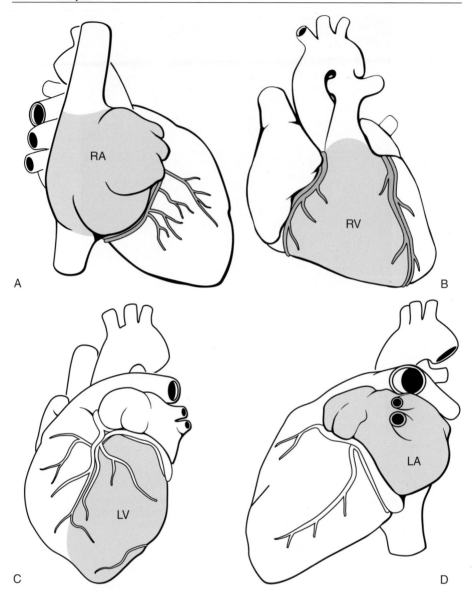

A

B

C

D

Figure 4-12. Topographic views of the surface of the fetal heart from the right anterior **(A),** anterior **(B),** left posterior **(C),** and posterior **(D)** angles showing the anatomic locations of the cardiac chambers. RA, right atrium; RV, right ventricle; LV, left ventricle; LA, left atrium.

cardiac chambers and outflow tracts. Figures 4-14 and 4-15 are the corresponding ultrasound images to planes A and B. The right ventricle, with its most anterior outflow tract (pulmonary artery), is the most anterior cardiac chamber in proximity to the anterior chest wall (Figs. 4-14 and 4-15). The left ventricle and its outflow tract (aorta) occupies the midsection of the fetal heart (Fig. 4-15). The left atrium, which receives blood from the pulmonary veins, is the most posterior cardiac chamber in proximity to the fetal spine (Fig. 4-15). The pulmonary artery emerges from the right ventricle, crosses over the aorta, and dips posteriorly into the chest. It divides into the right and left pulmonary arteries and the ductus arteriosus. The

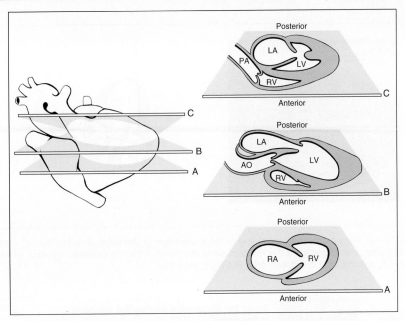

Figure 4-13. Anatomic sections (parasternal long axis) through the fetal heart from right to left (**A, B,** and **C,** respectively) showing the spatial relationships of cardiac chambers and outflow tracts (see text). PA, pulmonary artery; AO, aorta; RA, right atrium; RV, right ventricle; LA, left atrium; LV, left ventricle.

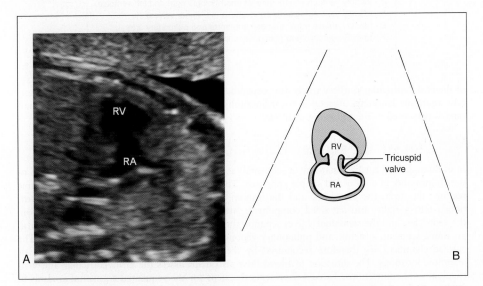

Figure 4-14. Parasternal long-axis view of the right side of the heart showing the right ventricle and atrium. RV, right ventricle; RA, right atrium.

aorta, with its long axis parallel to the long axis of the left ventricle, angles anteriorly and points toward the fetal right shoulder as it exits from the left ventricle and before it arches and descends along the left side of the spine. Three arteries originate from the aortic arch: the brachiocephalic (innominate), the left common carotid, and the left subclavian. The long axes

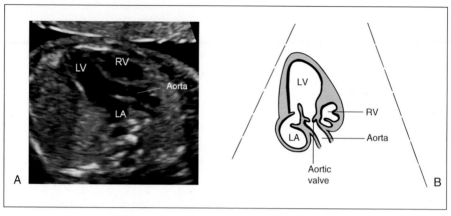

Figure 4-15. Parasternal long-axis view of the midsection of the heart showing the left ventricular outflow tract as it occupies the midsection of the heart. Note the posterior location of the left atrium. LA, left atrium; LV, left ventricle; RV, right ventricle.

	Steps for Sequential Segmental Analysis in the Fetus

1. Identify visceral situs
2. Identify atrial arrangement (morphologic right and left atrium)
3. Identify atrioventricular (AV) connections (AV valves)
4. Identify ventricular arrangement (morphologic right and left ventricle)
5. Identify ventriculoarterial connections (semilunar valves)
6. Identify arterial trunk arrangement (aorta and pulmonary artery)
7. Identify systemic and pulmonary venous connections

of the two ventricular outflow tracts are perpendicular to each other (Fig. 4-13B,C), an important anatomic landmark in fetal echocardiography. Detailed evaluation of fetal cardiac anatomy is presented in the following chapters.

SEQUENTIAL SEGMENTAL ANALYSIS

In evaluating fetal cardiac anatomy, a sequential segmental approach helps in the description of the abnormality in a clear and simple approach. The segmental analysis involves three anatomic regions: the atria, the ventricles, and the arterial trunks. Each anatomic region is also partitioned into a right- and left-sided component. Atrioventricular valves separate the atria from the ventricles, and the semilunar valves separate the ventricles from the arterial trunks. A fourth anatomic segment, systemic and pulmonary venous connections, should also be evaluated. The cardiac chambers are therefore recognized by their morphologic structures rather than their anatomic locations. The direction of blood flow also helps assess the atrioventricular and ventriculoarterial connections. Table 4-3 presents the steps for the sequential segmental analysis in fetal cardiac evaluation. Detailed anatomic evaluation of cardiac chambers, arterial trunks, and valvular structures will be presented in the following chapters.

■ KEY POINTS: GENERAL ANATOMIC LANDMARKS OF THE FETAL HEART

- ■ Situs solitus refers to the normal arrangements of vessels and organs within the body.
- ■ Situs inversus refers to a mirror-image arrangement of vessels and organs to situs solitus and is associated with a slight increase in CHD and with Kartagener syndrome in 20% of cases.

- Situs ambiguous (heterotaxy) refers to visceral malpositions and malformations and is commonly associated with CHD.
- The position of the aorta and inferior vena cava below the diaphragm is the most reliable criterion for determination of right or left isomerism.
- A four-chamber view of the fetal heart is obtained in almost the same plane as a transverse plane of the chest at the level of the fourth rib.
- The authors define a cardiac axis between 25 and 65 degrees in the left chest as normal.
- Dextrocardia describes a heart that is located in the right chest.
- Dextroposition, a form of dextrocardia, describes a heart that is located in the right chest with the apex pointing medially or to the left.
- Dextroversion describes a heart that is located in the right chest with the cardiac axis pointing to the right side.
- Levocardia, a term denoting the normal position of the heart, is often used when visceral situs abnormalities are present.
- Levoposition refers to the condition where the heart is displaced farther toward the left chest, usually in association with a space-occupying lesion.
- Mesocardia indicates an atypical location of the heart with the apex pointing toward the midline of the chest.
- The cardiothoracic circumference is fairly constant throughout gestation, with a mean value of 0.45 at 17 weeks and 0.50 at term.
- The cardiothoracic area is an alternate method for assessing cardiac dimensions and normal values are fairly constant throughout gestation, with a mean value between 0.25 and 0.35.
- Holosystolic tricuspid regurgitation with right atrial enlargement is a common pathogenetic feature and is seen in almost 90% of fetal cardiomegaly cases.
- An increased C/T circumference can also be observed in the presence of reduced chest volume primarily due to skeletal dysplasias or pulmonary hypoplasia.
- The right ventricle is the most anterior chamber and the left atrium is the most posterior chamber.
- The right atrium is right anterior and the left ventricle is left posterior in location.
- The sequential segmental analysis of the fetal heart involves three anatomic regions: the atria, the ventricles, and the arterial trunks.

References

1. DeVore GR, Sarti DA, Siassi B, et al. Prenatal diagnosis of cardiovascular malformations in the fetus with situs inversus viscerum during the second trimester of pregnancy. *J Clin Ultrasound* 1986;14:454–457.
2. Holzmann D, Ott PM, Felix H. Diagnostic approach to primary ciliary dyskinesia: a review. *Eur J Pediatr* 2000;159(1–2):95–98.
3. Salomon LJ, Baumann C, Delezoide AL, et al. Abnormal abdominal situs: what and how should we look for? *Prenat Diagn* 2006;26:282–285.
4. Cordes TM, O'Leary PW, Seward JB, et al. Distinguishing right from left: a standardized technique for fetal echocardiography. *J Am Soc Echo* 1994;7:47–53.
5. Bronshtein M, Gover A, Zimmer EZ. Sonographic definition of the fetal situs. *Obstet Gynecol* 2002;99(6): 1129–1130.
6. O'Rahilly R, Muller F. *Human embryology and teratology*. New York: Wiley-Liss, 1992;241.
7. Agur AM. *Grant's atlas of anatomy*. Baltimore: Williams and Wilkins, 1991;8–9.
8. Snider RA, Serwer GA. *Echocardiography in pediatric heart disease*. St. Lous: Mosby, 1990;23.
9. Isaacson G, Mintz MC, Crelin ES. *Atlas of fetal sectional anatomy with ultrasound and magnetic resonance imaging*. New York: Springer-Verlag, 1986;64.
10. Abuhamad AZ, Sedule-Murphy SJ, Kolm P, et al. Prenatal ultrasonographic fetal rib length measurement: Correlation with gestational age. *Ultrasound Obstet Gynecol* 1996;7:193–196.
11. Comstock CH. Normal fetal heart axis and position. *Obstet Gynecol* 1987;70:255.
12. Crane JM, Ash K, Fink N, et al. Abnormal fetal cardiac axis in the detection of intrathoracic anomalies and congenital heart disease. *Ultrasound Obstet Gynecol* 1997;10:90–93.
13. Smith RS, Comstock CH, Kirk JS, et al. Ultrasonographic left cardiac axis deviation: a marker for fetal anomalies. *Obstet Gynecol* 1995;85:187–191.
14. Comstock CH, Smith R, Lee W, et al. Right fetal cardiac axis: clinical significance and associated findings. *Obstet Gynecol* 1998;91:495–499.
15. Boulton SL, McKenna DS, Cly GC, et al. Cardiac axis in fetuses with abdominal wall defects. *Ultrasound Obstet Gynecol* 2006;28:785–788.
16. Bernasconi A, Azancot A, Simpson JM, et al. Fetal dextrocardia: diagnosis and outcome in two tertiary centres. *Heart* 2005;91:1590–1594.

17. Walmsley R, Hishitani T, Sandor GGS, et al. Diagnosis and outcome of dextrocardia diagnosed in the fetus. *Am J Cardiol* 2004;94:141–143.
18. Winer-Muram HT, Tonkin ILD. The spectrum of heterotaxic syndromes. *Radiol Clin North Am* 1989;27:1147–1170.
19. Paladini D, Chita SK, Allan LD. Prenatal measurement of cardiothoracic ratio in evaluation of heart disease. *Arch Dis Child* 1990;65:20–23.
20. Tongsong T, Tatiyapornkul T. Cardiothoracic ratio in the first half of pregnancy. *J Clin Ultrasound* 2004;32(4):186–189.
21. Chaoui R, Bollmann R, Goldner B, et al. Fetal cardiomegaly: echocardiographic findings and outcome in 19 cases. Fetal Diagn Ther 1994;9(2):92–104.

THE RIGHT ATRIUM

The right atrium is located anteriorly and to the right of the left atrium. The posterior portion of the right atrium (sinus venarum) has a smooth wall and receives the superior and inferior venae cavae and the coronary sinus (Fig. 5-1). The anterior portion of the right atrium is lined with coarse muscle bundles, named pectinate muscle (Fig. 5-1). The smooth and coarse regions within the right atrium are separated by a ridge called the crista terminalis (Fig. 5-1), which runs inferiorly and parallel to the openings of the inferior and superior venae cavae. The inferior vena cava enters the right atrium at its lowest part, near the interatrial septum (Fig. 5-1). The Eustachian valve, which represents a flap of endocardium, is located at the opening of the inferior vena cava (Fig. 5-1). This valve serves a critical function in the fetus as it directs highly oxygenated blood originating from the ductus venosus within the inferior vena cava to the foramen ovale in a caudal-to-cranial flow pattern. On occasions, the Eustachian valve can be imaged on fetal echocardiography in a four-chamber-view plane that is posterior to the optimal plane, where it can be mistaken for the flap of the foramen ovale. The coronary sinus, which delivers venous return from the heart, runs across the atrioventricular groove posteriorly and enters the right atrium inferiorly in proximity to the atrial septum and the inferior vena cava opening (1) (Figs. 5-1 and 5-2). The opening of the coronary sinus is also guarded by a valve called the Thebesian valve (Fig. 5-1). The superior vena cava (SVC) enters the right atrium anteriorly and has no flap at its opening. The sinoatrial (SA) node is located on the epicardium of the right atrial wall superiorly, just below the SVC (Fig. 5-1). The atrioventricular (AV)

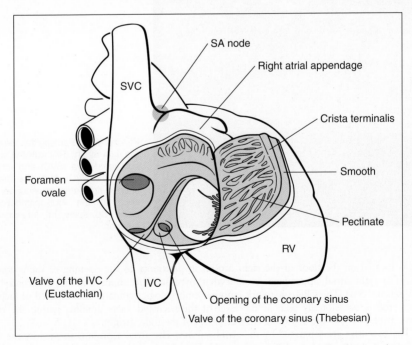

Figure 5-1. Right atrial internal anatomy. The posterior wall is smooth; the anterior wall is coarse. Note the openings of the inferior vena cava (IVC), superior vena cava (SVC), and coronary sinus. See text for details. RV, right ventricle; SA, sinoatrial.

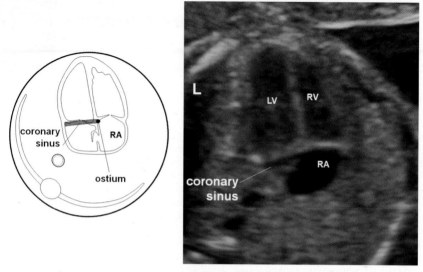

Figure 5-2. Transverse view of the fetal chest in a plane slightly caudal to the four-chamber-view plane showing the coronary sinus at the floor of the right atrium (RA). RV, right ventricle; LV, left ventricle; L, left.

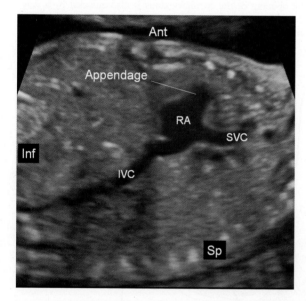

Figure 5-3. Parasagittal view of the right atrium (RA) with the superior vena cava (SVC) and inferior vena cava (IVC). Note the broad-shaped right atrial appendage, not seen at the four-chamber-view plane. Sp, spine; Inf, inferior; Ant, anterior.

node is located on the floor of the right atrium in proximity to the opening of the coronary sinus. The right atrial appendage is somewhat pyramidal in shape and has a broad base (Figs. 5-1 and 5-3). The Chiari network, another embryologic remnant, is composed of lacelike strands and is occasionally seen at the level of the tricuspid valve annulus within the right atrium. Table 5-1 lists the anatomic characteristics of the right atrium.

The two atria are separated by the atrial septum. The atrial septum is formed by the septum primum and secundum. The foramen ovale is formed as a perforation in the septum secundum (Fig. 5-4). The septum primum, embryologically the first atrial septum to develop, forms the leaflet of the foramen ovale. Atrial septal defects are categorized according to the

TABLE 5-1	Anatomic Characteristics of the Right Atrium

Anteriorly located, to the right of the left atrium
Posterior portion is smooth; anterior portion is trabeculated
Receives the inferior vena cava, superior vena cava, and coronary sinus
Contains the sinoatrial and atrioventricular nodes
Right atrial appendage is pyramidal in shape with broad base

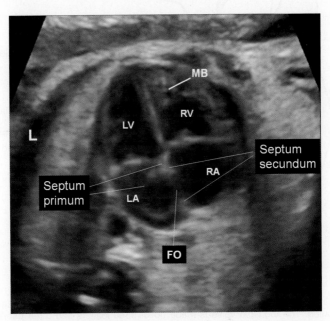

Figure 5-4. Apical four-chamber view of the fetal heart with the right atrium (RA), left atrium (LA), right ventricle (RV), and left ventricle (LV). At the apex of the heart in the right ventricle the typical thickened moderator band (MB) is recognized. Between both atria the interatrial septum is formed by both the septum primum and secundum. The flap of the foramen ovale is formed by the septum primum, while the foramen ovale (FO) is an opening in the midportion of the septum secundum. L, left.

anatomic location of the defect within the septum. Defects in the lower one third of the atrial septum are referred to as septum primum defects, defects in the middle one third are referred to as septum secundum defects, and defects in the posterior and superior portions of the septum are referred to as sinus venosus defects.

 THE TRICUSPID VALVE

The tricuspid valve prevents the blood from flowing back into the right atrium from the right ventricle during ventricular systole. This valve has three leaflets—anterior, septal, and posterior—named based on their orientation within the right ventricle. The valves are anchored by chordae tendineae, which prevents the leaflets from prolapsing into the right atrium during systole. Chordae tendineae insert into three papillary muscles. The anterior papillary muscle, the largest of the three and commonly seen on ultrasound, is located in the apex of the right ventricle and receives chordae tendineae insertions from the anterior and posterior leaflets (Fig. 5-5). The posterior papillary muscle is located in the posterior lateral wall and receives

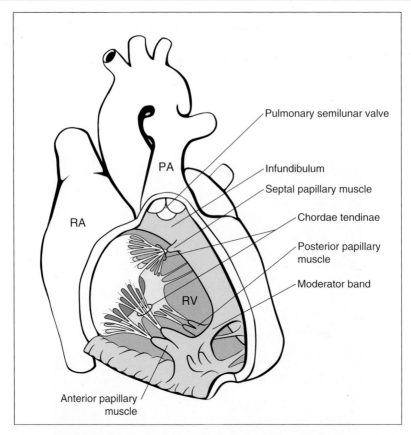

Figure 5-5. Internal anatomy of the right ventricle (RV), which is made up of an inlet, apical, and outlet portion. The tricuspid valve is made up of three leaflets and three papillary muscles. The moderator band occupies the apex of the RV. See text for details. RA, right atrium; PA, pulmonary artery.

chordae tendineae insertions from the posterior and septal leaflets (Fig. 5-5). The septal papillary muscle has attachments to the septal and anterior leaflets. Chordae tendineae from the valve leaflets insert directly into the septal wall, a feature found only in the right ventricle (Figs. 5-5 and 5-6). The tricuspid valve inserts more apically than the mitral valve on the interventricular septum (2) (Fig. 5-4). This anatomic finding is extremely useful in determining ventricular situs and in recognizing atrioventricular canal abnormalities. Unlike the mitral valve, a subpulmonic conus separates the tricuspid valve from the pulmonary valve, resulting in no fibrous continuity between the two (Fig. 5-5).

 THE RIGHT VENTRICLE

The right ventricle is the closest cardiac chamber to the anterior chest wall, anatomically located behind the sternum. The right ventricle is made up of three portions: The inlet and apical portions, which are heavily trabeculated, and the outlet portion, which is smooth (Fig. 5-5). One of the main ultrasound characteristics of the right ventricle is the coarse trabeculation with the moderator band (septoparietal muscle bundle) occupying the apical portion (Fig. 5-5). When compared to the left ventricle, the right ventricle shows on ultrasound evaluation, at the level of the four-chamber view, an increased echogenicity of its walls. The right ventricle is crescent shaped as it curves over the interventricular septum. The right and left ventricles are nearly equal in size in the fetus (Fig. 5-4). Table 5-2 lists the anatomic characteristics of the right ventricle.

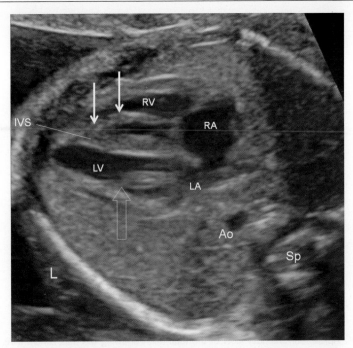

Figure 5-6. Axial view of the fetal heart at the level of the four-chamber view. Note in the right ventricle (RV) the apical insertion of the chordae tendineae of the tricuspid valve to the right ventricular wall and apex of the heart (*two solid arrows*). Open arrow in the left ventricle (LV) points to the free wall attachment of the papillary muscle of the mitral valve. RA, right atrium; LA, left atrium; IVS, interventricular septum; Ao, aorta; Sp, spine; L, left.

TABLE 5-2	Anatomic Characteristics of the Right Ventricle

Inlet and apical regions are heavily trabeculated
Crescent shaped, most anterior chamber, located below sternum
Outlet (infundibulum) is smooth
Moderator band located in apical region
Tricuspid atrioventricular valve
Tricuspid valve is more apically inserted on the septum than the mitral valve
Ventricular wall receives direct chordae tendineae insertions
Three papillary muscles

 ## THE LEFT ATRIUM

The left atrium is posteriorly located, anatomically in proximity to the spine, and receives the right and left pulmonary veins. A total of four pulmonary veins, a superior and an inferior pair, anchor the heart to the lungs and enter the left atrium on its upper posterolateral surface (see Fig. 4-4B in Chapter 4). At the level of the four-chamber view, two of the four pulmonary veins are seen: the two inferior pulmonary veins, as slitlike openings in the posterior wall of the left atrium (Fig. 5-7). The two inferior pulmonary veins enter the left atrium to either side of the descending aorta and esophagus (Fig. 5-7). The left atrial chamber is round and has smooth walls with the exception of the left atrial appendage, which is narrow and fingerlike in shape and contains numerous pectinate muscles. The leaflet of the foramen ovale, which beats from right to left, is located within the left atrium (Fig. 5-4). The left atrium is nearly equal in size to the right atrium in the fetus. Figure 5-8 shows an autopsy specimen of

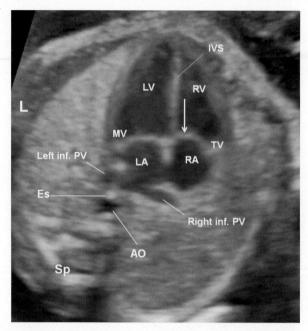

Figure 5-7. Apical four-chamber view of the fetal heart showing the right atrium (RA), left atrium (LA), right ventricle (RV), left ventricle (LV), and interventricular (IVS) septum. Note (*arrow*) the more apical insertion of the tricuspid valve (TV) in relation to the mitral valve (MV). In the apical four-chamber view the septum appears very thin in comparison to the lateral view (compare with Fig. 5-6). The right and left inferior (inf) pulmonary veins (PV), are seen to enter the left atrium posteriorly on either side of the descending aorta (AO) and esophagus (Es). Sp, spine; L, left.

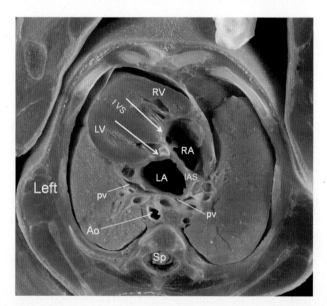

Figure 5-8. Autopsy specimen of a transverse chest at the level of the four-chamber view of the fetal heart showing the right atrium (RA), left atrium (LA), right ventricle (RV), left ventricle (LV), interventricular septum (IVS), and interatrial septum (IAS). Note (*arrows*) the more apical insertion of the tricuspid valve in relation to the mitral valve. The pulmonary veins (pv) are seen to enter the left atrium posteriorly. Sp, spine; Ao, descending aorta.

TABLE 5-3	Anatomic Characteristics of the Left Atrium

Posteriorly located, over the spine
Anterior and posterior portion is smooth
Receives four pulmonary veins
Left atrial appendage is narrow, fingerlike with coarse walls

a transverse view of the fetal chest at the level of the four-chamber view. Table 5-3 lists the anatomic characteristics of the left atrium.

 ## THE MITRAL VALVE

The mitral valve prevents the blood from flowing back into the left atrium from the left ventricle during ventricular systole. This valve has an anterior and a posterior leaflet with no septal attachment. Chordae tendineae from each leaflet insert into the two anterolateral and posteromedial papillary muscles, which attach to the free wall of the left ventricle, a differentiating feature from those in the right ventricle (Fig. 5-9). The anterior leaflet, which is sometimes referred to as the septal or anteromedial leaflet, attaches primarily to the anterolateral papillary muscle and is in fibrous continuity with the aortic valve (Fig. 5-10). The posterior leaflet, which is sometimes referred to as the posterolateral leaflet, attaches to the posteromedial papillary muscle. Unlike the right ventricular wall, the left ventricular wall receives no direct chordae tendineae insertions from the mitral valve (Fig. 5-6).

 ## THE LEFT VENTRICLE

The left ventricle is conical in shape and is posterior to the right ventricle. It occupies most of the left lateral surface of the fetal heart. It is anatomically narrower and longer than the right

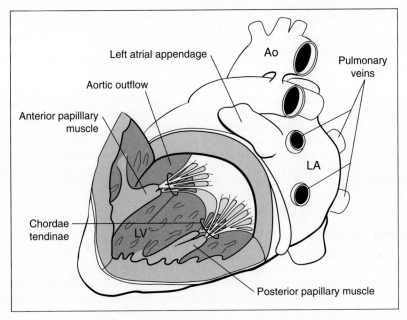

Figure 5-9. Internal anatomy of the left ventricle (LV). The mitral valve is made of two leaflets and two papillary muscles. Note the close proximity of the anterior (anteromedial) leaflet of the mitral valve to the aortic outflow. See text for details. Ao, aorta; LA, left atrium.

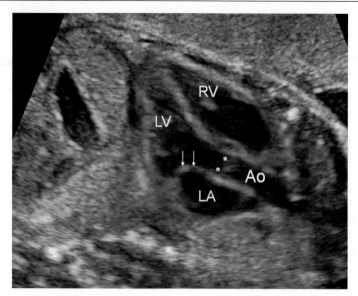

Figure 5-10. Five-chamber view of the fetal heart showing the anatomic proximity of the anterior leaflet of the mitral valve (*arrows*) to the aortic valve (*asterisks*). LV, left ventricle; LA, left atrium; RV, right ventricle; Ao, aorta.

TABLE 5-4	Anatomic Characteristics of the Left Ventricle

Conical in shape, posterolateral location with a smooth inlet
Bicuspid atrioventricular valve (mitral)
Close anatomic relationship of inlet and outlet (mitral and aortic valves)
Two prominent papillary muscles that insert into the free ventricular wall
No moderator band
Ventricular wall receives no direct chordae tendineae insertions

ventricle (2). The left ventricular wall, which is less echogenic than the right ventricular wall in the fetus, is generally smooth with no septoparietal muscle bundles. Unlike the right ventricle, the inlet and outlet of the left ventricle are in close anatomic relationship and are separated by the anterior leaflet of the mitral valve (Fig. 5-10).

The ventricles are separated by the ventricular septum. The apical portion (near the cardiac apex) is muscular in origin, and the basal portion (near the atrioventricular valves) is membranous. Table 5-4 lists the anatomic characteristics of the left ventricle.

THE FOUR-CHAMBER VIEW

Scanning Technique

1. Determine the fetal situs, as previously described in Chapter 4.
2. Obtain a transverse plane of the fetal abdomen. In a perfect transverse plane of the fetal abdomen, a complete fetal rib is imaged along each of the two lateral abdominal walls (Fig. 5-11A). When multiple ribs are imaged along the two lateral abdominal walls, an oblique rather than a transverse view is obtained (Fig. 5-11B).
3. From a transverse view of the fetal abdomen, slide the transducer toward the fetal chest, maintaining the transverse plane, until the four-chamber view is imaged (see Fig. 4-2 in Chapter 4). The optimum plane for the visualization of the four-chamber view requires the

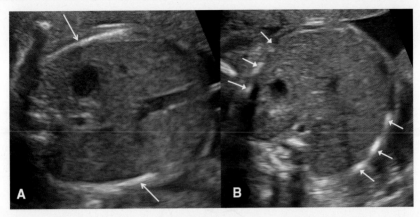

Figure 5-11. A: Transverse view of the fetal abdomen at the level of the stomach. Note the presence of a significant portion of one rib at each lateral abdominal wall (*arrows*). This ensures a near-perfect transverse plane of the abdomen. **B:** Oblique view of the fetal abdomen at the level of the stomach. Note the presence of multiple segments of ribs at each lateral abdominal wall (*arrows*).

following anatomic markers: one complete rib on each side of the fetal lateral chest wall, the two inferior pulmonary veins noted along the posterior wall of the left atrium, and the apex of the heart (Fig. 5-7). Table 5-5 lists the anatomic characteristics of the four-chamber view.

Types of Four-chamber View

Three types of four-chamber views of the fetal heart can be obtained, according to the orientation of the fetus to the ultrasound beam (Fig. 5-12). When the fetal position within the uterus is such that the left anterior chest wall is closest to the transducer, an *apical* four-chamber view is obtained (Fig. 5-7). In this fetal position, the ultrasound beam is nearly parallel to the ventricular septum, and it insonates the apical portion of the fetal heart first. When the fetal right posterior chest wall is closest to the transducer, a *basal* four-chamber view is obtained (Fig. 5-13). In this fetal position, the ultrasound beam enters the fetal chest inferior to the right shoulder, nearly parallel to the ventricular septum, and it insonates the base of the fetal heart first. When the fetal spine is neither anterior nor posterior but closer to the right or left lateral uterine walls, a *long-axis* or *axial* four-chamber view is obtained (Fig. 5-6). In this fetal position, the ultrasound beam is nearly perpendicular to the ventricular septum.

Evaluation of all the anatomic details that the four-chamber view provides often requires examination of more than one type of four-chamber view. This is usually accomplished by

TABLE 5-5	Anatomic Characteristics of the Normal Four-chamber View

Normal-size heart in chest
Transverse plane of fetal chest with one complete rib on each side of fetal lateral chest wall
Descending aorta in front and to the left of the fetal spine
Apex of fetal heart pointing to the left upper chest at about a 45-degree angle
Atria equal in size
Foramen ovale in midsection of atrial septum with leaflet of foramen ovale in left atrium
Two inferior pulmonary veins, seen as slitlike opening in posterior wall of left atrium
Patent atrioventricular valves
Tricuspid valve septal leaflet more apically inserted on the septum than mitral valve
Ventricles equal in size and contractility
Intact ventricular septum
Moderator band in right ventricular apex

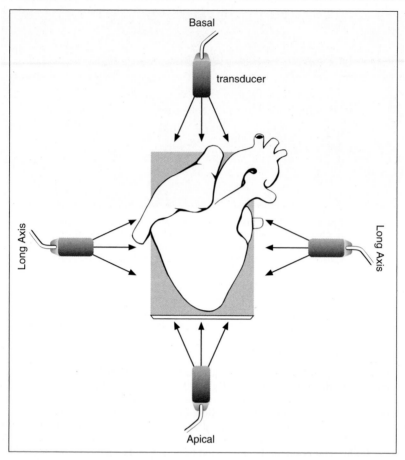

Figure 5-12. Four-chamber-view planes of the heart. The orientation of the ultrasound beam to the fetal chest determines the type of four-chamber view imaged. See text for details.

insonating the fetal heart from opposite sides of the maternal abdomen (3). An apical and a long-axis or axial four-chamber view or a basal and a long-axis or axial four-chamber view can usually be obtained in this manner. The apical view allows optimal visualization of the apex of the heart, the ventricles, the atrioventricular valves, and longitudinal atrial and ventricular dimensions. The primum area of the atrial and ventricular septae, however, are usually inadequately imaged by the apical view. This is due to the longitudinal orientation of the ultrasound beam to the septae in the apical view, making it appear thinner than it actually is with the potential for false diagnosis. The basal view allows adequate visualization of the atria and the atrioventricular valves. The long-axis or axial view allows adequate visualization of the atrial and ventricular septae, atrial and ventricular walls, and septal thickness.

An echogenic intracardiac focus is occasionally seen in the four-chamber view, primarily but not exclusively located within the papillary muscles of the left ventricle (Fig. 5-14A). The echogenic focus can be single or multiple and can also be located in the right ventricle (Fig. 5-14B) or in both the right and left ventricles. There is current controversy on the clinical significance of an echogenic intracardiac focus, especially when seen as an isolated finding in the fetus (4–7). The authors recommend genetic counseling for patients with a fetal intracardiac echogenic focus in pregnancies at increased background risk for Down syndrome and a targeted cardiac examination to rule out associated cardiac malformations. A racial difference in the incidence of echogenic intracardiac focus exists, with a significant increase for fetuses

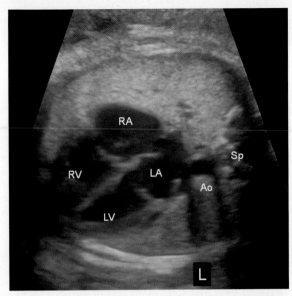

Figure 5-13. Basal four-chamber view of the fetal heart. Note that the fetal spine is anterior and the ultrasound beam enters the chest from the right posterior chest wall. LV, left ventricle; LA, left atrium; RV, right ventricle; RA, right atrium; Ao, aorta; L, left; Sp, spine.

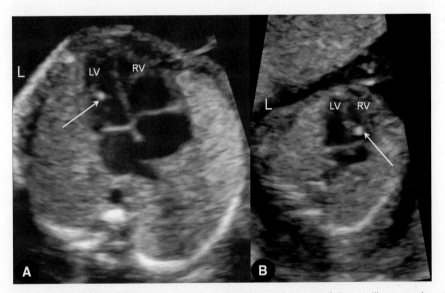

Figure 5-14. A: Single echogenic intracardiac focus located in one of the papillary muscles of the left ventricle (*arrow*). **B:** Single echogenic intracardiac focus located in one of the papillary muscles of the right ventricle (*arrow*). LV, left ventricle; RV, right ventricle.

born to Asian mothers (8). This racial difference should be taken into account when counseling patients about the potential association with Down syndrome.

The four-chamber view represents the inlet of the heart. Several cardiac abnormalities are associated with an abnormal four-chamber view of the heart. Tables 3-1 and 3-2 in Chapter 3 list cardiac abnormalities commonly associated with a normal and an abnormal four-chamber view, respectively.

SHORT-AXIS VIEWS OF THE HEART

Scanning Technique

Short-axis views of the heart, also referred to as parasternal short-axis views, can be obtained as follows:

1. Determine the fetal situs (see Chapter 4).
2. Obtain a four-chamber-view plane of the heart (see previously).
3. From a four-chamber-view plane (Fig. 5-15, plane A), rotate the transducer 90 degrees to obtain short-axis views of the heart (Fig. 5-15, plane B).

Minor adjustments are often required to avoid shadowing by the upper extremities of the fetus. Serial short-axis views of the heart, from the apex of the left ventricle to the pulmonary artery bifurcation, can be obtained by slight anterior-to-posterior (apical-to-basal) angulation of the transducer (Fig. 5-16). Note that short-axis views of the heart are obtained in an oblique plane of the chest.

Anatomic Features of the Short-axis Views

Short-axis views of the heart provide detailed anatomic evaluation of the spatial relationship of cardiac chambers. They are useful in the evaluation of ventricular size, ventricular wall, and septal thickness. The orientation of the great vessels and their divisions can also be accurately assessed by obtaining short-axis views of the base of the heart (discussed in Chapter 6).

In the most apical short-axis view (Fig. 5-16A), the left ventricle is circular in shape and posterior to the right ventricle (Fig. 5-17). The left ventricular wall is smooth when compared to the trabeculated right ventricular apex. The papillary muscles of the left ventricle are seen in a more posterior (basal) section (Fig. 5-16B). The posteromedial and anterolateral papillary muscles of the left ventricle are imaged in the same short-axis plane at 8 and 5 o'clock, respectively (Fig. 5-18). The muscular part of the ventricular septum separates the two ventricular

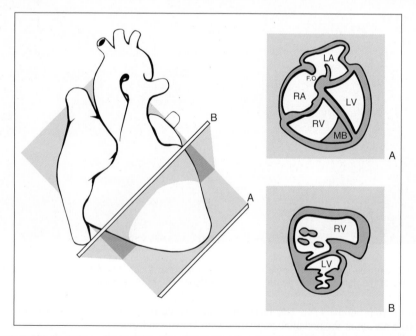

Figure 5-15. Technique for imaging the short-axis views of the heart. From a four-chamber-view plane of the fetal heart **(plane A),** rotate the transducer 90 degrees in order to obtain short-axis views (parasternal views) of the heart **(plane B).** LA, left atrium; LV, left ventricle; FO, foramen ovale; RA, right atrium; RV, right ventricle; MB, moderator band.

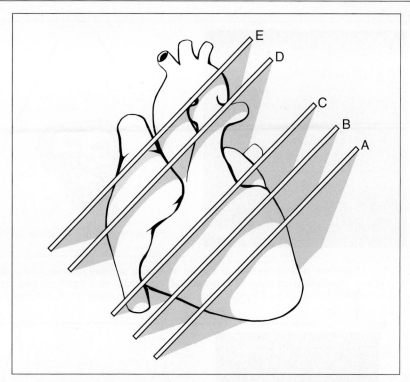

Figure 5-16. Short-axis (parasternal) views of the heart. Serial short-axis views can be obtained by slight anterior-to-posterior angulation of the transducer.

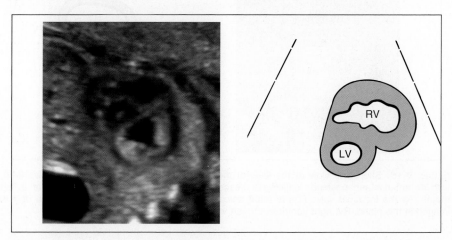

Figure 5-17. Short-axis view of the apex of the heart. The left ventricle is circular in shape and posterior to the right. The left ventricular wall is smooth when compared to the trabeculated right ventricular apex. LV, left ventricle; RV, right ventricle.

cavities at this level. The mitral and tricuspid valves can be imaged in a more posterior (basal) plane (Fig. 5-16C). The mitral valve, with its anterior and posterior leaflets, is crescent shaped and has the appearance of a fish mouth (Fig. 5-19). The tricuspid valve is more apically placed in the heart than the mitral valve, and thus a portion of it is imaged in the same short-axis plane as that imaging the mitral valve (Fig. 5-19).

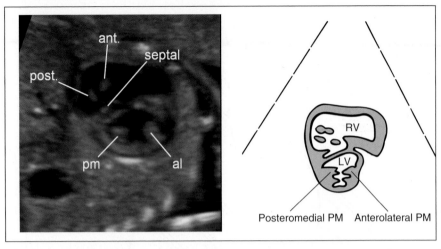

Figure 5-18. Short-axis view at the level of the left ventricular papillary muscles. The postero-medial (pm) and anterolateral (al) papillary muscles (PM) are imaged at 8 and 5 o'clock, respectively. Note the three leaflets of the tricuspid valve: anterior (ant), posterior (post), and septal.

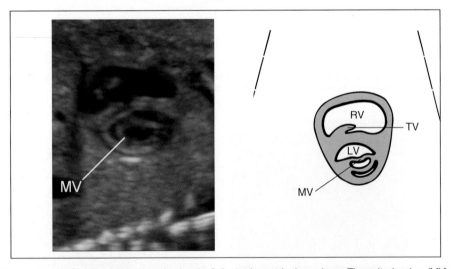

Figure 5-19. Short-axis view at the level of the atrioventricular valves. The mitral valve (MV), with its anterior and posterior leaflets, is crescent shaped and has the appearance of a fish mouth. As the tricuspid valve (TV) is more apically placed in the heart, a small portion of it is imaged in this plane. RV, right ventricle; LV, left ventricle.

Planes D and E in Figure 5-16 represent short-axis views at the level of the right ventricular outflow tract and at the base of the heart, respectively. These planes will be discussed in more detail in Chapter 6.

■ KEY POINTS: THE CARDIAC CHAMBERS

■ The right atrium receives the superior vena cava, inferior vena cava, and coronary sinus.
■ The Eustachian valve, located at the opening of the inferior vena cava, directs ductus venosus blood toward the foramen ovale.

- The tricuspid valve has three leaflets and three papillary muscles.
- Chordae tendineae from the tricuspid valve leaflets insert directly into the right ventricular wall.
- The tricuspid valve inserts more apically than the mitral valve on the interventricular septum.
- The right ventricle is the closest chamber to the anterior chest wall.
- The inlet and apical portions of the right ventricle are heavily trabeculated, with the moderator band occupying the apical portion.
- A subpulmonic conus separates the tricuspid valve from the pulmonary valve.
- The left atrium is the most posterior cardiac chamber.
- The left atrium receives four pulmonary veins; the two inferior ones are seen at the level of the four-chamber view.
- The leaflet of the foramen ovale is imaged in the left atrium and beats from right to left.
- The mitral valve has two leaflets and two papillary muscles, which insert on the left ventricular free wall.
- The anterior leaflet of the mitral valve is in fibrous continuity with the aortic valve.
- The left ventricular wall receives no direct chordae tendineae insertions from the mitral valve.
- A single fetal rib is imaged along each of the two lateral chest walls in an optimal four-chamber view of the heart.
- The four-chamber view represents the inlet of the heart.
- In short-axis view, the mitral valve appears crescentic and has the appearance of a fish mouth.

References

1. Chaoui R, Heling KS, Kalache KD. Caliber of the coronary sinus in fetuses with cardiac defects with and without left persistent superior vena cava and in growth-restricted fetuses with heart-sparing effect. *Prenat Diagn* 2003;23(7):552–557.
2. Chaoui R. The examination of the normal fetal heart using two-dimensional echocardiography. In: Yagel S, Silvermann N, Gembruch U, eds. *Fetal cardiology.* London, New York: Martin Dunitz, 2003;141–149.
3. Abuhamad AZ. *A practical guide to fetal echocardiography.* Philadelphia: Lippincott–Raven Publishers, 1997;35.
4. Benacerraf BR. The role of the second trimester genetic sonogram in screening for Down syndrome. *Semin Perinatol* 2005;29(6):386–394.
5. Filly RA, Benacerraf BR, Nyberg DA, et al. Chorioid plexus cyst and echogenic intracardiac focus in women at low risk for chromosomal anomalies. *J Ultrasound Med* 2004;23(4):447–449.
6. Coco C, Jeanty P, Jeanty C. An isolated echogenic heart focus is not an indication for amniocentesis in 12,672 unselected patients. *J Ultrasound Med* 2004;23(4):489–496.
7. Smith-Bindman R, Hosmer W, Feldstein VA, et al. Second-trimester ultrasound to detect fetuses with Down syndrome: a meta- analysis. *JAMA* 2001;285(8):1044–1055.
8. Borgida AF, Maffeo C, Gianferarri EA, et al. Frequency of echogenic intracardiac focus by race/ethnicity in euploid fetuses. *J Matern Fetal Neonatal Med* 2005;18(1):65–66.

6   **THE GREAT VESSELS**

 THE PULMONARY ARTERY

The pulmonary artery (main pulmonary artery, pulmonary trunk) arises from the right ventricle in the anterior aspect of the heart. It crosses over the aorta and points toward the fetal left shoulder as it emerges from the right ventricle. The pulmonary artery, which dips posteriorly into the chest shortly after it crosses over the aorta, divides into the right and left pulmonary arteries and the ductus arteriosus. The ductus arteriosus, which is patent in the fetus, connects with the descending aorta. The division of the pulmonary artery into the right and left pulmonary arteries is an important anatomic characteristic that differentiates it from the ascending aorta. The left pulmonary artery continues posteriorly and inferiorly and courses over the left bronchus into the left lung hilum; the right pulmonary artery originates at a right angle from the pulmonary artery and crosses under the aortic arch, superior to the roof of the left atrium and behind the superior vena cava, before it dips into the right lung hilum. During right ventricular diastole, blood is prevented from flowing back into the ventricle by the pulmonary semilunar valve. The pulmonary semilunar valve is closest to the anterior chest wall, near the left sternal border, and is made of three leaflets: right, left (septal), and anterior. The pulmonary semilunar valve is anatomically separated from the tricuspid valve by a subpulmonic conus. This anatomic separation results in the inability to image both right ventricular inflow and outflow tracts in the same ultrasound plane in long-axis views. In fetal life, the pressure in the pulmonary circulation is near systemic due to the patency of the ductus arteriosus. Prenatally, the thickness of the muscular layer within the wall of the pulmonary tree is similar to that of systemic vessels. Attenuation of this muscular layer is noted in postnatal life due to a decrease in pulmonary arterial pressure that follows closure of the ductus arteriosus.

THE AORTA

The aorta is anatomically divided into four segments: the ascending aorta, the aortic arch, the thoracic aorta, and the abdominal aorta. The ascending aorta arises from the left ventricle in the central portion of the heart and to the right of the pulmonary artery. It angles anteriorly, pointing toward the fetal right shoulder and parallel to the long axis of the left ventricle as it emerges from the heart. Within the heart, the ascending aorta is bordered anteriorly by the interventricular septum and posteriorly by the anterior leaflet of the mitral valve. This continuity between the anterior wall of the ascending aorta and the interventricular septum is an important anatomic finding. When there is overriding of the aorta, as in tetralogy of Fallot or double outlet right ventricle, there is a disruption in this normal continuity. The inflow and outflow portions of the left ventricle can be imaged in the same long-axis ultrasound plane because of fibrous continuity between the aortic valve and the anterior leaflet of the mitral valve. The ascending aorta passes between the right and left atrium and inferior to the pulmonary artery before it emerges from the heart and curves posteriorly from the aortic arch. The aortic arch crosses over the right pulmonary artery and bronchus, defining a normal left aortic arch. The aortic arch gives rise to three arterial branches: the brachiocephalic (innominate), the left common carotid, and the left subclavian artery. The brachiocephalic artery divides into the right common carotid and the right subclavian artery. The aortic arch therefore provides the majority of blood supply to the head, neck, and upper extremities. Aortic arch branches provide an important anatomic characteristic as they distinguish the aortic arch from the ductal arch, which gives no branches as it connects with the descending aorta. The thoracic aorta lies posterior to the left atrium and adjacent to the esophagus, and the abdominal aorta lies to the left of the midline right over the spine. During left ventricular diastole, blood is prevented from flowing back into the ventricle by the aortic semilunar valve. The aortic semilunar valve has three leaflets: right and left coronary cusps giving rise to the right

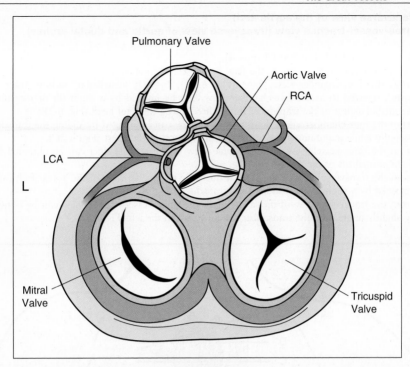

Figure 6-1. Anatomic relationship of the semilunar valves to the atrioventricular valves. Note the location of the pulmonary valve, anterior and slightly to the left of the aortic valve. The aortic valve is located in the central portion of the heart, between the right and left atrioventricular valves. Right and left coronary arteries (RCA, LCA) are seen to arise from the ascending aorta behind the right and left coronary cusps. L, left.

and left coronary arteries, respectively, and a posterior or noncoronary cusp. The anatomic relationships of the semilunar valves to the atrioventricular valves are shown in Figure 6-1. The directions of flow out of the pulmonary and aortic semilunar valves are at an almost 90-degree angle to each other as they arise from their respective chambers, an important anatomic orientation that is disrupted in fetuses with transposition of the great vessels or double outlet right ventricle.

Scanning Technique

The orientation and access to the fetal heart differ from postnatal scanning. In this section, we will rely on the anatomic approach of various diagnostic planes as it relates to the anatomic long axis of the fetus (fetal spine), rather than the long axis of the heart itself. Transverse views are therefore obtained from a transverse, or near-transverse, orientation of the ultrasound transducer to the fetal chest, and sagittal views are obtained from a sagittal or parasagittal orientation of the ultrasound transducer to the fetal chest. Cardiac views that are neither near transverse nor near sagittal are referred to as oblique views. The authors believe that this approach is best adapted to fetal cardiac imaging (1,2).

Scanning Technique for Transverse Views

- **Abdominal circumference** (see Chapter 4)
- **Four-chamber view** (see Chapter 5)
- **Five-chamber view**
- **Three-vessel view**
- **Transverse view of the arterial duct (ductus arteriosus)**

■ **Transverse view of the aortic arch**
■ **Three-vessel-trachea view (transverse view of aortic and ductal arches)**

1. Determine the fetal situs (see Chapter 4).
2. Obtain a four-chamber view of the fetal heart (see Chapter 5).
3. From the four-chamber-view plane (Fig. 6-2A), the left ventricular outflow tract (the aorta), referred to as the five-chamber view, can be imaged by a slight tilt or rotation of the medial aspect of the transducer in the direction of the fetal head (Fig. 6-2B).
4. From the four-chamber view, the three-vessel view can be imaged by sliding the transducer cranially while maintaining the transverse orientation in the chest (Fig. 6-2C).
5. From the three-vessel view, the transverse view of the arterial duct can be obtained by a slight cranial tilt of the transducer (Fig. 6-2D).
6. From the transverse view of the arterial duct, the transverse view of the aortic arch can be obtained by a slight cranial slide of the transducer (Fig. 6-2E).
7. From the transverse view of the aortic arch, the three-vessel-trachea view can be obtained by slightly angulating the transducer caudally and to the left (Fig. 6-2F).

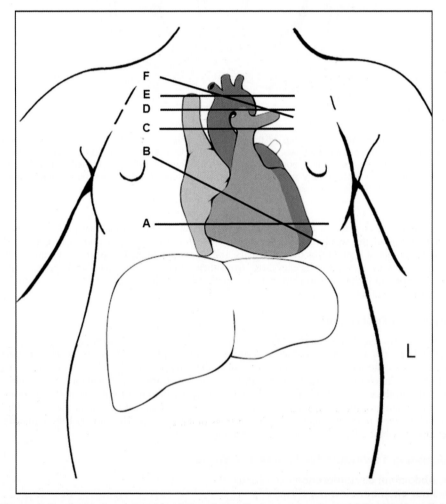

Figure 6-2. Anatomic relationship of the diagnostic transverse planes of the fetal heart. **A:** Four-chamber view. **B:** Five-chamber view. **C:** Three-vessel view. **D:** Transverse view of arterial duct. **E:** Transverse view of aortic arch. **F:** Three-vessel-trachea view. L, left. See text for details.

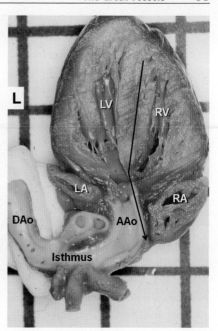

Figure 6-3. Anatomic specimen of the five-chamber view of the fetal heart demonstrating the wide angle between the direction of the ventricular septum and the anterior wall of the ascending aorta (AAo). The entire ascending aorta is seen in this view. LV, left ventricle; RV, right ventricle; LA, left atrium; RA, right atrium; DAo, descending aorta; L, left.

The Five-chamber View

The five-chamber view is obtained in a transverse plane cephalad to the four-chamber view with a slight angulation of the transducer toward the fetal head (Fig. 6-2B), thus allowing for a full display of the ascending aorta (Fig. 6-3). The aortic outflow accounts for the fifth component of the five-chamber view, which demonstrates the left ventriculoarterial connection and the perimembranous and muscular ventricular septum. The ascending aorta arises in the midportion of the heart between the two atrioventricular valves (Fig. 6-1) in a left-to-right orientation (in the direction of right shoulder). A wide angle is seen between the direction of the ventricular septum and the anterior wall of the ascending aorta (Figs. 6-3 and 6-4), an important anatomic observation that is commonly absent in conotruncal anomalies (more parallel orientation with the ventricular septum). The ascending aorta runs between the two atria before it forms the transverse aortic arch. A critical anatomic component of the five-chamber view is the continuity of the posterior wall of the aorta with the mitral valve (fibrous–fibrous continuity) and the continuity of the anterior wall of the aorta with the ventricular septum (fibrous–muscular continuity) (Fig. 6-5). This continuity is disrupted in the presence of aortic override (see Chapter 17). The five-chamber view displays the inflow, trabecular, and outflow components of the left ventricle and a portion of the trabecular right ventricle (Fig. 6-5). Tricuspid valve and right ventricular inflow are not seen in the five-chamber view. The two superior pulmonary veins enter the posterior wall of the left atrium at the five-chamber-view level (Fig. 6-5).

The Three-vessel View

The three-vessel view is obtained in a transverse plane of the fetal upper thorax (Fig. 6-2C). The three-vessel view demonstrates the main pulmonary trunk in an oblique section and the ascending aorta and the superior vena cava in transverse sections (Fig. 6-6). These three vessels are arranged in an oblique line with the pulmonary artery in the most anterior position, the superior vena cava in the most posterior position, and the aorta in between (Fig. 6-6). The pulmonary artery is the largest in size and the superior vena cava is the smallest. Measuring for pulmonary artery dimensions in this plane is not advisable given an oblique orientation of the vessel. The pulmonary artery arises anteriorly in the chest and angles posteriorly to the left of the spine (Fig. 6-6). The pulmonary artery divides into the left and right pulmonary arteries

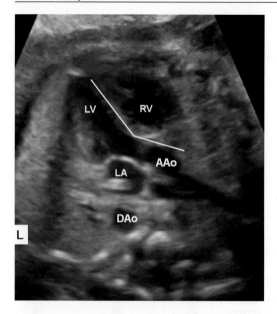

Figure 6-4. Five-chamber view of the fetal heart demonstrating the wide angle between the direction of the ventricular septum and the anterior wall of the ascending aorta (AAo). This important anatomic observation is commonly absent in conotruncal malformations. LV, left ventricle; RV, right ventricle; LA, left atrium; DAo, descending aorta; L, left.

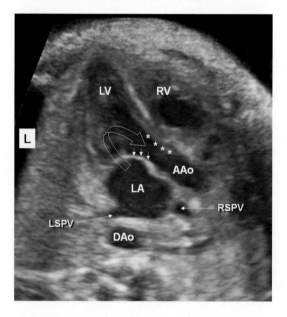

Figure 6-5. Five-chamber view of the fetal heart demonstrating the continuity of the posterior wall of the aorta with the mitral valve (*small arrows*) and the continuity of the anterior wall of the ascending aorta (AAo) with the ventricular septum (*asterisks*). The inflow and outflow components of the left ventricle (LV) are seen in one view (*open arrow*). The right and left superior pulmonary veins (RSPV, LSPV) enter the posterior wall of the left atrium at this level. RV, right ventricle; LA, left atrium; DAo, descending aorta; L, left.

(Fig. 6-6). The left pulmonary artery follows the same course as the main trunk, whereas the right pulmonary artery originates at a right angle and runs behind the ascending aorta and the superior vena cava (Fig. 6-6). In the posterior aspect of the three-vessel-view plane, the descending aorta is to the left of the spine, a small normal azygos vein is to the right of the spine, and the two main bronchi are noted slightly anterior to the esophagus when imaging is obtained in high resolution (Fig. 6-6). The trachea is not seen at the three-vessel-view plane as it is located at a slightly higher level in the mediastinum. The three-vessel-view plane is helpful in the assessment of conotruncal abnormalities. Abnormalities may involve vessel size, vessel alignment, vessel arrangement, vessel number, and location of descending aorta (3).

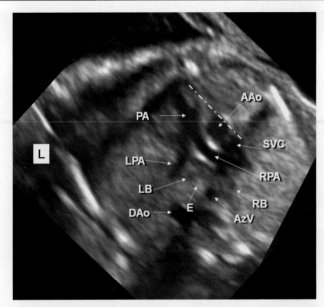

Figure 6-6. Three-vessel view of the fetal heart demonstrating the pulmonary artery (PA), the ascending aorta (AAo), and the superior vena cava (SVC) in the upper chest arranged in an oblique line (see *dashed line*) with the PA most anterior, SVC most posterior, and AAo in between. The PA divides into the left (LPA) and right (RPA) pulmonary arteries. The RPA originates at a right angle and runs behind the AAo and the SVC. E, esophagus; RB, right bronchus; LB, left bronchus; AzV, azygos vein; DAo, descending aorta; L, left.

Color Doppler can also be used to evaluate flow patterns in the great vessels. The utility of the three-vessel view in the diagnosis of various cardiac abnormalities is discussed in respective chapters.

The Transverse View of the Arterial Duct

This plane is obtained from a slight cranial tilt of the three-vessel view (Fig. 6-2D). It displays the main pulmonary artery with the ductal branch joining the descending aorta to the left of the spine (Fig. 6-7). The ascending aorta and superior vena cava are seen in cross section on the right (Fig. 6-7). The oblique line arrangement of the vessels and their size is similar to that in the three-vessel view (see three-vessel-view section). The trachea and esophagus are seen in the midline posteriorly (Fig. 6-7). The azygos vein can be seen on occasions as it enters the superior vena cava posteriorly. Normally, the azygos vein can be seen in about 50% of fetuses in the second trimester and in about 98% in the third trimester of pregnancy (4). Figure 6-8 shows the relationship of the arterial duct, the ascending aorta, and the superior vena cava in an anatomic specimen.

The Transverse View of the Aortic Arch

This plane is obtained in a slight cranial slide from the transverse arterial duct view (Fig. 6-2E) and demonstrates the transverse aortic arch, which is the most superior vessel in the thorax. In this view, two vessels are seen: the transverse aortic arch and the superior vena cava (Fig. 6-9). The transverse aortic arch is seen to arise from the midchest, halfway between the sternum and spine (in contrast to the main pulmonary artery in the three-vessel view), and has an oblique course, which crosses the midline from the right anterior to left posterior chest (Fig. 6-9). The superior vena cava is seen to the right of the aortic arch (Fig. 6-9). In the posterior chest, the trachea and the esophagus are seen as midline structures above the spine (Fig. 6-9). Color Doppler demonstrates flow in an anterior-to-posterior direction. Given that this plane demonstrates two vessels only, it should not be mistaken for abnormal anatomy. A left caudal tilt of the

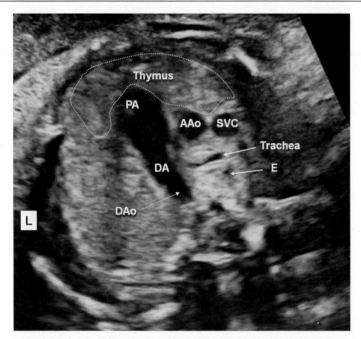

Figure 6-7. Transverse view of the arterial duct showing the pulmonary artery (PA) with the ductal branch (DA) joining the descending aorta (DAo) to the left of the spine. The ascending aorta (AAo) and superior vena cava (SVC) are seen in cross section on the right. The thymus is anterior to the three vessels and is marked with a dashed line. E, esophagus; L, left.

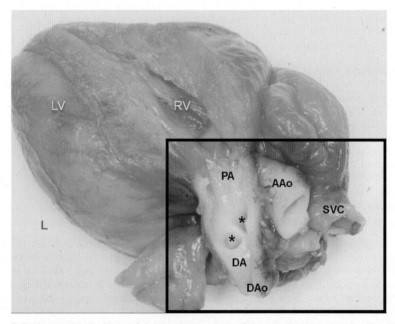

Figure 6-8. Anatomic specimen of the transverse view of the arterial duct showing the relationship of the pulmonary artery (PA), ascending aorta (AAo), and superior vena cava (SVC). Asterisk shows the origin of both left and right pulmonary arteries. DAo, descending aorta; LV, left ventricle; RV, right ventricle; L, left.

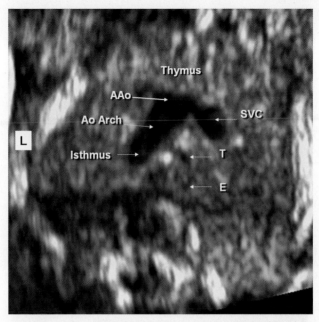

Figure 6-9. Transverse view of the aortic arch (Ao Arch) demonstrating the aortic arch with an oblique course, which crosses the midline from right anterior to left posterior chest. The superior vena cava (SVC) is seen to the right of the aortic arch. The thymus gland is seen anteriorly. The trachea (T) and the esophagus (E) are seen as midline structures above the spine. AAo, ascending aorta; L, left.

transducer will bring to view the three-vessel-trachea-view plane. The thymus gland is best seen in this plane in the anterosuperior section of the mediastinum (Fig. 6-9). It appears hypoechoic when compared to lung tissue, and the borders can be clearly seen when the fetal spine is closer to the posterior uterine wall. The thymus may be absent or hypoplastic in association with microdeletion 22q11.2 (5). Normal dimensions of the fetal thymus have been established (6,7).

Three-vessel-trachea View (Transverse Duct and Aortic Arch View)

This view is more cranial to the three-vessel view and is obtained in a left and caudal angulation from a transverse aortic arch view (Fig. 6-2F). This view demonstrates the aortic arch and ductal arch merging together into the descending aorta with an acute angle between them (8) (Figs. 6-10 and 6.11). Both arches are located to the left of the spine and trachea, an important anatomic landmark because no vessel is seen to the right of the trachea in normal cardiovascular anatomy (Figs. 6-10 and 6.11). The superior vena cava is seen in a cross section and is located to the right of the aortic arch (8) (Figs. 6-10 and 6.11). The oblique line orientation of the three vessels is maintained with the ductal arch, the largest of the three, assuming a more anterior position, the aortic arch in the middle, and the superior vena cava more inferior (Fig. 6-11). Color Doppler reveals anteroposterior flow in both arches. Figure 6-12 shows the relationship of the aortic and ductal arch in an anatomic specimen where the superior vena cava has been removed.

Scanning Technique for Sagittal Views

- Inferior and superior vena cava view
- Aortic arch view
- Ductal arch view

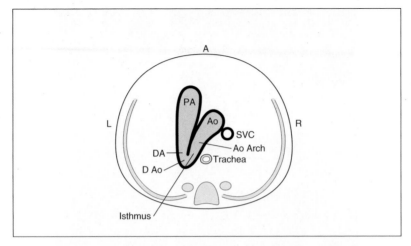

Figure 6-10. Drawing of the three-vessel-trachea view illustrating the aortic arch (Ao Arch) and ductal arch (DA) merging together into the descending aorta (D Ao) to the left of the spine and trachea. The superior vena cava (SVC) is seen in a cross section and is located to the right of the aortic arch. L, left; A, anterior; R, right.

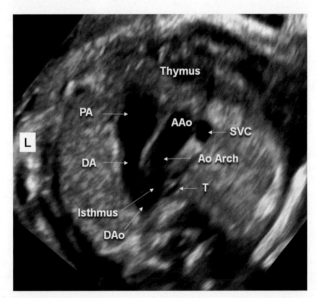

Figure 6-11. Three-vessel-trachea view demonstrating the aortic arch (Ao arch) and ductal arch (DA) merging together into the descending aorta (DAo) to the left of the spine and trachea (T). The superior vena cava (SVC) is seen in a cross section and is located to the right of the aortic arch. PA, pulmonary artery; AAo, ascending aorta; L, left.

1. Determine the fetal situs (see Chapter 4).
2. Obtain a sagittal view of the thoracic fetal spine.
3. By sliding the transducer from the right parasagittal to the left parasagittal chest while maintaining a sagittal orientation, three ultrasound planes can be imaged: the superior and inferior venae cavae (Fig. 6-13A), the aortic arch (Fig. 6-13B), and the ductal arch (Fig. 6-13C), in that order.

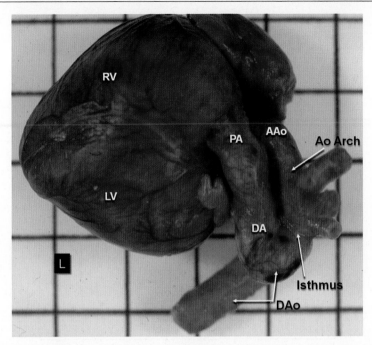

Figure 6-12. Anatomic specimen of the three-vessel-trachea view demonstrating the aortic arch (Ao arch) and ductal arch (DA) merging together into the descending aorta (DAo). The superior vena cava is not seen in this specimen as it was removed. PA, pulmonary artery; AAo, ascending aorta; RV, right ventricle; LV, left ventricle; L, left.

4. These ultrasound planes are difficult to image when the fetal spine is in an anterior or lateral position within the uterus. Furthermore, slight adjustment of the transducer is often required in order to image the aortic and ductal arches in their entirety. The ductal arch view can be imaged from two planes, a sagittal and a parasagittal approach.

The Inferior and Superior Vena Cava View

The inferior and superior vena cava view, also called the bicaval view, is obtained in a right parasagittal plane (Fig. 6-13A). This plane shows the inferior and superior venae cavae as they enter the posterior aspect of the right atrium (Fig. 6-14). The right atrial appendage with its broad base is seen anteriorly (Fig. 6-14). A portion of the left atrium and a cross section of the right pulmonary artery are seen posterior to the right atrium (Fig. 6-14). The left and right atria are bordered by the upper portion of the atrial septum (Fig. 6-14). The superior vena cava, which is formed by the merger of right and left brachiocephalic veins, lies anterior to the right pulmonary artery and against the posterolateral aspect of the ascending aorta (Fig. 6-14). The azygos vein, which empties into the superior vena cava posteriorly after it crosses over the right bronchus, can be occasionally seen in this view with optimal ultrasound imaging. The inferior vena cava is widened as it enters the right atrium due to the confluence of the ductus venosus and suprahepatic veins (Fig. 6-14). The Eustachian valve is seen at the junction of the inferior vena cava with the right atrium (Fig. 6-14). A portion of the thymus gland is seen anteriorly, bordered by the anterior thoracic wall and the superior vena cava (Fig. 6-14). The inferior and superior vena cava view does not allow for color or pulsed Doppler interrogation of the vessels due to the direction of caval blood flow perpendicular to the ultrasound beam.

The Aortic Arch View

The aortic arch view is obtained by sliding the transducer to the left parasagittal plane (Fig. 6-13B). In this view, the aorta is seen to arise from the central portion of the chest with an acute circular curvature (aortic arch), which has been likened to a candy or a walking cane

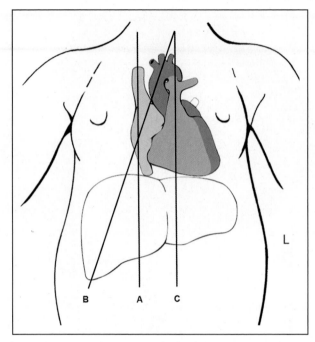

Figure 6-13. Anatomic relationship of the diagnostic sagittal planes of the fetal heart. **A:** Inferior and superior vena cava view. **B:** Aortic arch view. **C:** Ductal arch view. L, left. See text for details.

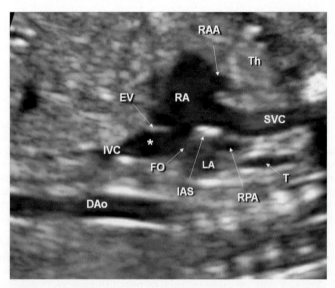

Figure 6-14. The inferior (IVC) and superior vena cava (SVC) view shows both the IVC and SVC entering the posterior aspect of the right atrium (RA). A portion of the left atrium (LA) and a cross section of the right pulmonary artery (RPA) are seen posterior to the right atrium. The IVC is widened as it enters the right atrium (*asterisk*) due to the confluence of the ductus venosus and suprahepatic veins. The Eustachian valve (EV) is seen at the junction of the inferior vena cava with the right atrium. IAS, interatrial septum; FO, foramen ovale; RAA, right atrial appendage; T, trachea; Th, thymus; DAo, descending aorta.

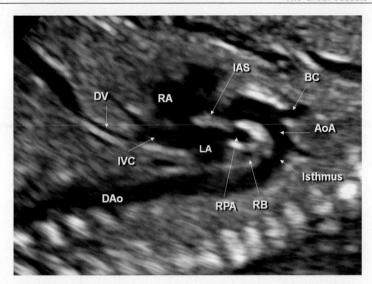

Figure 6-15. The aortic arch (AoA) view shows the aorta arising from the central portion of the chest with an acute circular curvature. The left atrium (LA), right pulmonary artery (RPA), and right bronchus (RB) are seen posteriorly. RA, right atrium; IAS, interatrial septum; BC, brachiocephalic; DAo, descending aorta; IVC, inferior vena cava; DV, ductus venosus.

(Fig. 6-15). Three arterial branches arise from the superior aspect of the aortic arch: the brachiocephalic (innominate), the left common carotid, and the left subclavian. The brachiocephalic artery divides into the right common carotid and subclavian arteries. The large innominate vein (largest vessel in mediastinum) is occasionally seen anterosuperiorly to the brachiocephalic artery, and a portion of the thymus gland is seen anteriorly in the upper mediastinum. A small portion of the left atrium, which lies between the ascending and descending aorta, is seen posterior to the right atrium (Fig. 6-15). The foramen ovale is seen in the atrial septum with its leaflet opening toward the left atrium. The right pulmonary artery and right bronchus are seen in cross section posterior to the aortic arch (Fig. 6-15). The aortic isthmus, which is located between the left common carotid artery and the junction of the ductus arteriosus, is seen in this view (Fig. 6-15). The aortic isthmus is implicated in the development of most aortic coarctations.

The Ductal Arch View(s)
The ductal arch view(s) can be imaged by sliding the transducer further to the left from the aortic arch view (Fig. 6-13C). The ductal arch can be imaged from a sagittal or parasagittal approach (Fig. 6-16A, B), which differs with regard to the display of intracardiac anatomy. In both approaches, the ductal arch is seen to arise from the anterior aspect of the chest, with a wide, angular curvature, almost perpendicular to the descending aorta (Figs. 6-17 and 6-18). The anatomic appearance of the ductal arch has been likened to a hockey stick. The ductal arch does not give rise to any branches and is seen in its entirety as it connects with the descending aorta. The left pulmonary artery is seen inferiorly.

In the sagittal plane, the spine is seen posteriorly in a midsagittal plane, the ascending aorta is seen in an oblique section centrally, the left atrium borders the aorta inferiorly by the anterior leaflet of the mitral valve, and the descending aorta is seen in its entirety (Fig. 6-17). The right ventricle, pulmonary valve, and main pulmonary artery are seen anteriorly (Fig. 6-17). The right atrium and tricuspid valve are not seen in the sagittal approach.

The parasagittal approach to the ductal arch view shows the left atrium, right atrium, right ventricle, tricuspid valve, and main pulmonary artery wrapping around a cross section

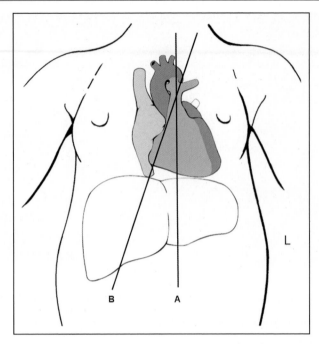

Figure 6-16. Anatomic relationship of the two long-axis views of the ductal arch. **A:** The sagittal approach. **B:** The parasagittal approach. L, left. See text and Figures 6-17 and 6-18 for details.

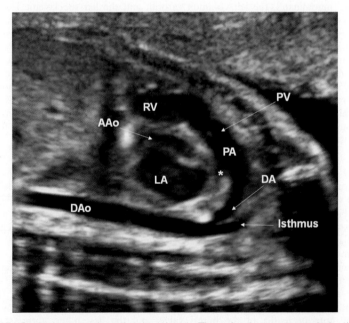

Figure 6-17. Sagittal approach to the ductal arch. The spine is seen posteriorly, the ascending aorta (AAo) is seen in an oblique section centrally, the left atrium (LA) is seen inferiorly, and the descending aorta (DAo) is seen in its entirety. Note the Y-shape confluence of the ductus arteriosus (DA) and the aortic isthmus into the descending aorta. Asterisk indicates the origin of the left pulmonary artery. RV, right ventricle; PA, pulmonary artery; PV, pulmonary valve.

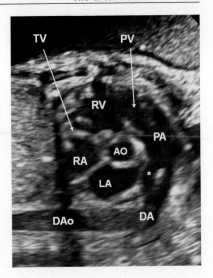

Figure 6-18. Parasagittal approach to the ductal arch. The left atrium (LA), right atrium (RA), right ventricle (RV), tricuspid valve (TV), and pulmonary artery (PA) are seen wrapping around a cross section of the aorta (Ao). Asterisk indicates the left pulmonary artery. PV, pulmonary valve; DAo, descending aorta; DA, ductus arteriosus.

of the aorta at the level of the aortic valve (Fig. 6-18). The cross section of the aorta is seen posterior to the right ventricle and anterior to the roof of the left atrium (Fig. 6-18). The pulmonary valve is seen in an anterior and superior position to the aortic valve (Fig. 6-18).

Several anatomic features distinguish the aortic from the ductal arch in the fetus. The aortic arch is more circular in shape, arises centrally and superiorly in the chest, and provides three arterial branches before it becomes the descending part of the aorta. The ductal arch, on the other hand, has a more angular curve, arises more anteriorly in the chest, and provides no branches. The ductal arch has the highest peak systolic velocities in the fetal cardiovascular system.

Scanning Technique for Oblique Views

- ■ *Right ventricular outflow view (short axis)*
- ■ *Left ventricular long-axis view*
- ■ *Ventricular short-axis views* (see Chapter 5)

1. Determine the fetal situs (see Chapter 4).
2. Obtain a midsagittal plane of the fetal chest.
3. The right ventricular outflow view is then obtained from the midsagittal plane of the chest by angling the transducer to an oblique plane that is oriented from the right iliac bone to the left shoulder of the fetus (Fig. 6-19A).
4. The left ventricle long-axis view is obtained from the midsagittal plane of the chest by angling the transducer to an oblique plane that is oriented from the left iliac bone to the right shoulder of the fetus (Fig. 6-19B).

Right Ventricular Outflow View

In the right ventricular outflow view, the right ventricular inflow and outflow tracts can be seen in the same plane and are typically at an almost perpendicular orientation to each other (Fig. 6-20). The right ventricular infundibulum is seen to occupy the most anterior anatomic location in the heart and the anterior and septal leaflets of the tricuspid valve are seen in this plane (Fig. 6-20). The main pulmonary artery with its anterior valve is seen as it crosses over the aorta and divides into the right pulmonary artery and ductus arteriosus (Fig. 6-20). The right pulmonary artery courses under the aorta and to the right (Fig. 6-20). The aorta is imaged in a cross section at the level of the aortic valve. The left atrium is seen posterior to

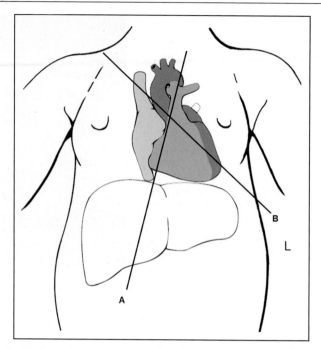

Figure 6-19. Anatomic approach to the right ventricular outflow **(A)** and left ventricular long-axis **(B)** views. L, left. See text for details.

the aorta and the leaflet of the foramen ovale can be imaged within it in optimal imaging conditions (Fig. 6-20).

Left Ventricle Long-axis View
In the long-axis view of the left ventricle, the left ventricular inflow and outflow tracts are demonstrated (Fig. 6-21). The continuity of the anterior wall of the aorta with the ventricular septum and the proximity of the posterior wall of the aorta with the anterior leaflet of the mitral valve are seen (Fig. 6-21). The perimembranous and muscular parts of the ventricular septum are seen. The left ventricular inflow and outflow tracts have a much narrower angle than those of the right ventricle (Fig. 6-21). Anteriorly, a portion of the right ventricle at its outflow tract level is seen (Fig. 6-21). Posterior to the heart, cross and oblique sections of the descending aorta, right pulmonary artery, right bronchus, and esophagus can be seen with optimal ultrasound imaging. A portion of the thymus gland is located between the anterior wall of the aorta and the anterior chest wall (Fig. 6-21). The large innominate (brachiocephalic) vein is occasionally seen on the inferior border of the thymus gland.

▥ KEY POINTS: THE GREAT VESSELS

- ■ The pulmonary artery (trunk) arises from the right ventricle in the anterior aspect of the heart, crosses over the aorta, and points toward the fetal left shoulder as it emerges from the right ventricle.
- ■ The division of the pulmonary artery into the right and left pulmonary arteries is an important anatomic characteristic that differentiates it from the ascending aorta.
- ■ The ascending aorta arises from the left ventricle in the central portion of the heart and to the right of the pulmonary artery.

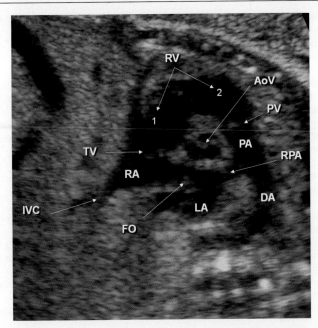

Figure 6-20. The right ventricular outflow view. Right ventricular inflow (*1*) and outflow (*2*) are seen in the same plane almost perpendicular to each other. The pulmonary artery (PA) with its pulmonary valve (PV) is seen as it crosses over the aortic valve (AoV) and divides into the right pulmonary artery (RPA) and ductus arteriosus (DA). The left atrium (LA) is seen posterior to the aorta. FO, foramen ovale; RA, right atrium; RV, right ventricle; TV, tricuspid valve; IVC, inferior vena cava.

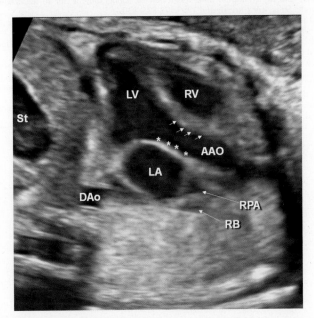

Figure 6-21. Long-axis view of the left ventricle (LV) demonstrating the continuity of the anterior wall of the ascending aorta (AAO) with the ventricular septum (*small arrows*) and the proximity of the posterior wall of the aorta with the anterior leaflet of the mitral valve (*asterisks*). Anteriorly, a portion of the right ventricle (RV) at its outflow tract level is seen. Posterior to the heart, the descending aorta (DAo), right pulmonary artery (RPA), and right bronchus (RB) are seen. LA, left atrium; St, stomach.

■ The ascending aorta angles anteriorly, pointing toward the fetal right shoulder and parallel to the long axis of the left ventricle as it emerges from the heart.

■ Aortic arch branches provide an important anatomic characteristic as they distinguish the aortic arch from the ductal arch, which gives no branches, as it connects with the descending aorta.

■ A critical anatomic component of the five-chamber view is the continuity of the posterior wall of the aorta with the mitral valve and the continuity of the anterior wall of the aorta with the ventricular septum.

■ A wide angle is seen between the direction of the ventricular septum and the anterior wall of the ascending aorta, an important anatomic observation that is commonly absent in transposition of the great arteries.

■ The three vessels in the three-vessel view are arranged in an oblique line, with the pulmonary artery in the most anterior position, the superior vena cava in the most posterior position, and the aorta in between.

■ The transverse aortic arch is the most superior vessel in the thorax.

■ The transverse aortic arch is seen to arise from the midchest and has an oblique course, which crosses the midline from the right anterior to the left posterior chest.

■ In the three-vessel-trachea view, both aortic and ductal arches are located to the left of the spine and trachea, an important anatomic landmark because no vessel is seen to the right of the trachea in normal cardiovascular anatomy.

■ The ductal arch, when compared to the aortic arch, has a more angular curve, arises more anteriorly in the chest, and provides no branches.

■ The ductal arch has the highest peak systolic velocities in the fetal cardiovascular system.

References

1. Abuhamad A. *A practical guide to fetal echocardiography*. Philadelphia: Lippincott–Raven Publishers, 1997;41–60.
2. Chaoui R, Bollmann R, Hoffmann H, et al. [Sonoanatomy of the fetal heart. Proposal of simple cross-sectional planes for the non-cardiologists]. *Ultraschall Klin Prax* 1991;6:59–67.
3. Yoo SJ, Lee YH, Cho KS. Abnormal three-vessel view on sonography: a clue to the diagnosis of congenital heart disease in the fetus. *Am J Roentgenol* 1999;172:825–830.
4. Belfar HL, Hill LM, Peterson C, et al. Sonographic imaging of the fetal azygous vein. Normal and pathologic appearance. *J Ultrasound Med* 1990;9(10):569–573.
5. Chaoui R, Kalache KD, Heling KS, et al. Absent or hypoplastic thymus on ultrasound: a marker for deletion 22q11.2 in fetal cardiac defects. *Ultrasound Obstet Gynecol* 2002;20:546–552.
6. Zalel Y, Gamzu R, Mashiach S, et al. The development of the fetal thymus: an in utero sonographic evaluation. *Prenat Diagn* 2002;22(2):114–117.
7. Cho JY, Min JY, Lee YH, et al. Diameter of the normal fetal thymus on ultrasound. *Ultrasound Obstet Gynecol* 2007;29:634–638.
8. Jeanty P, Chaoui R, Tihonenko I, et al. A review of findings in fetal cardiac section drawings. Part 3: the 3-vessel-trachea view and variants. *J Ultrasound Med* 2008;27:109–117.

COLOR DOPPLER IN FETAL ECHOCARDIOGRAPHY 7

INTRODUCTION

Color and pulsed Doppler ultrasound was introduced to clinical practice about two decades ago and its clinical application in fetal echocardiography was quickly accepted (1–7). Color and pulsed Doppler ultrasound is currently available on almost all mid- and high-end ultrasound equipment involved in obstetric sonography. When imaging the fetal heart on ultrasound, some examiners recommend limiting the use of color Doppler to high-risk conditions such as the presence of a suspected anatomic or functional cardiac abnormality. Other examiners recommend the routine use of color Doppler as an integral component of fetal cardiac evaluation in every fetus, arguing that its routine use increases both the accuracy and speed of the examination (8–10). There is general agreement, however, that when the fetal heart is examined in detail as part of a fetal echocardiogram, the routine application of color Doppler is warranted. In a recent consensus statement, the International Society of Ultrasound in Obstetrics and Gynecology stated that color Doppler ultrasonography is an important component of the fetal echocardiogram and recommended its mandatory use in that setting and that the additional use of power Doppler is optional (11). We recommend the liberal use of color Doppler in the ultrasound examination of the fetal heart and that color Doppler should be part of fetal echocardiography.

In this book, the use of color Doppler as it pertains to the diagnosis of cardiac malformations is described in the respective chapters on cardiac anomalies. Table 7-1 summarizes the clinical information that can be provided by color Doppler in normal and abnormal hearts. This chapter will focus on the optimization of color Doppler in fetal imaging and on the targeted anatomic cardiac planes evaluated by color Doppler ultrasonography.

OPTIMIZING COLOR DOPPLER FOR THE FETAL CARDIAC EXAMINATION

Color Doppler examination of the fetal heart is enhanced when the proper settings of the ultrasound equipment are applied. The examiner should familiarize himself or herself with the standard features of the ultrasound equipment prior to the application of color Doppler. Improper use of color Doppler in the cardiac ultrasound examination may lead to false-negative or false-positive diagnoses. Steps in the optimization of the color Doppler ultrasound image in fetal cardiac examination are hereby discussed.

Size of the Color Box

The optimum color Doppler image is a compromise between its quality and its frame rate. The color box, when activated, slows the frame rate of the ultrasound examination to a significant degree. When examining the fetal heart with color Doppler, a rapid frame rate with an acceptable image quality is essential given the small and complex anatomy of the fetal heart and its rapid rate in utero. We recommend choosing the smallest color box possible to maintain the frame rate as high as possible (Figs. 7-1 and 7-2). Frame rates greater than 20 to 25 images/sec are perceived by the human eye as "real time." The image quality can be improved further by optimizing the use of the velocity range, the wall filter, the persistence, the gain, and color line density.

Velocity Scale

Velocity scale or pulse repetition frequency (PRF) is used to determine the range of mean velocities in the region of interest or within the color box. For color Doppler interrogation of the atrioventricular valves, the semilunar valves, and the great vessels, high-velocity range

TABLE 7-1	Clinical Information Provided by Color Doppler

Information from color Doppler	Clinical impact
Blood flow information demonstrated (yes/no)	Demonstration of blood flow over a region of interest (e.g., perfusion across an "atretic" or dysplastic valve) Better demonstration of small structures (e.g., narrow pulmonary artery recognized, shunt over a detected VSD) Identification of cardiac structures in early gestation
Direction of blood flow is demonstrated (antegrade/retrograde)	Demonstration of antegrade or retrograde flow in the aortic arch, in the pulmonary artery, across the ductus arteriosus, across the foramen ovale, in a left superior vena cava or a confluent vein, etc.
Detection of unexpected blood flow events (laminar flow, turbulent flow, etc.)	Detection of shunting across a small VSD, regurgitation across the tricuspid valve, turbulent flow across the aorta or the pulmonary artery with valve stenosis, detection of ventriculo-coronary fistula in pulmonary atresia
Demonstration of small vessels	Pulmonary veins, peripheral pulmonary arteries, anomalous tortuous ductus arteriosus, abnormal vessels as MAPCAs, LSVC, dilated azygos vein, etc.
Optimizing placement of the sample volume for spectral Doppler evaluation	Stenosis or regurgitation of a valve, Doppler of small vessels, Doppler of fetal veins (ductus venosus, pulmonary veins, inferior vena cava, azygos vein, abnormal draining pulmonary veins)

VSD, ventricular septal defect; MAPCAs, major aorto-pulmonary collateral arteries; LSVC, left superior vena cava.

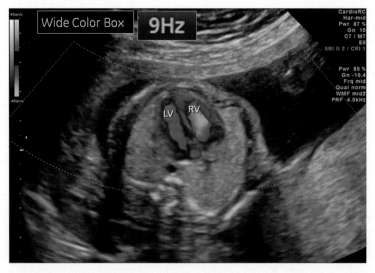

Figure 7-1. Apical four-chamber view in color Doppler showing a slow frame rate of 9 Hz (9 frames/sec) when a large color box is chosen. A slow frame rate impedes visualization of the fetal heart on color Doppler. Compare with Figure 7-2. LV, left ventricle; RV, right ventricle.

($> \pm30$ cm/sec) is selected. Figure 7-3A shows an improper use of low-velocity scale color setting resulting in aliased colors, which gives the impression of "turbulences" within the cardiac chambers. Increasing the color velocity scale to the appropriate level as shown in Figure 7-3B enhances the image quality. Low- to mid-velocity scales, in the order of 10 to 20 cm/sec, are suitable for the pulmonary and caval veins given their low-velocity flow.

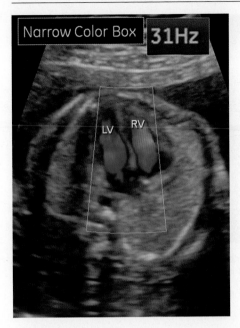

Figure 7-2. Apical four-chamber view in color Doppler of the same fetus as in Figure 7-1 but now the size of the box is chosen appropriately to cover the four-chamber view, providing the necessary color information with a frame rate of 31 Hz (31 frames/sec). LV, left ventricle; RV, right ventricle.

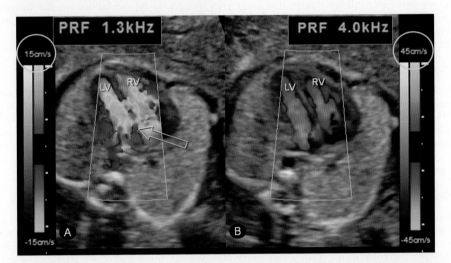

Figure 7-3. Effect of velocity scale (pulse repetition frequency [PRF]) on color Doppler display. **A:** The color Doppler velocity scale that is chosen is too low (±15 cm/sec) for the assessment of flow across the atrioventricular valves (high-velocity flow), which leads to color aliasing, mimicking turbulences (open arrow). **B:** The color velocity scale is appropriately increased (±45 cm/sec), resulting in accurate display of blood flow at the four-chamber view in diastole. LV, left ventricle; RV, right ventricle.

Color Filter

The color filter allows for the elimination of signals from wall motion and other low velocities. A high filter should therefore be selected for the color evaluation of the atrioventricular valves and flow across the aorta, and low color filter should be used for the evaluation of the pulmonary arteries and veins given their low flow settings.

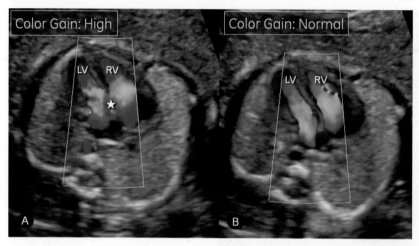

Figure 7-4. Effect of color gain on color Doppler display. **A:** The color gain at the level of the four-chamber view in diastole is set at high, resulting in color overlap over the septum, mimicking the presence of an atrioventricular septal defect (*star*). Reducing color gain to the appropriate low setting in **B** shows the normal flow pattern without color overlap. LV, left ventricle; RV, right ventricle.

Color Persistence

Color persistence allows information from prior images to be overlapped on the current image, superimposing color signals from different phases of the cardiac cycle and thus reducing the impression of pulsation. Low color persistence settings should be generally selected for fetal cardiac assessment.

Color Gain

Color gain demonstrates the amount of color exhibited on the screen, similar to the gray-scale gain function. Artifacts occur when the color gain setting is too high in fetal cardiac imaging (Fig. 7-4A,B). Gain settings in the midrange may also lead to superimposition of color over the border of a structure of interest, particularly when the atrioventricular valves are examined, giving the false impression of a septal defect. The color gain in cardiac imaging should therefore be initially set on low and gradually increased until the color information is optimized.

Color Doppler Image Resolution and Color Line Density

Color Doppler image resolution is related to the axial and lateral resolution as it relates to the number of color Doppler lines and sample volumes within the chosen color box. An increase in color resolution results in slow frame rate. A compromise should therefore be sought between the color image quality and frame rate. We opt for a high color resolution when peripheral pulmonary vessels are imaged or in fetal echocardiography in early gestation where the region of interest (color box) is usually small. The smallest color box is chosen in both these conditions in order to get the highest frame rate possible.

CARDIAC PRESETS AND STEP-BY-STEP EXAMINATION

Most of the previously described features for optimizing the fetal cardiac examination on color Doppler can be stored on the ultrasound machine under two cardiac presets for "low and high velocities" where they can be quickly retrieved for the corresponding examination. A step-by-step examination of the fetal heart using color Doppler is hereby suggested:

1. Adjust the two-dimensional image of the targeted region such as the four-chamber view.
2. Insonate the heart in an angle that is nearly parallel to the direction of blood flow.

3. Try to get a high image frame rate on two-dimensional (2-D) image by optimizing the 2-D image (minimizing depth and sector width). Reduce the 2-D gain in order to darken the image slightly.

4. Activate color Doppler and choose the smallest size possible of the color box that provides the targeted information.

5. For the color Doppler assessment of the atrioventricular and semilunar valves, adjust the following parameters:
   - Increase the color wall filter and pulse repetition frequency (velocity scale).
   - Reduce color persistence and choose a low to middle resolution.
   - Increase color gain until the region of interest is best visualized on color Doppler.
   - Maintain a parallel orientation to the direction of blood flow as you insonate different planes within the heart.

6. For assessing the pulmonary veins and small vessels, reduce the wall filter and the pulse repetition frequency and increase the color gain and persistence.

 ## COLOR DOPPLER IN FETAL ECHOCARDIOGRAPHY

The use of color Doppler in cardiac imaging can be of help in confirming normal anatomy and also in the full anatomic description of complex cardiac malformations. In a review of the application of color Doppler, we showed that three planes, namely, the four-chamber view, the five-chamber view, and the three-vessel-trachea view, are sufficient in describing most cardiac anomalies (9).

In the following section, the anatomic information that is provided by the application of color Doppler in standard diagnostic planes in the fetus will be described.

Upper Abdomen

The upper abdomen is best examined by color Doppler in a transverse or parasagittal orientation. In the transverse orientation, color Doppler is optimized when the plane is slightly angled superiorly demonstrating the hepatic veins, the umbilical veins, and the cross section of the ductus venosus as it merges into the inferior vena cava (Fig. 7-5A). In the parasagittal view, color Doppler demonstrates the course of the umbilical vein, the ductus venosus, and the inferior vena cava as it courses toward the right atrium (Fig. 7-5B). This plane is also useful to describe vein anomalies in suspected heterotaxy (see Chapters 22 and 23) and to rule

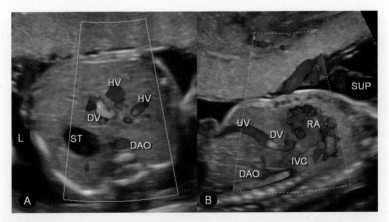

Figure 7-5. Assessment of the upper abdomen by color Doppler in a cross section plane **(A)** and a longitudinal plane **(B)**. A: Confluence of hepatic veins (HV) and ductus venosus (DV) can be demonstrated. B: The course of the umbilical vein (UV) toward the DV is seen as well as the course of the inferior vena cava (IVC) toward the right atrium (RA). DAO, descending aorta; ST, stomach; L, left; SUP, superior.

out agenesis of ductus venosus. It is an ideal plane for the examination of the ductus venosus by pulsed Doppler.

Four-Chamber View

The best approach to the four-chamber view on color Doppler is through an apical (Fig. 7-6A) or a basal insonation (Fig. 7-6B). These transverse planes enable simultaneous demonstration of the left and right atria and ventricles, the interatrial and interventricular septa, and a transverse section of the descending aorta. Diastolic perfusion from both atria into the ventricles across the mitral and tricuspid valves can then be easily assessed and typically shows two red (apical) or blue (basal) stripes of equal size separated by the interventricular septum. In systole, no color Doppler stripes should be visualized over the atrioventricular valves, unless a tricuspid or mitral regurgitation is present. Table 7-2 lists typical cardiac abnormalities recognized by color Doppler in the four-chamber-view plane.

Five-chamber View

The five-chamber view in color Doppler is a very important plane that shows simultaneously the left ventricular inflow and outflow tracts. The origin of the aortic root from the left ventricle can be visualized and the laminar flow confirmed. This view can be obtained either from an apical view demonstrating aortic blood flow in blue color within the ascending aorta (Fig. 7-7A) or from a basal view (right side of fetus) demonstrating aortic blood flow in red color within the ascending aorta (Fig. 7-7B). Color Doppler of the five-chamber view in the normal fetus shows the septo-aortic continuity, the absence of turbulences in systole, and insufficiency in diastole across the aortic valve. Table 7-3 lists typical cardiac abnormalities recognized by color Doppler in the five-chamber-view plane.

Short-axis or Three-vessel View

In the short-axis or three-vessel view the origin of the pulmonary artery from the right ventricle is visualized on color Doppler. An apical insonation will show pulmonary blood flow in blue color demonstrating the nonturbulent flow across the pulmonary valve and the bifurcation into the right and left pulmonary arteries (Fig. 7-8). When the plane is slightly inclined, the connection of the pulmonary artery to the ductus arteriosus is demonstrated.

Three-vessel-trachea View

Color Doppler of the three-vessel-trachea view is considered one of the most informative planes in the assessment of the fetal heart (9). In this plane, the main pulmonary artery,

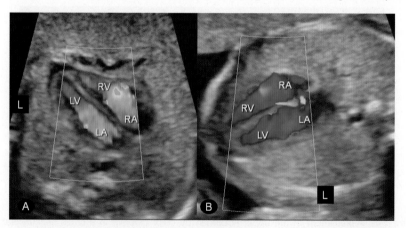

Figure 7-6. The four-chamber plane in color Doppler is best visualized from an apical **(A)** or a basal **(B)** view in order to demonstrate ventricular filling either in red (A) or in blue (B). In these orientations, the course of blood flow is nearly parallel to the angle of insonation. RV, right ventricle; LV, left ventricle; RA, right atrium; LA, left atrium; L, left.

TABLE 7-2	Four-chamber View in Color Doppler during Diastole: Some Abnormal Signs and Possible Underlying Cardiac Abnormality	
Color flow sign	Possible cardiac defect	Corresponding figures
Two separate AV valves with a small connection across the septum	Ventricular septal defect	15-11B, 15-13, 15-15
Two separate AV valves with discrepant ventricular width and narrow left ventricle	Coarctation of the aorta	12-6, 12-10
Two separate AV valves draining into one ventricle	Double inlet ventricle (single ventricle)	16-4
One common AV valve draining two atria into two separate ventricles	AV septal defect	15-27–15-30
Only right-sided inflow and left side with absent or minimal flow	Hypoplastic left heart syndrome, mitral atresia	11-11, 11-18, 11-20
Only left ventricular inflow and right side with absent or minimal flow	Tricuspid atresia with VSD, pulmonary atresia with intact septum	16-11, 13-13

AV, atrioventricular; VSD, ventricular septal defect.

ductus arteriosus, transverse aortic arch, aortic isthmus, and superior vena cava are demonstrated, with the aortic and ductal arches forming a "V-configuration," which points toward the posterior spine on the left (Fig. 7-9). The trachea may be identified as a bright-walled structure lying to the right of the great vessels and posterior to the superior vena cava. This important plane also provides information related to flow patterns within the right and left ventricular outflow tracts during systole and diastole. Color Doppler provides a rapid assessment of the size of great vessels in this plane with the pulmonary artery being slightly larger and more anterior than the transverse aortic arch. Turbulent flow, reversal flow, size discrepancy, or even absence or interruption of a vessel can be easily assessed (9). Color Doppler at the three-vessel-trachea view is very helpful in early gestation as it easily identifies size, location, and flow patterns within the great vessels. Table 7-4 lists typical cardiac abnormalities recognized by color Doppler in the three-vessel-trachea-view plane.

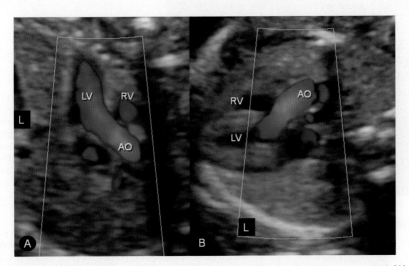

Figure 7-7. The five-chamber view in color Doppler is best visualized from an apical **(A)** or a transverse (lateral) **(B)** view in order to align the flow within the ascending aorta in a near-parallel course with the angle of insonation. LV, left ventricle; AO, aorta; RV, right ventricle; L, left.

TABLE 7-3	**Five-chamber View in Color Doppler During Systole and Diastole: Some Abnormal Signs and Possible Underlying Cardiac Abnormality**

Color flow sign	Possible cardiac defect	Corresponding figures
Turbulent flow with intact interventricular septum	Valvular aortic stenosis	11-8, 11-12
No flow across the aortic valve	Aortic atresia and hypoplastic left heart syndrome	11-23
VSD with aorta clearly arising from the left ventricle	Perimembranous VSD Aortic coarctation Interruption of the aortic arch	15-15
VSD with overriding aortic root	Tetralogy of Fallot Pulmonary atresia with VSD Absent pulmonary valve syndrome Common arterial trunk (double outlet right ventricle)	17-5, 17-9, 17-16, 18-7
Larger vessel arising from the left ventricle (with or without VSD)	Transposition of the great arteries	20-6, 20-8, 20-9
Aortic regurgitation in diastole (extremely rare event)	Common arterial trunk Valvular dysplasia (i.e., trisomy 18) Primary endocardial fibroelastosis of the left ventricle Cardiomyopathy Aorto-left ventricular tunnel Marfan syndrome	18-8

VSD, ventricular septal defect.

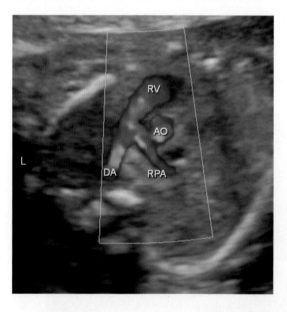

Figure 7-8. Color Doppler at the three-vessel view demonstrating the main pulmonary artery (PA) with its bifurcation into the left and right pulmonary arteries (here right pulmonary artery [RPA] is seen), aorta (AO) in the middle, and the connection of the PA with the ductus arteriosus (DA). RV, right ventricle; L, left.

Longitudinal Views of Aortic and Ductal Arches

Aortic and ductal arches can be visualized on color Doppler in a longitudinal parasagittal plane (Fig. 7-10). The aortic arch shows its three branches on color Doppler. Often it is difficult to adjust conventional color Doppler to demonstrate the aortic arch and its branches given different velocity ranges. Power Doppler or bidirectional high-definition color is often used for displaying the aortic arch and its branches given a higher sensitivity and more

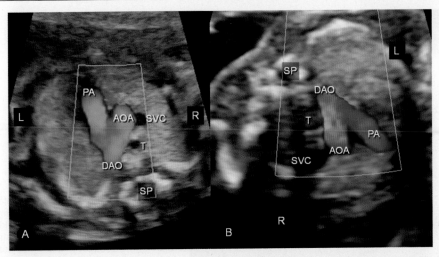

Figure 7-9. Color Doppler at the three-vessel-trachea view demonstrating the two best approaches to this view: an apical approach **(A)** when the fetus is in a dorso-posterior position or an approach from the left dorsal side **(B)** when the fetus is in a dorso-anterior position. The transverse aortic arch (AOA) and pulmonary artery (PA) merge toward the descending aorta (DAO). SVC, superior vena cava; T, trachea; SP, spine; L, left; R, right.

TABLE 7-4	Three-vessel-trachea View in Color Doppler during Systole and Diastole: Some Abnormal Signs and Possible Underlying Cardiac Abnormality	
Color flow sign	**Possible cardiac defect**	**Corresponding figures**
Antegrade flow in both PA and aortic arch, but dilated PA with turbulent flow	Pulmonary stenosis	13-4, 13-5
Antegrade flow in both PA and aortic arch, but dilated aortic arch with turbulent flow	Aortic stenosis	11-8
Antegrade flow in both PA and aortic arch, but narrow PA	Pulmonary stenosis in tetralogy of Fallot, Ebstein anomaly, DORV, tricuspid atresia with VSD and others	17-6, 17-10, 17-11
Antegrade flow in both PA and aortic arch, but narrow arch	Coarctation of the aorta	12-7, 12-10
Antegrade flow in PA but no aortic arch continuity	Interrupted arch, severe coarctation	
Antegrade flow in PA but aortic arch tiny and retrograde flow	Hypoplastic left heart syndrome	11-19, 11-23
Antegrade flow in aortic arch but PA tiny and retrograde flow	Pulmonary atresia with intact septum or with VSD	13-14
Only one large vessel with antegrade flow, another vessel not visualized	Aorta in D-TGA, cc-TGA, DORV with great vessel malposition, some fetuses with pulmonary atresia and VSD (other vessel hidden under the large vessel)	20-6, 20-9

PA, pulmonary artery; DORV, double outlet right ventricle; VSD, ventricular septal defect; D-TGA, D-transposition of great arteries; cc-TGA, congenitally corrected transposition of great arteries.

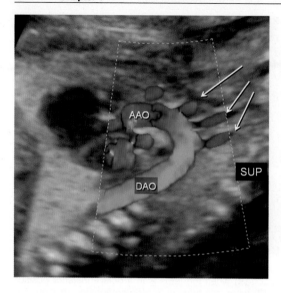

Figure 7-10. Aortic arch in color Doppler visualized from a ventral approach demonstrating the ascending aorta (AAO), the transverse aortic arch with the origin of the three brachiocephalic vessels (*arrows*), and the descending aorta (DAO). SUP, superior.

uniformity in color display. The ductal arch shows the main pulmonary artery, the ductus arteriosus, and in some views the left pulmonary artery. The ductal arch plane is more easily obtained from a ventral view in the fetus and can confirm laminar flow within the ductus arteriosus during systole.

Pulmonary Veins

There are four pulmonary veins, two inferior and two superior, entering the left atrium on the right and left sides posteriorly. It is generally difficult to image all four pulmonary veins on color Doppler in the fetus (12). Using color Doppler, the right and left inferior pulmonary veins can be visualized in red color from an apical approach as they enter the left atrium posteriorly (Fig. 7-11A). The right inferior pulmonary vein is easily recognized, since it has a course along a fictive line extending along the direction of the interatrial septum, and the course of the left inferior pulmonary vein points directly toward the foramen ovale (Fig. 7-11A). The right superior pulmonary vein can also be seen in blue color from a dorso-anterior approach (Fig. 7-11B). Newer color Doppler applications such as power Doppler ultrasound or dynamic flow can be helpful in visualizing the pulmonary veins, especially when the angle of insonation is perpendicular in orientation.

 POWER DOPPLER AND SENSITIVE DIGITAL BIDIRECTIONAL POWER DOPPLER

Color Doppler ultrasound utilizes the frequency shift generated by the velocity of flow of the red blood cells within a vessel to generate the color image. This frequency shift is dependent on the angle of insonation of the ultrasound beam with the direction of flow within the vessel, which creates a major limitation, especially when vascular structures are imaged at an angle to the direction of flow. The amplitude of the Doppler signal, generated by the signal intensity of the red blood cells within a vessel, can generate a color image independent of the angle of insonation (13,14). This technique is known as "power Doppler ultrasound." Power Doppler has several advantages over conventional color Doppler:

- Enhanced sensitivity: Since amplitude of Doppler signals instead of their frequency shift is analyzed, power Doppler is shown to be three to five times more sensitive than conventional color Doppler in visualizing small vessels and low flows.
- Improved noise differentiation: In power Doppler, noise signals are encoded in a uniform color (Fig. 7-12C). Hence, it is possible to turn the gain all the way up, which fills the entire image with noise, and the vascular signal will still be distinguishable.

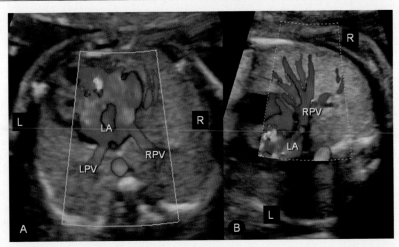

Figure 7-11. Color Doppler of an apical four-chamber view demonstrating in **A** the connection of right inferior (RPV) and left inferior (LPV) pulmonary veins into the left atrium (LA). **Plane B** shows in a right lateral view the superior right pulmonary vein (RPV) entering the left atrium. L, left; R, right.

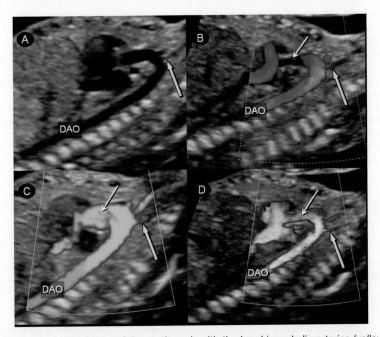

Figure 7-12. Parasagittal view of the aortic arch with the brachiocephalic arteries (*yellow arrow*) on two-dimensional image **(A),** (conventional) color Doppler **(B),** power Doppler **(C),** and bidirectional high-definition flow **(D).** In plane B, color Doppler information lacks display of all flow events in the aortic arch and the brachiocephalic vessels (missing color display in part of aorta due to the angle of insonation [*white arrow*] and suboptimal blood flow display in the brachiocephalic vessels). In plane C, blood flow is uniform in power Doppler, laminar flow is displayed, and filling of brachiocephalic vessels can be identified. Plane D demonstrates the most sensitive Doppler feature with clear borders of the aortic arch and brachiocephalic vessels. DAO, descending aorta.

- Enhanced edge definition: Power Doppler has better edge definition when displaying flow. This is because color signals, which extend partially beyond the edges, have lower signal amplitude due to the lack of moving erythrocytes and are thus not displayed.
- Flow detection irrespective of angle insonation (Fig. 7-12C, white arrow): Power Doppler is able to detect flow at right angles to the beam. The amplitudes of the positive and negative components of the flow tend to add up, resulting in a powerful signal.

Several studies have demonstrated the utility of power Doppler in fetal cardiology and in the reconstruction of three-dimensional volumes (13,14). Disadvantages of power Doppler in fetal cardiology include the lack of information on direction of blood flow and on the presence or absence of turbulence. By combining the Doppler frequency shifts with signal amplitude, digital broadband assessment of Doppler signals is applied providing a very sensitive tool known as advanced dynamic flow (15) or "high-definition (HD) flow" (Fig. 7-12D). This relatively new technique has been shown to be superior to conventional color Doppler as it demonstrates higher resolution, good lateral discrimination, and higher sensitivity (15). Figure 7-12 shows the aortic arch on 2-D, color Doppler, power Doppler, and high-definition flow. HD flow color maps can be chosen by the examiner either as a bidirectional color flow map or as a uniform color.

■ KEY POINTS: COLOR DOPPLER IN FETAL ECHOCARDIOGRAPHY

- Use of color Doppler is recommended in fetal echocardiography.
- Color optimization is critical in order to display the best image.
- The smaller the color box, the higher the frame rate.
- Color presets for the atrioventricular and semilunar valves include high-velocity scale, high filter, low gain, and low color persistence.
- Color presets for the pulmonary veins and other small vessels include low-velocity scale, low filter, high gain, and high persistence.
- A near parallel insonation to the direction of blood flow helps to optimize the image when color Doppler is used.
- Color Doppler of the three-vessel-trachea view is considered one of the most informative planes in the assessment of the fetal heart.
- Power Doppler utilizes the amplitude of the Doppler signal, generated by the signal intensity of the red blood cells within a vessel, in generating a color image independent of the angle of insonation.
- For small vessels, power Doppler and bidirectional digital Doppler (high-definition color) are more sensitive techniques for demonstrating vessel course on color Doppler without aliasing.

References

1. De Vore GR, Horenstein J, Siassi B, et al. Fetal echocardiography. VII. Doppler color flow mapping: a new technique for the diagnosis of congenital heart disease. *Am J Obstet Gynecol* 1987;156:1054–1064.
2. Sharland GK, Chita SK, Allan LD. The use of colour Doppler in fetal echocardiography. *Int J Cardiol* 1990;28:229–236.
3. Gembruch U, Chatterjee MS, Bald R, et al. Color Doppler flow mapping of fetal heart. *J Perinat Med* 1991;19:27–32.
4. Copel JA, Morotti R, Hobbins JC, et al. The antenatal diagnosis of congenital heart disease using fetal echocardiography: is color flow mapping necessary? *Obstet Gynecol* 1991;78:1–8.
5. De Vore GR. Color Doppler examination of the outflow tracts of the fetal heart: a technique for identification of cardiovascular malformations. *Ultrasound Obstet Gynecol* 1994;4:463–471.
6. Chaoui R, Bollmann R. [Fetal color Doppler echocardiography. Part 1: General principles and normal findings]. *Ultraschall Med* 1994;15:100–104.
7. Chaoui R, Bollmann R. [Fetal color Doppler echocardiography. Part 2: Abnormalities of the heart and great vessels]. *Ultraschall Med* 1994;15:105–111.
8. Chaoui R. Color Doppler sonography in the assessment of the fetal heart. In: Nicolaides K, Rizzo G, Hecher K, eds. *Placental and fetal Doppler.* Abingdon, UK: Parthenon, 2000;171–186.
9. Chaoui R, McEwing R. Three cross-sectional planes for fetal color Doppler echocardiography. *Ultrasound Obstet Gynecol* 2003;21:81–93.
10. Abuhamad A. Color and pulsed Doppler in fetal echocardiography. *Ultrasound Obstet Gynecol* 2004;24:1–9.
11. Lee W, Allan L, Carvalho JS, et al.; ISUOG Fetal Echocardiography Task Force. ISUOG consensus statement: what constitutes a fetal echocardiogram? *Ultrasound Obstet Gynecol* 2008;32(2):239–242.
12. Chaoui R, Lenz F, Heling KS. Doppler examination of the fetal pulmonary venous circulation. In: Maulik D, ed. *Doppler ultrasound in obstetrics and gynecology.* New York: Springer Verlag, Heidelberg, 2003;451–463.

13. Chaoui R, Kalache KD. Three-dimensional power Doppler ultrasonography of the fetal cardiovascular system. In: Maulik D, ed. *Doppler ultrasound in obstetrics and gynecology.* New York: Springer Verlag, Heidelberg, 2003.
14. Chaoui R, Kalache KD, Hartung J. Application of three-dimensional power Doppler ultrasound in prenatal diagnosis. *Ultrasound Obstet Gynecol* 2001;17:22–29.
15. Heling KS, Chaoui R, Bollmann R. Advanced dynamic flow—a new method of vascular imaging in prenatal medicine. A pilot study of its applicability. *Ultraschall Med* 2004;25(4):280–284.

DOPPLER PRINCIPLES

The concept of color and pulsed Doppler ultrasonography is derived from the Doppler effect, which is based on the apparent variation in frequency of a light or a sound wave as its source approaches or moves away, relative to an observer (1). When an ultrasound wave with a certain transmitted frequency insonates a blood vessel, the reflected frequency or frequency shift is directly proportional to the speed with which the red blood cells are moving (blood flow velocity) within that particular vessel (Fig. 8-1). This frequency shift is also proportional to the cosine of the angle that the ultrasound beam makes with this vessel (the angle of incidence) and to the frequency of the insonating ultrasound wave (see Fig. 8-1). The Doppler frequency shift therefore reflects but does not actually measure the velocity of blood flow.

In spectral Doppler ultrasonography, the frequency spectrum is displayed in a graphic form (Fig. 8-2). In this display, the vertical axis represents the frequency shift, and the horizontal axis represents the temporal change of this frequency shift as it relates to the events of the cardiac cycle (see Fig. 8-2). The frequency shift can therefore be easily measured at any point along the cardiac cycle.

In clinical applications, Doppler velocimetry is mostly used to assess for the downstream resistance to the flow of blood (2). This is based on the concept that the mean flow is proportional to the mean pressure and inversely proportional to the mean downstream resistance ($Qm = Pm/Rm$). This concept, however, only applies to steady nonpulsatile flow conditions. In a medical setting where flow is pulsatile, vascular impedance rather than vascular resistance describes opposition to flow (3). Downstream resistance is just one component of vascular impedance which is also dependent on the pulse frequency, blood inertia, distensibility of the vessel wall, and wave reflection (3). In a laboratory setting where the ability to measure vascular impedance is present, Doppler indices correlate well with impedance to pulsatile flow, pressure pulsatility, and vascular resistance (4). The frequency shift therefore provides information on the downstream impedance to flow of whichever vascular bed is being studied.

 DOPPLER WAVEFORM QUANTIFICATION

Several Doppler indices are available for waveform quantification (5–7). Doppler indices are ratios of frequency shifts obtained from the same cardiac cycle and are thus independent of the angle of insonation. Figure 8-3 lists the three most commonly used Doppler indices in obstetrics. Although Doppler indices are widely used in the evaluation of the fetal peripheral circulation, Doppler waveform quantification at the cardiac level has mostly relied on measurements of absolute frequencies which, unlike Doppler indices, are angle dependent. In order to obtain accurate Doppler indices in fetal echocardiography, the sample volume is placed distal to the respective valves, the insonating angle should be within 15–20 degrees of the direction of blood flow, Doppler waveforms should be obtained during fetal apnea, and multiple measurements should be made. Obtaining several measurements at different cardiac cycles will also ensure reproducibility of results. Color Doppler is used to direct placement of the sample volume; placing the sample volume at the brightest colors of the blood flow segment will ensure the best measurements. Table 8-1 lists the optimum approach to Doppler echocardiography. The following is a list of waveform measurements that are commonly used in Doppler echocardiography:

> *Peak velocity:* The maximum velocity on the Doppler spectrum (cm/sec) (Fig. 8-4).
> *Time-to-peak velocity (TPV):* The time from onset to peak velocity (msec), also referred to as acceleration time (see Fig. 8-4).

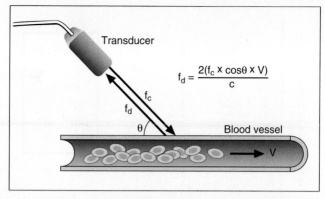

Figure 8-1. Doppler effect in ultrasonography. When an ultrasound wave insonates a blood vessel, the frequency shift of the reflected ultrasound wave (f_d) is directly proportional to the frequency of the insonating ultrasound wave (f_c); the velocity of blood flow within the vessel (V); the cosine of the angle that the ultrasound beam makes with this vessel (theta); and inversely proportional to a constant (C), which reflects the milieu that the ultrasound beam is traversing.

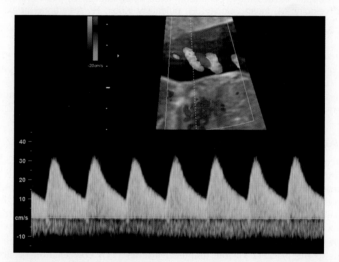

Figure 8-2. Spectral Doppler ultrasonography of the umbilical artery. The vertical axis represents the frequency shift (velocity scale) (cm/sec) and the horizontal axis represents time. In this spectrum, the temporal change of the frequency shift is displayed as it relates to the events of the cardiac cycle.

Deceleration time: The time from the peak of the waveform to the intersection of the descending slope with the baseline (msec) (see Fig. 8-4).

Time-velocity integral (TVI): The measurement of the area under the Doppler waveform over one cardiac cycle (cm) (see Fig. 8-4).

Time-averaged velocity (TAV): TVI divided by the period time (cm/sec) (see Fig. 8-4).

E/A ratio: A measurement used to quantify Doppler waveforms across the atrioventricular valves. E represents peak velocity during early ventricular filling, and A represents peak velocity during the atrial contraction (Fig. 8-5).

Filling time: The diastolic time of the cardiac cycle (msec) (see Fig. 8-5).

Ejection time: The systolic time of the cardiac cycle (msec) (see Fig. 8-5).

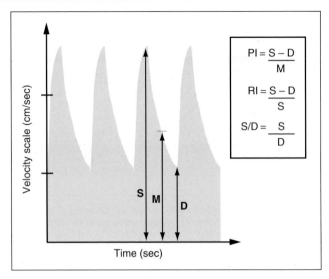

Figure 8-3. Doppler indices most commonly used in obstetrics: S, peak systolic velocity; D, end diastolic velocity; M, mean velocity; PI, pulsatility index; RI, resistance index; S/D, S/D or A/B ratio.

Percent reverse flow: A measurement used to quantify Doppler waveforms in the inferior vena cava. It represents TVI of the reverse flow segment (atrial contraction) divided by the TVI of the total forward flow and multiplied by 100 (Fig. 8-6).

S/A: A measurement used to quantify Doppler waveforms in the ductus venosus. S represents maximum systolic velocity and A represents the atrial nadir (Fig. 8-7).

 FETAL CARDIOVASCULAR PHYSIOLOGY

The fetal circulation is different from the adult circulation in many respects. The fetal circulation is in parallel rather than in series and the right ventricular cardiac output is greater than the left ventricular cardiac output (8,9). The patency of the foramen ovale and the ductus arteriosus in the fetus allows blood to flow from the right to the left circulation, bypassing the lung. The majority of blood that is ejected from the right ventricle is directed through the ductus arteriosus into the thoracic aorta with a minute amount entering the lungs through the right and left pulmonary arteries (10). About 50% of the blood flowing through the thoracic aorta returns to the placenta via the umbilical arteries (11). Oxygenation occurs in the placenta and the highly oxygenated blood returns to the fetus through the umbilical vein. About half of the blood in the umbilical vein enters the ductus venosus with the remainder entering the portal system and hepatic veins (11). Blood from the ductus venosus and left hepatic veins enters the inferior vena cava, the right atrium, and is then preferentially streamed into the left atrium through the foramen ovale. From the left atrium, blood enters the left ventricle and is then ejected into the aorta during systole. The presence of right to left shunts at the level of

TABLE 8-1	**Optimum Approach to Pulsed Doppler Echocardiography**

- Place sample volume distal to targeted valves.
- Keep insonating angle at less than 20 degrees from direction of blood flow.
- Place sample volume at brightest colors of blood flow segment.
- Obtain Doppler waveforms during fetal apnea.
- Obtain multiple measurements.

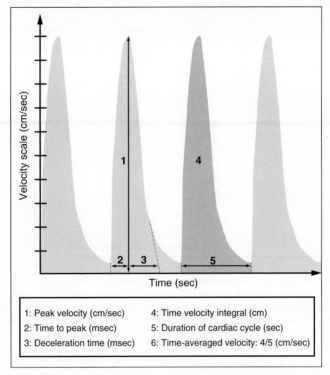

Figure 8-4. Doppler waveform quantification in echocardiography. See text for further details.

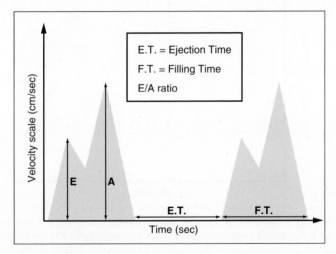

Figure 8-5. Doppler waveform quantification across the atrioventricular valves. E/A is used for measurement where E represents peak velocity during early ventricular filling and A represents peak velocity during the atrial contraction. Ejection time represents systolic time and filling time represents diastolic time of the cardiac cycle.

the foramen ovale and ductus arteriosus has a significant impact on cardiac flow patterns and affects the distribution of blood and oxygen to various organs. This shunting mechanism ensures the delivery of blood with high oxygen content to the coronary and cerebral circulations.

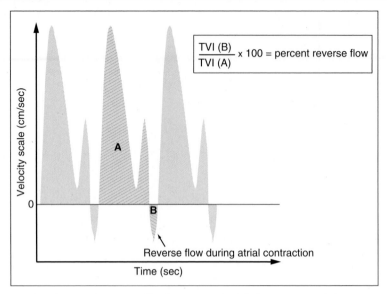

Figure 8-6. Doppler waveform quantification across the inferior vena cava. Percent reverse flow is used for measurement. It represents time velocity integral of the reverse flow segment (atrial contraction) (B) divided by the time velocity integral of the total forward flow segment (A) and multiplied by 100.

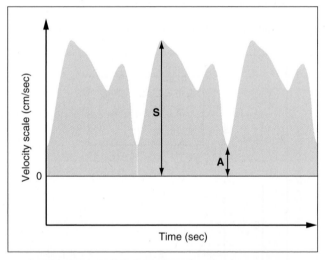

Figure 8-7. Doppler waveform quantification across the ductus venosus. S/A is used for measurement where S represents maximum systolic velocity and A represents the atrial nadir.

Right ventricular volume flow exceeds left ventricular volume flow in the fetus by a ratio of 1.3:1 (12). The combined ventricular output of the fetus at term is approximately 1735 mL/min, whereas flow indicated for estimated fetal weight is constant at a mean value of 553 ± 153 mL/min/kg (13). Stroke volume increases exponentially with advancing gestation (14). It increases from 0.7 mL at 20 weeks to 7.6 mL at term for the right ventricle and 0.7 mL at 20 weeks to 5.2 mL at term for the left ventricle (14). Doppler studies in humans confirm that the Frank-Starling mechanism is operational in the fetal heart where an increase in preload results in an increase in ventricular stroke volume (15).

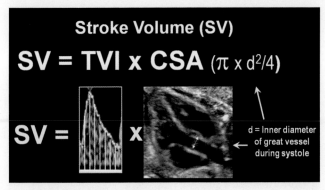

Figure 8-8. Stroke volume (SV) of left or right ventricle is equal to time-velocity integral (TVI) of the left or right ventricular outflow multiplied by the cross-sectional area (CSA) of the aortic or pulmonary artery respectively. Cross-sectional area is equal to π times the square of the internal diameter of the aorta or pulmonary artery divided by 4.

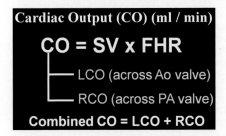

Figure 8-9. Cardiac output (CO) (mL/min) is equal to stroke volume (SV) times the fetal heart rate (FHR). In the fetus cardiac output is equal to the combined left (LCO) and right (RCO) cardiac output; Ao, aorta; PA, pulmonary artery.

The progressive development of organs during gestation influence blood distribution and vascular impedance (8). With advancing gestation, ventricular compliance is increased, total peripheral resistance is decreased, preload is increased, and combined cardiac output is increased (8). Compliance of the fetal left heart increases more rapidly than compliance of the fetal right heart with advancing gestation (8). The pulmonary vascular resistance is high in the fetus and the pulmonary arterial pressure is almost systemic (16,17). Flow to the pulmonary vascular bed is maintained at a low rate with a noted increase toward the end of gestation (9,16). Cardiac output in the fetus is mainly affected by preload and ventricular compliance (8). Stroke volume and cardiac output calculations are shown in Figures 8-8 and 8-9.

ATRIOVENTRICULAR VALVES

Doppler Technique

Obtain an apical or a basal four-chamber view. Make sure that your angle of insonation is less than 20 degrees from the direction of blood flow across the atrioventricular valves. Use color Doppler in order to identify blood flow across the atrioventricular valves. Place the Doppler sample volume within the ventricles and on the apical side of the mitral or tricuspid valves, at the brightest colors of the blood flow segment.

Doppler Waveforms

Figure 8-10 shows typical Doppler waveforms obtained across the atrioventricular valves. These Doppler waveforms, which correspond to ventricular filling during diastole, are biphasic. The first phase of the waveform is known as the E wave: it corresponds to early ventricular filling of diastole. The second phase of the waveform is known as the A wave: it corresponds to active ventricular filling of diastole (atrial contraction or atrial kick). Because

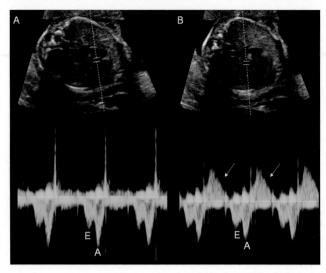

Figure 8-10. Doppler waveforms across the atrioventricular valves. The Doppler waves are biphasic with the first phase corresponding to early ventricular filling (E) and the second phase corresponding to the atrial contraction (A). Doppler waveforms across the mitral valve **(B)** show aortic flow during the systolic component (*arrows*) because of fibrous continuity between the mitral and aortic valves. Pulmonic flow is not evident across the tricuspid valve **(A)**.

of leaflet continuity between the mitral and aortic valve annuli, the Doppler waveform across the mitral valve shows aortic flow during the systolic component (see Fig. 8-10B). Pulmonic flow on the other hand is not evident across the tricuspid valve (see Fig. 8-10A) because of the presence of a subpulmonic conus separating the tricuspid valve annulus from the pulmonary valve annulus. The E/A ratio is used for Doppler waveform quantification across the atrioventricular valves (see Fig. 8-5).

Doppler waveforms across the atrioventricular valves are dependent on the compliance of the ventricular muscle, preload, and afterload (18,19). The E/A ratio is an index of ventricular diastolic function. Unlike in postnatal life, in the fetus the velocity of the A wave is higher than that of the E wave. This observation, which is thought to be secondary to an increased cardiac muscle stiffness during fetal life (20), highlights the importance of the role that atrial systole plays in cardiac filling in the fetus. As ventricular stiffness decreases with advancing gestation, E/A ratio increases from 0.53 ± 0.05 in the first trimester to about 0.70 ± 0.02 in the second half of pregnancy (21,22). Indeed E/A ratios around 0.82 ± 0.04 are noted at term (23). The rise in E/A ratio with advancing gestation suggests a shift of blood flow from late to early diastole. This shift of blood flow may be secondary to an increase in ventricular compliance, a rise in ventricular relaxation rate, or a reduction in afterload with decreased placental resistance, all of which occur with advancing gestation (24). When the mitral and tricuspid Doppler waveforms are compared, peak flow velocities in both early and late diastole are higher across the tricuspid valve (22–24). This finding is in keeping with previous studies suggesting greater blood flow across the tricuspid valve than the mitral valve in the fetus (12,13,25) and thus supporting the concept of right heart dominance in the fetus. Shifting to left ventricular dominance starts in utero toward the end of gestation (8). The E/A ratio is an index of ventricular preload and compliance (8). Figures 8-11 and 8-12 display normal values of E/A ratios across the mitral and tricuspid valves, respectively.

Abnormal Findings
Abnormal diastolic filling with small waveform pattern across the mitral valve is found in the presence of hypoplastic left heart syndrome with patent mitral valve and in critical aortic

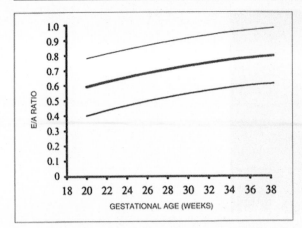

Figure 8-11. Normal values (95% confidence intervals) for E/A ratios across the mitral valve with advancing gestation. (Reproduced from Arduini D, Rizzo G, Romanini C. *Fetal cardiac function.* New York: Parthenon, 1995; 38–39, with permission.)

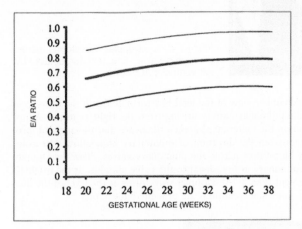

Figure 8-12. Normal values (95% confidence intervals) for E/A ratios across the tricuspid valve with advancing gestation. (Reproduced from Arduini D, Rizzo G, Romanini C. *Fetal cardiac function.* New York: Parthenon, 1995; 38–39, with permission.)

stenosis. Abnormal waveform across the tricuspid valve is seen in pulmonary atresia with intact septum associated with a hypoplastic right ventricle. Dilated and hypertrophic cardiomyopathies are commonly associated with abnormal Doppler waveforms in both atrioventricular valves. Abnormal findings on the atrioventricular valves in systole are mainly related to mitral and tricuspid regurgitation. Mitral regurgitation is mainly found in endocardial fibroelastosis in association with critical aortic stenosis, in some forms of hypoplastic left heart syndrome, or in volume overload in combination with a tricuspid regurgitation. Tricuspid regurgitation is a fairly common finding and is discussed in detail in Chapter 14.

SEMILUNAR VALVES

Doppler Technique

Aorta: Obtain an apical or basal four-chamber view of the heart. Rotate the medial aspect of the transducer slightly cephalad in order to view the aorta arising from the left ventricle (five-chamber view). Adjust your transducer's orientation on the maternal abdomen to ensure that the angle of insonation is less than 20 degrees from the direction of the aortic blood flow. Use color Doppler in order to identify blood flow across the aortic valves. Place the Doppler sample volume within the aorta, distal to the valve annulus, at the brightest colors of the blood flow segment (Fig. 8-13).

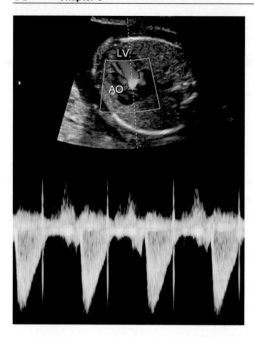

Figure 8-13. Doppler waveforms across the aortic valve. See text for details. LV, left ventricle; AO, aorta.

Pulmonary artery: From a five-chamber view of the fetal heart, rotate or tilt the transducer cephalad in order to view the pulmonary artery arising from the right ventricle. Adjust your transducer's orientation on the maternal abdomen to ensure that the angle of insonation is less than 20 degrees from the direction of pulmonary blood flow. Use color Doppler in order to identify blood flow across the pulmonary valves. Place the Doppler sample volume within the pulmonary artery, distal to the valve annulus, at the brightest colors of the blood flow segment (Fig. 8-14). Doppler waveforms at the level of the ductus arteriosus in normal and abnormal conditions are presented in Chapter 13.

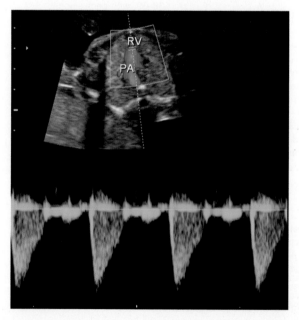

Figure 8-14. Doppler waveforms across the pulmonary valve. See text for details. RV, right ventricle; PA, pulmonary artery.

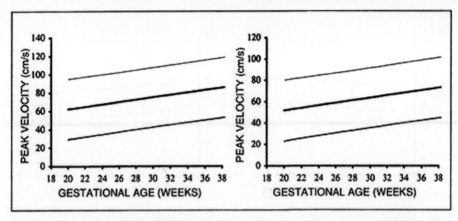

Figure 8-15. Normal values (95% confidence intervals) for peak systolic velocities across the aortic (*left*) and pulmonary (*right*) valves with advancing gestation. (Reproduced from Arduini D, Rizzo G, Romanini C. *Fetal cardiac function*. New York: Parthenon, 1995;38–39, with permission.)

Doppler Waveforms

Figures 8-13 and 8-14 show typical Doppler waveforms obtained across the aortic and pulmonary valves, respectively. Peak systolic velocity and time-to-peak velocity are the most commonly used indices for Doppler waveform quantification (see Fig. 8-4). These Doppler indices reflect ventricular contractility, arterial pressure, and afterload (26,27). Peak systolic velocity is a function of myocardial contractility, valve annulus size, preload, and afterload (28,29), while time-to-peak velocity is a function of mean arterial pressure (30). In the aorta and pulmonary artery, peak systolic velocity and time-to-peak velocity increase with advancing gestation (31–34). Peak systolic velocity is greater in the aorta than in the pulmonary artery (25,35). A slightly larger valve annulus in the pulmonary artery or a decreased afterload in the aorta secondary to the cerebral circulation may account for a higher peak systolic velocity in the aorta (25,36). Time-to-peak velocity is shorter in the pulmonary artery than in the aorta, which suggests a higher mean arterial pressure in the pulmonary artery in the fetus (37). Aortic and pulmonary artery normal peak systolic velocities and time-to-peak velocities are displayed in Figures 8-15 and 8-16, respectively.

Abnormal Findings

Abnormal Doppler waveforms across the aortic valve are seen in critical aortic stenosis and in coarctation of the aorta. Abnormal Doppler waveforms across the pulmonary artery occur in pulmonary stenosis and in pulmonary regurgitation.

 INFERIOR VENA CAVA

Doppler Technique

Obtain a sagittal view of the fetal chest and abdomen with color Doppler. By sliding the transducer to the right parasagittal plane, the inferior vena cava can be imaged as it enters into the right atrium (Fig. 8-17). The inferior vena cava can be studied at two locations; at the inlet into the right atrium or in the segment between the entrance of the renal vein and the ductus venosus. A good correlation coefficient exists between these two measurement sites, and the location that provides the smallest angle of insonation with the blood flow should be chosen (38).

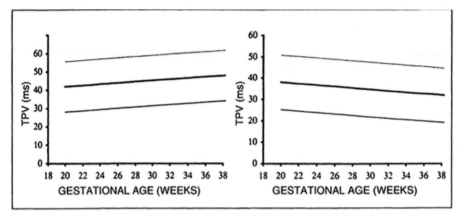

Figure 8-16. Normal values (95% confidence intervals) for time-to-peak velocities (TPV) across the aortic (left) and pulmonary (right) valves with advancing gestation. (Reproduced from Rizzo G, Arduini D, Romanini C, et al. Doppler echocardiographic assessment of time to peak velocity in the aorta and pulmonary artery of small for gestational age fetuses. *Br J Obstet Gynaecol* 1990;97:603–607, with permission.)

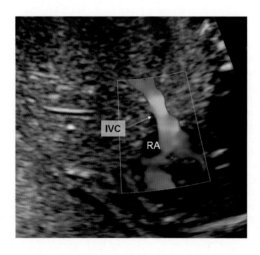

Figure 8-17. Color Doppler of a right parasagittal plane showing the inferior vena cava (IVC) as it enters into the right atrium (RA). This represents an optimal plane for the Doppler interrogation of the IVC as it is oriented almost parallel to the ultrasound beam.

Doppler Waveforms

Figure 8-18 shows a Doppler spectrum obtained at the level of the inferior vena cava. These Doppler waveforms are triphasic in shape with the first phase corresponding to atrial diastole and ventricular systole, the second phase corresponding to early diastole, and the third phase corresponding to late diastole or the atrial contraction (38,39). Typically, flow during late diastole is reversed in the inferior vena cava (38–40). The percentage of reverse flow, which is a ratio of the time velocity integral during the atrial contraction divided by the time velocity integral during total forward flow, is used for Doppler waveform quantification in the inferior vena cava (39) (see Fig. 8-6). This index of flow is a reflection of the pressure gradient between the right atrium and the right ventricle at end diastole, which is dependent on ventricular compliance and end diastolic pressure within the right ventricle (38,41–43). The percentage of reverse flow in the inferior vena cava decreases linearly with advancing gestation from a mean of 14.7 ± 2.55% at 20 weeks to a mean of 4.7 ± 2.55% at term (38). This decrease is probably related to an improved ventricular compliance and a decreased peripheral resistance with advancing gestation. Although forward flow in the inferior vena cava is not

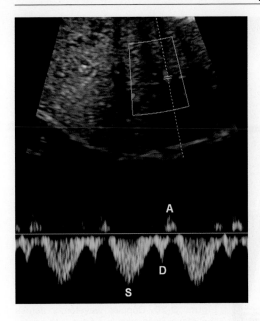

Figure 8-18. Doppler waveforms across the inferior vena cava. These waveforms are triphasic with the first phase corresponding to ventricular systole (S); the second phase corresponding to early diastole (D); and the third phase (reverse flow) corresponding to the atrial contraction (A).

significantly different from the superior vena cava, the relative amount of blood moving in a reverse direction during the atrial contraction is greater in the inferior vena cava than in the superior vena cava (39). Figure 8-19 displays normal values of the percentage reverse flow in the inferior vena cava with advancing gestation.

Abnormal Findings

Abnormal findings in the inferior vena cava Doppler waveforms occur in the presence of severe intrauterine growth restriction and primarily involve an increase in the reverse flow segment of the waveform, which corresponds to late diastole (Fig. 8-20).

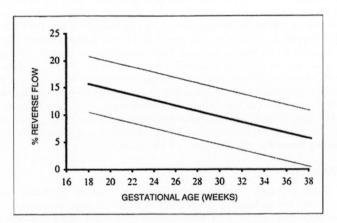

Figure 8-19. Normal values (95% confidence intervals) of the percentage reverse flow in the inferior vena cava with advancing gestation. (Reproduced from Rizzo G, Arduini D, Romanini C. Inferior vena cava flow velocity waveforms in appropriate- and small-for-gestational-age fetuses. *Am J Obstet Gynecol* 1992;166:1271–1280, with permission.)

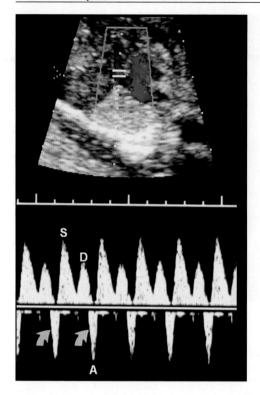

Figure 8-20. Doppler waveforms across the inferior vena cava in a fetus with severe growth restriction. Note the increased reverse flow during the atrial contraction (A) (*arrows*). S corresponds to ventricular systole, and D corresponds to early diastole.

DUCTUS VENOSUS

Doppler Technique

Obtain a coronal view of the fetal abdomen at the level of the diaphragm. Slight adjustments are required in order to view the inferior vena cava as it enters the right atrium. By superimposing color flow Doppler to the gray-scale image, the ductus venosus can be identified connecting the umbilical vein to the inferior vena cava just before it enters the right atrium (Fig. 8-21A). Color Doppler turbulence is often noted within the ductus venosus. The left hepatic vein is seen adjacent to the ductus venosus. The ductus venosus can also be imaged from a parasagittal approach to the fetal abdomen as seen in Figure 8-21B. A technically easier approach to the ductus venosus is obtained through a transverse/oblique view of the abdomen at the level of the abdominal circumference (Fig. 8-21C). Start by obtaining a transverse view of the abdomen at the level of the abdominal circumference. Add color Doppler to the gray-scale image and angle slightly cephalad while following the course of the umbilical vein within the abdomen. The ductus venosus, with color flow aliasing, is seen branching off the umbilical vein and coursing upward in the abdomen (see Fig. 8-21C).

Doppler Waveforms

Figure 8-22 shows a Doppler spectrum obtained at the level of the ductus venosus. These Doppler waveforms are biphasic in morphology with a first peak concomitant with systole (S); a second peak concomitant with early diastole (D); and a nadir concomitant with the atrial contraction (A) (44). Unlike the inferior vena cava, forward flow is present throughout the entire cardiac cycle in the ductus venosus in the normal human fetus (40). The ductus venosus is a small vein about 2 cm long and 2 mm wide at term (45,46). Because of its narrow lumen, a high velocity jet is projected across the ductus venosus toward the foramen

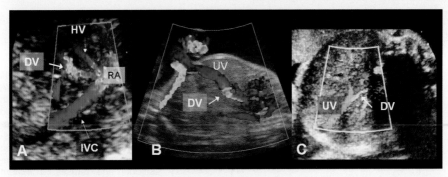

Figure 8-21. Approach to imaging of the ductus venosus (DV) on color Doppler. In **A,** a coronal plane of the chest shows the DV as it joins the inferior vena cava (IVC) toward the right atrium (RA). The hepatic vein (HV) is also seen in this plane. In **B,** a parasagittal plane shows the DV originating from the umbilical vein (UV), and in **C,** a transverse plane of the abdomen shows the DV as it originated from the UV. Note the presence of color aliasing in the DV in the three planes.

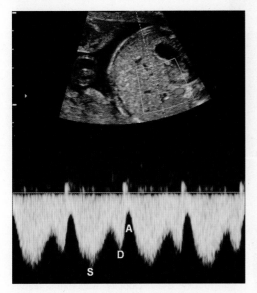

Figure 8-22. Doppler waveforms across the ductus venosus. These waveforms are biphasic with the first phase corresponding to cardiac systole (S) and the second phase corresponding to cardiac diastole (D). The nadir in the second phase corresponds to the atrial contraction (A).

ovale (47). The mean peak velocity in the ductus venosus increases from 65 cm/sec at 18 weeks to 75 cm/sec at term (47). As the peak velocity measurement is angle dependent, other indices were developed to quantify flow velocity waveforms in the ductus venosus. Two such indices were developed based on peak velocities during systole and during the atrial contraction (S/A, S-A/S) (48,49) (see Fig. 8-7). These indices change with advancing gestation and are in general a good reflection of right ventricular preload. Figure 8-23 displays normal values of the S/A ratio in the ductus venosus with advancing gestation.

Abnormal Findings
Abnormal findings in the ductus venosus Doppler waveforms occur in the presence of severe intrauterine growth restriction and primarily involve reduced, absent, or reversed flow in the atrial contraction portion of the waveform (A) (Fig. 8-24). Abnormal DV waveforms may also be seen in obstructive lesions of the right heart.

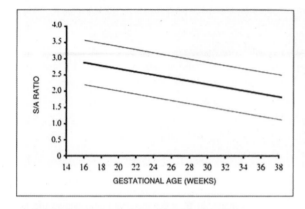

Figure 8-23. Normal values (95% confidence intervals) of the S/A ratio in the ductus venosus with advancing gestation. (Reproduced from Rizzo G, Pietropolli A, Bufalino L, et al. Ductus venosus systolic to atrial peak velocity ratio in appropriate and small for gestational age fetuses. *J Matern Fetal Invest* 1993;3:198, with permission.)

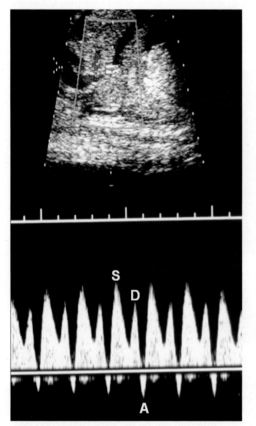

Figure 8-24. Doppler waveforms across the ductus venosus in a fetus with severe growth restriction. Note the presence of reverse flow during the atrial contraction (A) phase of the waveform. S corresponds to ventricular systole, and D corresponds to early diastole.

PULMONARY VEINS

Doppler Technique

The pulmonary veins can be visualized at their entrance to the left atrium. The right inferior pulmonary vein can be imaged in a basal four-chamber view and the left inferior pulmonary vein from a transverse four-chamber view (see Fig. 7-11). Using color Doppler on the described approach, the right and left inferior pulmonary veins can be visualized with a flow

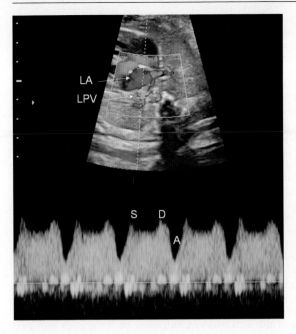

Figure 8-25. Doppler waveforms across one of the pulmonary veins. These Doppler waveforms are triphasic in shape and are similar to those obtained at the ductus venosus (DV). A systolic peak (S) is followed by a diastolic peak (D) and during atrial systole the A wave is at its nadir; LPV, left pulmonary vein; LA, left atrium.

parallel to the insonation angle. The Doppler sample volume should be placed in the lung parenchyma just before the entrance into the left atrium.

Doppler Waveforms

The flow velocity waveforms of the pulmonary veins reflect pressure changes in the left atrium during the cardiac cycle. The pulmonary vein Doppler waveforms are similar to those in the ductus venosus with a triphasic shape. A systolic peak (S) is followed by a diastolic peak (D) and during atrial systole the A wave is at its nadir (Fig. 8-25).

Abnormal Findings

Abnormal pulmonary vein Doppler waveforms are seen in fetuses with hypoplastic left heart syndrome with narrow interatrial communication showing flow reversal during late diastole (see Fig. 11-25). In fetuses with anomalous venous connections, Doppler of the pulmonary veins shows absence of the typical triphasic shape.

 ## CARDIAC ADAPTATION TO FETAL GROWTH RESTRICTION

Intrauterine growth restriction (IUGR) is associated with several changes at the level of the fetal heart involving preload, afterload, ventricular compliance, and myocardial contractility. An increase in afterload is seen at the level of the right ventricle due to increased placental impedance (50). A decrease in afterload is noted at the level of the left ventricle due to decreased cerebral impedance associated with the brain sparing reflex (50). These changes in afterload result in a redistribution of the cardiac output from the right to left ventricles (50). Preload is reduced at both atrioventricular valves due to hypovolemia and decreased filling associated with IUGR (32,51–53). This decrease in preload is reflected by a decrease in the E/A ratio, decreased atrial peak, and decreased time velocity integral at the mitral and tricuspid valves (32,51,52). Other investigators, however, reported an unchanged E/A ratios in the compromised fetus (53). These controversial data may have resulted from different study populations or due to internal variability of results. Although the reduction in E/A ratio in IUGR fetuses may result from a reduced preload, overall diastolic function impairment is related to a dysfunction in myometrial relaxation at the cellular level (54,55). Ventricular compliance, assessed by the ratio of the time-velocity integral of the A wave over the time-velocity integral of the total wave of the atrioventricular valve, is decreased in IUGR fetuses (8,50). The right ventricle is more affected by reduced compliance than the left ventricle (8,50).

Reduced peak-systolic velocity at the level of the semilunar valves is also noted in many IUGR fetuses (56). This may result from a reduced preload and an increased afterload of the right ventricle (56). An increase in time-to-peak velocity across the aorta is seen in IUGR fetuses and suggests a decrease in mean arterial pressure in that vessel (31). In contrast, a decrease in time-to-peak velocity across the pulmonary artery is noted in IUGR fetuses and may result from an increase in pulmonary and peripheral impedance in those fetuses (31).

Evidence of reduced myocardial contractility in the presence of severe IUGR has also been reported. Ventricular ejection force, an index of ventricular systolic function that is independent of preload and afterload, is decreased at the level of the right and left ventricles in fetal growth restriction (57). IUGR fetuses with reduced ventricular ejection force have a shorter time to delivery, a higher incidence of nonreassuring fetal heart rate tracing, and a lower pH at birth when compared to controls (57). A significant correlation between the severity of fetal acidosis at cordocentesis and ventricular ejection force values validates the association of this index and the severity of fetal compromise (57). Myocardial cell damage, demonstrated by elevated levels of cardiac troponin-T, is seen in some fetuses with severe growth restriction (50). This advanced stage of fetal compromise is associated with signs of increased systemic venous pressure, a change in the distribution of cardiac output, a rise in right ventricle afterload, and a high incidence of tricuspid regurgitation (50). These findings suggest that Doppler abnormalities in the proximal venous system of the growth restricted fetus suggest fetal myocardial cell damage and increased systemic venous pressure (50).

The fetal heart plays a central role in the adaptive mechanisms for hypoxemia and placental insufficiency. Longitudinal data on the hemodynamic sequence of the natural history of fetal growth restriction show that the umbilical artery and middle cerebral artery are the first variables to become abnormal (54). These arterial Doppler abnormalities are followed by abnormalities in the right cardiac diastolic indices, followed by the right cardiac systolic indices, and finally by both left diastolic and systolic cardiac indices (54). Preserving the left systolic function as the last variable to become abnormal ensures an adequate left ventricular output, which supplies the cerebral and coronary circulations.

Several of the Doppler changes seen in association with fetal IUGR in the peripheral circulation are directly related to the adaptation of the fetal heart. The current management of IUGR involves Doppler at the peripheral arterial circulation (middle cerebral and umbilical arteries); central venous vessels (ductus venosus and inferior vena cava); and cardiotocography. Adding cardiac Doppler may improve management of the IUGR fetus, but studies are lacking on the prospective clinical evaluation of the IUGR fetus with cardiac Doppler. It is becoming more obvious, however, that these changes in the central venous circulation reflect an advanced stage of fetal compromise, commonly associated with myocardial dysfunction and damage.

■ KEY POINTS: PULSED DOPPLER ECHOCARDIOGRAPHY

- ■ The Doppler frequency shift is directly proportional to the velocity of blood flow within the targeted vessel, the cosine of the insonating angle, and to the frequency of the insonating ultrasound wave.
- ■ The Doppler frequency shift provides information on the downstream impedance to flow of the vascular bed studied.
- ■ Most Doppler waveform quatification at the cardiac level relies on absolute frequencies which are angle dependent.
- ■ The fetal circulation is in parallel rather than in series and the right ventricular cardiac output is greater than the left ventricular cardiac output.
- ■ Blood from the ductus venosus is preferentially streamed into the left atrium through the formane ovale.
- ■ Right ventricular volume flow exceeds left ventricular volume flow in the fetus.

■ With advancing gestation, ventricular compliance is increased, total peripheral resistance is decreased, preload is increased, and combined cardiac output is increased.

■ The pulmonary vascular resistance is high in the fetus.

■ Doppler waveforms across the atrioventricular valves are biphasic in shape.

■ In the fetus, the velocity of the A wave is higher than that of the E wave across the atrioventricular valves.

■ Peak systolic velocity and time-to-peak velocity are indices used for waveform quantification across the semilunar valves.

■ Inferior vena cava Doppler waveforms are triphasic in appearance.

■ Flow during late diastole is reversed in the inferior vena cava in the normal fetus.

■ Ductus venosus Doppler waveforms are biphasic in appearance.

■ Forward flow is present during the entire cardiac cycle in the ductus venosus in the normal fetus.

■ The flow velocity waveforms of the pulmonary veins reflect pressure changes in the left atrium during the cardiac cycle.

■ The pulmonary vein Doppler waveforms are similar to those in the ductus venosus with a triphasic shape.

■ In IUGR fetuses, afterload is increased across the right ventricle and decreased across the left ventricle.

■ Preload is reduced in both ventricles in IUGR fetuses.

■ Sequence of adaptive changes in the fetal heart in IUGR includes right cardiac diastolic abnormalities followed by right cardiac systolic abnormalities and finally by both left diastolic and systolic cardiac abnormalities.

References

1. Doppler C. Über das farbige Licht der Doppelsterne und einiger anderer Gestirne des Himmels. *Abh König Böhm Ges Wiss* 1843;2:466.
2. Schulman H, Winter D, Farmakides G, et al. Doppler examinations of the umbilical and uterine arteries during pregnancy. *Clin Obstet Gynecol* 1989;32(4):738–745.
3. Nichols WW, O'Rourke MF. *McDonald's blood flow in arteries*. London: Edward Arnold, 1990:283.
4. Adamson SL, Langille BL. Factors determining aortic and umbilical blood flow pulsatility in fetal sheep. *Ultrasound Med Biol* 1992;18(3):255–266.
5. Gosling RG, King DH. Ultrasound angiology. In: Harcus AW, Adamson J, eds. *Arteries and veins*. Edinburgh: Churchill-Livingstone, 1975.
6. Pourcelot L. Applications clinique de l'examen Doppler transcutane. In: Pourcelot L, ed. *Velocimetric ultrasonore Doppler*. Paris: INSERM, 1974;213.
7. Stuart B, Drumm J, FitzGerald DE, et al. Fetal blood velocity waveforms in normal pregnancy. *Br J Obstet Gynaecol* 1980;87:780.
8. Chang CH, Chang FM, Yu CH, et al. Systemic assessment of fetal hemodynamics by Doppler ultrasound. *Ultrasound Med Biol* 2000;26:777–785.
9. Mielke G, Norbert B. Cardiac output and central distribution of blood flow in the human fetus. *Circulation* 2001;103:1662–1668.
10. Itskovitz J. Maternal-fetal hemodynamics. In: Maulik D, McNellis D, eds. *Reproductive and perinatal medicine*. VIII. Doppler ultrasound measurement of maternal-fetal hemodynamics. Ithaca: Perinatology, 1987;13.
11. Griffin D, Cohen-Overbeek T, Campbell S. Fetal and uteroplacental blood flow. *Clin Obstet Gynecol* 1983;10(3):565–602.
12. Reed KL, Meijboom EJ, Sahn DJ, Scagnelli SA, Valdes-Cruz LM, Schenker L. Cardiac Doppler flow velocities in human fetuses. *Circulation* 1986;73:41–46.
13. de Smedt MCH, Visser GHA, Meijboom EJ. Fetal cardiac output estimated by Doppler echocardiography during mid- and late gestation. *Am J Cardiol* 1987;60:338–348.
14. Kenny JF, Plappert T, Doubilet P, et al. Changes in intracardiac blood flow velocities and right and left ventricular stroke volumes with gestational age in the normal human fetus: a prospective Doppler echocardiographic study. *Circulation* 1986;74(6):1208–1216.
15. Reed KL, Sahn DJ, Marx GR, et al. Cardiac Doppler flows during fetal arrhythmias: physiologic consequences. *Obstet Gynecol* 1987;70(1):1–6.
16. Mielke G, Benda N. Blood flow velocity waveforms of the fetal pulmonary artery and the ductus arteriosus: reference ranges from 13 weeks to term. *Ultrasound Obstet Gynecol* 2000;15:213–218.
17. Hong Y, Choi J. Doppler study on pulmonary venous flow in the human fetus. *Fetal Diagn Ther* 1999;14:86–91.
18. Stoddard MF, Pearson AC, Kern MJ, et al. Influence of alteration in preload on the pattern of left ventricular diastolic filling as assessed by Doppler echocardiography in humans. *Circulation* 1989;79:1226–1236.
19. Labovitz AJ, Pearson AC. Evaluation of left ventricular diastolic function: clinical relevance and recent Doppler echocardiographic insights. *Am Heart J* 1987;114:836–851.

20. Romero T, Covell J, Friedman WF. A comparison of pressure-volume relations of the fetal, newborn, and adult heart. *Am J Physiol* 1972;222:1285.
21. Wladimiroff JW, Huisman TWA, Stewart PA. Fetal cardiac flow velocities in the late 1st trimester of pregnancy: a transvaginal Doppler study. *J Am Coll Cardiol* 1991;17(6):1357–1359.
22. Van der Mooren K, Barendregt LG, Wladimiroff JW. Fetal atrioventricular and outflow tract flow velocity waveforms during normal second half of pregnancy. *Am J Obstet Gynecol* 1991;165(3):668–674.
23. Reed KL, Sahn DJ, Scagnelli S, et al. Doppler echocardiographic studies of diastolic function in the human fetal heart: changes during gestation. *J Am Coll Cardiol* 1986;8:391–395.
24. Wladimiroff JW, Stewart PA, Burghouwt MT, et al. Normal fetal cardiac flow velocity waveforms between 11 and 16 weeks of gestation. *Am J Obstet Gynecol* 1992;167:736–739.
25. Allan LD, Chita SK, Al-LGhazali W, et al. Doppler echocardiographic evaluation of the normal human fetal heart. *Br Heart J* 1987;57:528–533.
26. Bennett ED, Barclay SA, Davis AL, et al. Ascending aortic blood velocity and acceleration using Doppler ultrasound in the assessment of left ventricular function. *Cardiovasc Res* 1984;18:632–638.
27. Sabbah HN, Khaja F, Brymer JF, et al. Noninvasive evaluation of left ventricular performance based on peak aortic blood acceleration measured with a continuous-wave Doppler velocity meter. *Circulation* 1986;74:323–329.
28. Gardin, JM. Doppler measurements of aortic blood flow velocity and acceleration: load-independent indexes of left ventricular performance? *Am J Cardiol* 1989;64:935–936.
29. Bedotto JB, Eichhorn EJ, Grayburn PA. Effects of left ventricular preload and afterload on ascending aortic blood velocity and acceleration in coronary artery disease. *Am J Cardiol* 1989;64:856–859.
30. Kitabatake A, Inoue M, Masato A, et al. Noninvasive evaluation of pulmonary hypertension by a pulsed Doppler technique. *Circulation* 1983;68(2):302–309.
31. Severi FM, Rizzo G, Bocchi C, et al. Intrauterine growth retardation and fetal cardiac function. *Fetal Diagn Ther* 2000;15:8–19.
32. Rizzo G, Arduini D, Romanini C. Doppler echocardiographic assessment of fetal cardiac function. *Ultrasound Obstet Gynecol* 1992;2:434–445.
33. Groenenberg IAL, Stijnen T, Wladimiroff JW. Flow velocity waveforms in the fetal cardiac outflow tract as a measure of fetal well-being in intrauterine growth retardation. *Pediatr Res* 1990;27:379–382.
34. Machado MVL, Chita SC, Allan LD. Acceleration time in the aorta an pulmonary artery measured by Doppler echocardiography in the midtrimester normal human fetus. *Br Heart J* 1987;58:15–18.
35. Reed KL, Anderson CF, Shenker L. Fetal pulmonary artery and aorta: two-dimensional Doppler echocardiography. *Obstet Gynecol* 1987;69:175–178.
36. Comstock CH, Riggs T, Lee W, Kirk J. Pulmonary-to-aorta diameter ratio in the normal and abnormal fetal heart. *Am J Obstet Gynecol* 1991;165:1038–1044.
37. Machado MVI, Chita SC, Allan LD. Acceleration time in the aorta and pulmonary artery measured by Doppler echocardiography in the midtrimester normal human fetus. *Br Heart J* 1987;58:15–18.
38. Rizzo G, Arduini D, Romanini C. Inferior vena cava flow velocity waveforms in appropriate- and small-for-gestational-age fetuses. *Am J Obstet Gynecol* 1992;166:1271–1280.
39. Reed KL, Appleton CP, Anderson CF, et al. Doppler studies of vena cava flows in human fetuses: insights into normal and abnormal cardiac physiology. *Circulation* 1990;81:498–505.
40. Huisman TWA, Stewart PA, Wladimiroff JW. Flow velocity waveforms in the fetal inferior vena cava during the second half of normal pregnancy. *Ultrasound Med Biol* 1991;17:679–682.
41. Reuss ML, Rudolph AM, Dae MW. Phasic blood flow patterns in the superior and inferior venae cavae and umbilical vein of fetal sheep. *Am J Obstet Gynecol* 1983;145:70–78.
42. Wexler L, Berger DH, Gabe IT, et al. Velocity of blood flow in normal human venae cavae. *Circ Res* 1968;23:349–359.
43. Brawley RK, Aldham NH, Vasko SS, et al. Influence of right atrial pressure on instantaneous vena caval blood flow. *Am J Physiol* 1966;211:347–353.
44. Soregaroli M, Rizzo G, Danti L, et al. Effects of maternal hyperoxygenation on ductus venosus flow velocity waveforms in normal third-trimester fetuses. *Ultrasound Obstet Gynecol* 1993;3:115–119.
45. Chako AW, Reynolds SR. Embryonic development in the human of the sphincter of the ductus venosus. *Anat Rec* 1953;115:151–173.
46. Barclay AE, Franklin KJ, Prichard MM. The mechanism of closure of the ductus venosus. *Br J Radiol* 1942;15:66–71.
47. Kiserud T, Eik-Nes SH, Blass HGK, et al. Ultrasonographic velocimetry of the fetal ductus venosus. *Lancet* 1991;338:1412–1414.
48. Rizzo G, Pietropolli A, Bufalino L, et al. Ductus venosus systolic to atrial peak velocity ratio in appropriate and small for gestational age fetuses. *J Matern Fetal Invest* 1993;3:198.
49. DeVore GR, Horenstein J. Ductus venosus index: a method for evaluating right ventricular preload in the second-trimester fetus. *Ultrasound Obstet Gynecol* 1993;3:338–342.
50. Makikallio K, Vuolteenaho O, Jouppila P, et al. Ultrasonographic and biochemical marker of human fetal cardiac dysfunction in placental insufficiency. *Circulation* 2002;105:2058–2063.
51. Reed KI, Anderson CF, Shenker L. Changes in intracardiac Doppler blood flow velocities in fetuses with absent umbilical artery diastolic flow. *Am J Obstet Gynecol* 1987;157:774–779.
52. Forouzan I, Graham E, Morgan MA. Reduction of right atrial peak systolic velocity in growth-restricted discordant twins. *Am J Obstet Gynecol* 1996;175:1033–1035.
53. Hecher K, Campbell S, Doyle P, et al. Assessment of fetal compromise by Doppler ultrasound investigation of the fetal circulation: arterial, intracardiac, and venous blood flow velocity studies. *Circulation* 1995;91:129–138.

54. Figueras F, Puerto B, Martinez JM et al. Cardiac function monitoring of fetuses with growth restriction. *Eur J Obstet Gynecol Reprod Biol* 2003;110:159–163.
55. Silverman HS, Ninomiya M, Blanck G, et al. A mechanism for impaired posthypoxic relaxation in isolated cardiac myocites. *Circ Res* 1991;69:196–208.
56. Groenenberg IAL, Wladimiroff JW, Hop WCJ. Fetal cardiac and peripheral flow velocity waveforms in intra-uterine growth retardation. *Circulation* 1989;80:1711–1717.
57. Rizzo G, Capponi A, Rinaldo D, et al. Ventricular ejection force in growth-retarded fetuses. *Ultrasound Obstet Gynecol* 1995;5:247–255.

THREE-DIMENSIONAL FETAL ECHOCARDIOGRAPHY: BASIC AND ADVANCED APPLICATIONS

INTRODUCTION

The introduction of three-dimensional ultrasound (3-D ultrasound or volume sonography) to obstetric imaging provided an advance in imaging technology. Unlike conventional two-dimensional ultrasound (2-D), 3-D ultrasound provides a volume of a target anatomic region, which contains an infinite number of 2-D planes. The technology of 3-D ultrasound is based on advanced mechanical and electronic transducers with the ability to acquire a volume by a sweep of elements within the transducers and on rapid computer processors able to display the acquired information within milliseconds. The acquired 3-D volume can then be displayed either in a multiplanar format of 2-D images or as a spatial volume projecting the external or internal anatomic features of a volume on the screen. Despite these obvious advances afforded by 3-D sonography, the acquisition, display, and manipulation of 3-D volumes are techniques that require a substantial learning curve. In obstetric sonography, the variable position of the fetus within the uterus further adds to this technical difficulty and limits the clinical applicability of 3-D sonography, especially as it involves complex anatomic structures such as the fetal heart. In this chapter, we will present the basic and advanced principles of 3-D ultrasound as it relates to the examination of the fetal heart. The potential applications of 3-D sonography in the evaluation of fetal cardiac anomalies are shown in the respective chapters on abnormal hearts later in this book.

THREE-DIMENSIONAL VOLUME ACQUISITION

The first step in 3-D volume acquisition is the optimization of the 2-D ultrasound examination, because the quality of the 3-D volume is dependent on the quality of the 2-D ultrasound examination. The operator should ensure optimum 2-D image quality when scanning the fetal heart by following the steps listed in Table 9-1 as acquisition of a 3-D volume initiates from a 2-D ultrasound examination. The term *reference plane* is used to designate the starting 2-D plane for a 3-D acquisition.

In the commonly used mechanical 3-D transducers, the optimum image quality within a volume is noted in the reference plane and in the parallel planes to the reference plane, whereas the reconstructed orthogonal or oblique planes to the reference plane have a reduced image quality. The reference plane should therefore be chosen based on the anatomic region of interest within the heart. The four-chamber plane is best suited as the 3-D volume reference plane for the evaluation of the transverse planes of the chest including the cardiac chambers, origin of great vessels, and the three-vessel and three-vessel-trachea views. On the other hand, optimal evaluation of the aortic, ductal arches and venous connections is best achieved from a sagittal 3-D volume acquisition of the fetal chest. Acquisitions are also best achieved from a near-ventral approach (spine posterior), avoiding shadowing from the ribs and spine.

Three important considerations should be taken into account when acquiring a 3-D volume: (a) the size of the region of interest (ROI—3-D box), (b) the angle of acquisition, and (c) the resolution or quality of acquisition.

1. **ROI box:** The ROI determines two parameters of a 3-D volume, the height and width, corresponding to the x and y axes (Fig. 9-1). It is recommended that the operator uses the smallest ROI size that includes all the anatomic components of a target volume. The smallest ROI size that contains all the anatomic components of the fetal heart and its vascular connections will ensure the fastest acquisition while minimizing artifact within the volume.
2. **Angle of acquisition:** The angle of acquisition is the sweep angle of the elements within the probe and is adjusted by the operator in the 3-D preset prior to the 3-D volume

TABLE 9-1	Steps to Optimize the Two-dimensional Ultrasound Examination of the Fetal Heart

- Use the fetal echocardiography presets on the ultrasound machine.
- Minimize the depth on the screen.
- Narrow the sector width.
- Adjust the focal zone(s) to the level of the fetal heart.
- Insonate the heart from an angle that avoids shadowing from the fetal skeleton.

acquisition. The angle of acquisition refers to the depth of a volume, corresponding to the z axis (Fig. 9-1). A basic knowledge of the anatomy of the target organ and the type of acquisition is required when choosing an angle for a 3-D volume. Current options for the acquisition angle of a volume vary from 10 to 120 degrees based on various equipment manufacturers and specific probes. Matrix transducers currently provide limited acquisition angles. Spatio-temporal image correlation (STIC) acquisition angles are typically chosen between 20 and 35 degrees. Static 3-D acquisition angles are between 35 and 45 degrees, which is generally sufficient for the examination of the fetal chest providing anatomic details extending from the stomach inferiorly to the transverse aortic arch (clavicles) superiorly. Ensuring the smallest angle of acquisition of a 3-D volume will enhance the speed of acquisition, reduce artifact, and optimize the quality of the 3-D volume.

3. **Quality of acquisition:** The quality of acquisition refers to the number of planes acquired within a volume (Fig. 9-2). In 3-D static acquisition the quality is referred to as low, medium, or high (Fig. 9-2), whereas in STIC acquisition, the quality of acquisition is reflected in the duration of acquisition: 7.5, 10, 12.5, or 15 seconds (Fig. 9-2). The ROI size, acquisition angle, and quality should be adapted based on the type of 3-D volume and the target anatomic region in order to optimize result.

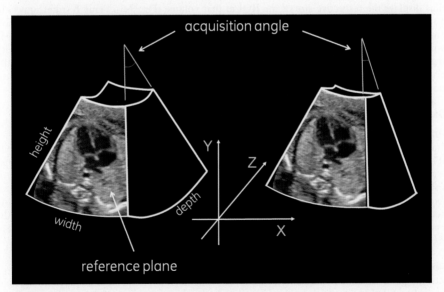

Figure 9-1. Prior to a volume acquisition, the reference plane is chosen by placing a box over the region of interest. The size of the box defines the width (x axis) and height (y axis) of a volume. The acquisition angle of a volume corresponds to its depth (z axis). This figure shows two volume acquisitions with the same width and height but with different depths (acquisition angles). The reference plane (four-chamber view) is located in the middle of the box. It is shown at the front in this figure for better illustration.

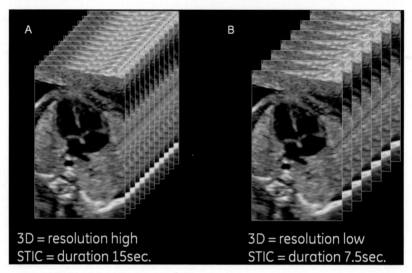

A

B

3D = resolution high
STIC = duration 15sec.

3D = resolution low
STIC = duration 7.5sec.

Figure 9-2. Three-dimensional (3-D) volume resolution is dependent on the resolution of the two-dimensional image prior to acquisition and on the number of slices (planes) within the acquisition box. A large number of slices is acquired when resolution is set on high in 3-D static acquisitions **(A)** and when the duration of acquisition is long in spatio-temporal image correlation (STIC) acquisitions (A). The resolution is set on "low" and the duration is short in **B.**

The multiplanar display of a 3-D volume provides information on the ROI and the angle of acquisition of the displayed volume. Plane A (left upper) in a multiplanar display corresponds to the reference plane, which is the starting anatomic 2-D plane of a 3-D volume and thus displays the respective size of the ROI in that volume (Fig. 9-3). Plane B (right upper) in a multiplanar display is a reconstructed orthogonal plane to plane A and shows the respective angle of acquisition of that volume (Fig. 9-3). In looking at the multiplanar display of a 3-D volume, one can gauge the appropriateness of the ROI and the angle of acquisition with regard to the target anatomic organ under study (Fig. 9-3). A proposed nomenclature for the clarification of 3-D terms was presented by Deng (1). Current options for 3-D volume acquisition are hereby presented.

Static Three-dimensional (Direct Volume Scan: Nongated)

Principle
Static 3-D acquisition refers to the acquisition of a 3-D volume in a nongated static mode (Fig. 9-4). The acquired volume contains an infinite number of 2-D still ultrasound planes with no regard to temporal or spatial motion. Currently, this is the most common mode of volume acquisition in obstetrics and gynecology and is frequently used for 3-D evaluation of fetal organs. The four-chamber plane is best used as the reference plane for the static 3-D acquisition when cardiac chambers and the origin of great vessels are under study. For the assessment of aortic or pulmonary arches, reference planes in parasagittal orientation are recommended.

Advantages
Advantages of static 3-D acquisition of the fetal heart include its speed of acquisition (0.5 to 2 seconds) and the ease of volume manipulation. Furthermore, static 3-D acquisition allows for the possibility to acquire large volumes, both in ROI and angle with minimal artifact. The static 3-D acquisition can also be combined with color, power Doppler, or B flow for vascular evaluation of volume content. The authors prefer the use of power Doppler or B flow in static 3-D acquisition given its uniform color display (2–4). Motion artifact is minimized when vessel pulsatility is reduced during volume acquisition with power Doppler (3,5).

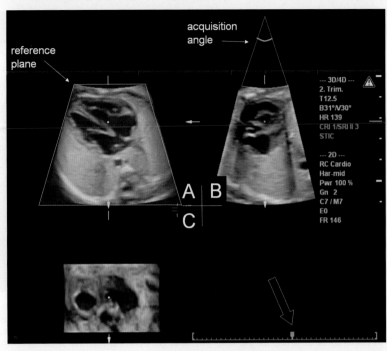

Figure 9-3. Orthogonal display of a spatio-temporal image correlation (STIC) volume acquired at the four-chamber view. The reference plane is depicted in the left upper image **(A)** with the chosen volume height and width. The acquisition angle 30[degree] is shown in **plane B,** in the right upper image. Plane B also provides information on acquisition artifacts (motion). The time-line of the STIC volume is shown in the right lower image **(C)** and the arrow points to the actual time of the orthogonal display within the cardiac cycle. Moving the cursor over the line allows scrolling through systole and diastole.

Disadvantages

Disadvantages of static 3-D acquisition include its inability to assess events related to the cardiac cycle, valve motion in the heart, and myocardial contractility.

Spatio-temporal Image Correlation (STIC) (Indirect Volume Scan, Motion Gated: Offline Four-dimensional)

Principle

STIC acquisition is an indirect, motion-gated, offline mode based on the concept of using tissue excursion concurrent with cardiac motion to extract the temporal information regarding the cardiac cycle. This concept was first suggested in 1996 (6) and later adapted to clinical ultrasound several years later (7–9). The acquisition of a STIC volume occurs over a duration of 7.5 to 15 seconds with an acquisition angle of 15 to 40 degrees. The acquired volume is processed internally, where the systolic peaks are used to calculate the fetal heart rate and the volume images are then rearranged according to their temporal events within the heart cycle, thus creating a cine-like loop of a single cardiac cycle.

Parameters that optimize the acquisition of a STIC volume include a clear 2-D reference plane with minimal shadowing by the fetal skeleton; an ROI that is set as narrow as possible, probably just outside the cardiac chambers; an angle of acquisition between 20 and 25 degrees in the second trimester; and a large acquisition time within the 7.5- to 15-second window if allowed by lack of fetal movements. These parameters will enhance the temporal and spatial resolution of the acquired volume and maximize the frame rate (Fig. 9-2).

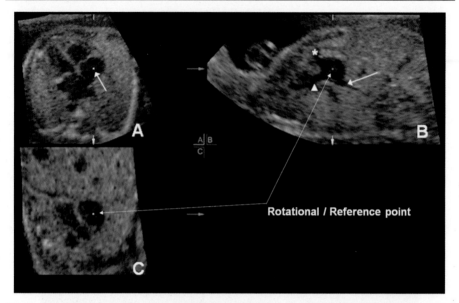

Figure 9-4. Static three-dimensional acquisition of a volume obtained from the transverse fetal chest at the level of the four-chamber view (reference plane—**plane A**). **Plane B** and **plane C** are two orthogonal planes to plane A. The reference (rotational point) is placed within the right atrium in plane A (*short arrow* in A and *long arrows* in B and C), thus showing the anatomy of the right atrium in three orthogonal planes. Note the right atrial appendage (*asterisk*), the inferior vena cava (*small arrow*), and the superior vena cava (*arrowhead*) entering the right atrium (plane B).

Advantages

Advantages of STIC volume acquisition include the ability to assess atrial and ventricular wall motion and valve excursion. The four-dimensional (4-D) information is available within seconds from the volume acquisition, thus facilitating its integration in clinical practice. Once the plane of interest is optimized, the STIC acquisition can be easily achieved. STIC acquisition can be obtained from 2-D gray-scale imaging combined with other imaging modalities, such as color, power, or high-definition flow Doppler and B flow.

Disadvantages

Disadvantages of STIC acquisition include a fairly delayed acquisition time, which can be hampered by fetal movements or maternal breathing movements, thus introducing artifact into the volume.

Real-time Three-dimensional (Direct Volume Scan, Real Time, Online Four-dimensional)

Principle

A real-time 3-D volume acquisition can be achieved with a mechanical transducer, but the rotation motor in current technology is a limiting factor in getting a large acquisition angle or good resolution (10). Real-time 3-D acquisition of cardiac volumes is now and in the future best obtained with matrix 3-D transducers allowing real-time dynamic 3-D evaluation.

Advantages

Postnatal studies have shown superiority of this approach to conventional 2-D ultrasound in the evaluation of congenital heart disease (11–14). Major advantages of real-time 3-D acquisitions are that gating of the heart rate is not required and volumes of the beating heart are displayed instantaneously without any transfer or postprocessing of the data. Other advantages include the ability to display on the ultrasound screen instantaneously 2-D and real-time 3-D volume. Color Doppler can also be added to a real-time 3-D acquisition as shown recently (15). This technology allows for the depiction of the shape, direction, and propagation of color flow jets in 3-D for analysis of various congenital heart abnormalities such as septal defects, valvar stenosis, and regurgitation (15,16).

Disadvantages
Although this technology holds significant promise for the future, current systems are limited by the size of the acquired volume, often too small for a complete evaluation of the fetal heart and great vessels, and the high cost of transducers (17).

VOLUME DISPLAY AND MANIPULATION

Once a volume is acquired, different options are available for its display and manipulation. Volume display can be performed by showing either (a) representative 2-D images from the volume, termed *multiplanar display* or *multiplanar reconstruction*, or (b) external or internal spatial views of the acquired volume, termed *volume rendering*.

Volume Display in Two-dimensional Planes

Single Two-dimensional Planes or Multiplanar Orthogonal Display
Principle Multiplanar mode is based on displaying a 3-D volume by three orthogonal 2-D planes conventionally termed planes A, B, and C (Figs. 9-3 and 9-4). Plane A, located in the left upper corner, is the reference plane for the acquisition, and planes B and C are orthogonal planes corresponding to the location of the reference point within the volume (Figs. 9-3 and 9-4). The operator can then display all three planes, two planes, or a single plane on the ultrasound display. Multiplanar display is commonly used for 3-D static and STIC acquisitions. STIC displays allow for the ability to play the loop in slow motion or stop at any time (open arrow in Fig. 9-3) for detailed analysis of specific phases of the cardiac cycle. The reference point, which corresponds to the intersection point of the three displayed planes in multiplanar display, can be used for volume manipulation. The authors recommend an easy approach that relies on moving the reference point in planes A or B to the desired anatomic structure within the heart for its display in three orthogonal planes and then performing minor rotations as needed across the *x*, *y*, or *z* axis for full display. Figure 9-4, for example, shows the anatomy of the right atrium in three orthogonal planes, which was obtained by placing the reference point inside the right atrium in plane A. Standardization of a 3-D volume in multiplanar display, by rotating the spine in plane A to the 6 o'clock position and placing the apex of the heart in the left upper chest, has been previously described in detail (18) (Fig. 9-5, Table 9-2). Once a static or a STIC volume obtained at the level of the four-chamber view is standardized as outlined, the diagnostic cardiac planes can be retrieved as has been described (19). Table 9-3 lists the spatial relationship of standard diagnostic cardiac planes in the fetal heart to the four-chamber-view plane in the second trimester of pregnancy (19).

Advantages Advantages of multiplanar display include familiarity with the displayed 2-D planes, the relative ease of manipulation of the volume given the acquaintance with the displayed 2-D anatomy, and the ability to view cardiac abnormalities from three orthogonal views simultaneously. By scrolling through an acquired STIC volume, the operator not only can sequentially display many diagnostic planes such as the abdominal plane and four-chamber, five-chamber, and three-vessel-trachea views (Fig. 9-6D–G), but can also review planes within a specific time within the cardiac cycle (Fig. 9-6B,C). Methods for examination of the fetal outflow tracts in 3-D static and STIC volumes have been described including the "spin" technique, which involves rotation along the *x* and *y* axes (20). The potential of color Doppler STIC volumes for the evaluation of normal and abnormal hearts was studied in a prospective design in experienced hands (21). Successful acquisition was possible in all cases and the display of the three transverse planes (four-chamber view, five-chamber view, and three-vessel-trachea view) was possible in 31 of 35 normal hearts and in 24 of 27 abnormal hearts (21).

Disadvantages Disadvantages of 2-D plane display are mainly related to the reconstructed planes in comparison to a live examination. Artifacts during acquisition may produce artifacts

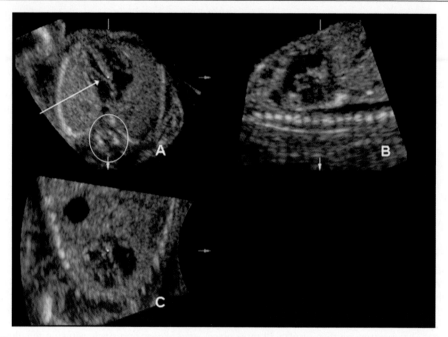

Figure 9-5. Static three-dimensional (3-D) acquisition of a volume obtained at the level of the four-chamber view (reference plane—**plane A**). Standardization of a 3-D volume of the fetal chest is achieved by rotating plane A along the z axis to place the spine at the 6 o'clock position (*circle*) and the apex of the heart in the left upper quadrant. Further standardization involves rotating **planes B** and **C** along the z axis to align the spine horizontally and vertically in planes B and C, respectively, and placing the rotational/reference point in the crux of the heart in plane A (*arrow*). See text and Table 9-2 for further details.

of the 2-D reconstructed plane with erroneous information. We recommend acquiring several volumes of the fetal heart in order to improve the accuracy of the offline analysis.

Application in Fetal Cardiac Anomalies The 2-D plane display can be applied in the evaluation of all cardiac anomalies as it can mimic a real-time examination of the fetal heart when the examiner scrolls through the volume in slow motion (Fig. 9-6). This application can be of help in the detection of atrioventricular septal defect (Fig. 9-7), when the plane at the level of the crux of the heart is carefully observed during systole and diastole (Fig. 9-7A,B). The reference point at the intersection of the three orthogonal planes can be used to confirm the presence of a ventricular septal defect as demonstrated in Figure 15-17. The reference point can also demonstrate the parallel orientation of the great arteries in transposition cases (20). An optimal view of the aortic arch can be reconstructed from a parasagittal acquisition of the fetal chest to confirm the presence of aortic coarctation as demonstrated in Chapter 12 and shown here in a normal fetus in Figure 9-6.

Multiplanar Tomographic Ultrasound Imaging
Principle Tomographic ultrasound imaging (TUI), or multislice analysis, is a modification to multiplanar imaging, where numerous parallel 2-D planes are simultaneously displayed, giving a sequential anatomic view of a region within the acquired volume (Fig. 9-8). The number of displayed planes, the interplane distance, and the thickness of the anatomic region can be manipulated (compare Figs. 9-8 and 9-9). The exact position of each plane within the target anatomic region is seen in the upper left plane of the TUI display (Fig. 9-8A).

Advantages Tomographic ultrasound display resembles the output of computed tomography and magnetic resonance imaging and thus has the advantage of displaying multiple planes in

TABLE 9-2	Standardization of Three-dimensional Volumes of the Fetal Chest (Cephalic Presentations[a])

Volume acquisition

- **Reference plane:** Obtain an axial view of the chest at level of the four-chamber view. Ensure that you have one full rib on each side.
- **Acquisition box:** Open the acquisition box wide enough to ensure that the fetal chest is contained within the box. The box boundaries should be placed just outside the fetal skin.
- **Acquisition angle:** Use an acquisition angle that is wide enough to include the stomach inferiorly and the lower neck superiorly.

Volume display

1. Rotate image in plane A (four-chamber view) along the z axis until the spine is at 6 o'clock and the apex of the heart is in the left upper chest.
2. Move the reference point in plane A to the spine (body of vertebra). This will bring a longitudinal view of the spine in planes B and C.
3. Rotate image in plane C (coronal view) along the z axis until the section of the midthoracic spine is aligned vertically.
4. Rotate image in plane B (sagittal view) along the z axis until the section of the midthoracic spine (posterior to the heart) is aligned horizontally.
5. Place the reference point in plane A at the crux of the heart, at the level of the insertion of the medial leaflet of the tricuspid valve into the septum.

[a]For breech presentations, start by rotating the three-dimensional volumes 180 degrees along the y axis, and then follow the steps above.
(From Abuhamad A. Standardization of 3-dimensional volumes in obstetric sonography: a required step for training and automation. *J Ultrasound Med* 2005;24:397–401, with permission.)

TABLE 9-3	Spatial Relationship of Cardiac Planes 1–3 to the Four-chamber View (4CV) Reference Plane and Tomographic Ultrasound Imaging (TUI) Display

Cardiac plane	Spatial relationship to 4CV	TUI image-to-image distance (mm)[a]
1	Parallel shift: −3.84 mm Y rotation: 26.5	0.56
2	Parallel shift: −9.00 mm	1
3	Parallel shift: +14.0 mm	2

[a]TUI output was set at seven images for each diagnostic cardiac plane.
Cardiac 1 = left ventricular outflow tract; cardiac 2 = right ventricular outflow tract; cardiac 3 = abdominal circumference.
(From Abuhamad A, Falkensammer P, Reichartseder F, et al. Automated retrieval of standard diagnostic fetal cardiac planes in the second trimester of pregnancy: a prospective evaluation of software. *Ultrasound Obstet Gynecol* 2008;31:30–36, with permission.)

longitudinal, transverse, and coronal orientation, providing a comprehensive picture of cardiac anatomy. Most fetal cardiac anomalies affect different segments of the heart, and a comprehensive examination should include the assessment of different planes, which can be demonstrated in one picture when displayed in TUI mode. The advantage of TUI in the evaluation of cardiac anomalies was analyzed in 103 confirmed cases of congenital heart malformation (22). A mean interslice distance of 2.7 (standard deviation [SD], 0.3) mm at 19 to 23 gestational weeks and 4.0 (SD, 0.4) mm at 30 to 33 weeks allowed a complete sequential analysis in all cases (22). Algorithms for the automatic display of diagnostic cardiac planes out of a 3-D static or STIC volume have been described following an initial standardization in plane A (23). This technology of automated sonography has the potential of standardizing and simplifying the ultrasound examination of the fetal heart by lessening the operator dependency on the conventional 2-D ultrasound modality. TUI is a significant component of automated

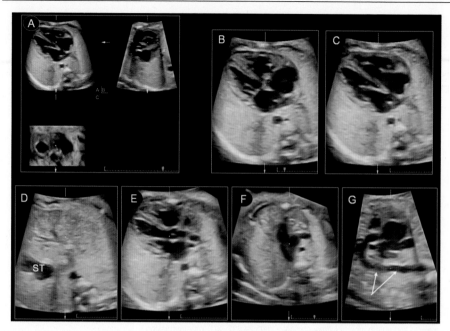

Figure 9-6. Manipulation of a spatio-temporal image correlation (STIC) volume. **A:** The original STIC data set is shown in an orthogonal plane display. The four-chamber plane as a "single plane" is demonstrated in systole **(B)** with closed atrioventricular valves and in diastole **(C)** with opened valves. Scrolling through the volume demonstrates the upper abdomen with the stomach (ST) **(D),** the slightly oblique five-chamber view **(E),** the three-vessel-trachea view in the upper thorax **(F),** and a reconstructed longitudinal plane **(G)** of the aortic arch. Reconstructed planes are generally of lower quality; note the presence of motion artifact in plane G on the descending aorta (*arrows* in G).

sonography as it controls for inherent variability in fetal cardiac anatomy (cardiac axis, cardiac position in chest, size of chest) by providing multiple planes for review (Figs. 9-8 and 9-9). In a study evaluating the automated software on STIC volumes of fetuses with transposition of great arteries, ventricular arterial connection anomaly was shown in all fetuses (24).

Disadvantages TUI involves reconstructed planes and thus has a lack of real-time imaging. Furthermore, the size of the acquisition box may limit the display of anatomic information. Another disadvantage of TUI is in its current limitation to display parallel planes that may not correspond to the required planes for diagnosis, especially in the presence of a cardiac anomaly. In these cases TUI assessment should be combined with a rotation of the x or y axis during evaluation.

Application in Fetal Cardiac Anomalies Since most cardiac defects involve multiple levels in the heart, TUI display can be used to demonstrate components of cardiac anomalies in more than one plane. Examples of such are shown in this book for hypoplastic left heart syndrome (Fig. 11-23), aortic coarctation (Fig. 12-11), tetralogy of Fallot (Fig. 17-10), absent pulmonary valve syndrome (Fig. 17-27), and transposition of the great arteries (Fig. 20-3 and 20-9).

Volume Display in Rendering

Volume rendering describes the display of external or internal surfaces of acquired volumes. In volume rendering, a box is displayed within the acquired volume with a reference border (rendered view direction, usually a colored line), which corresponds to the direction of rendering (Fig. 9-10). The operator can adjust the rendering direction and the thickness of the rendering box over a target anatomic region within the volume.

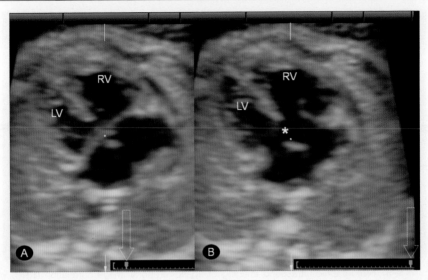

Figure 9-7. Spatio-temporal image correlation (STIC) volume in a fetus with an atrioventricular septal defect. In **plane A,** the defect is not clearly demonstrated as the valve leaflets are closed. By scrolling through the cursor (*open arrow*), the interventricular septal defect is clearly demonstrated (*asterisk*) in **plane B** when the valve leaflets are open. LV, left ventricle; RV, right ventricle.

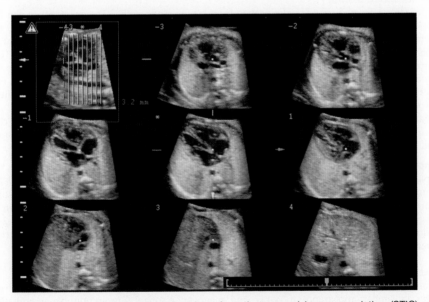

Figure 9-8. Tomographic ultrasound imaging of spatio-temporal image correlation (STIC) volume of the fetal heart in gray scale. In the upper left image, the orientation plane A is seen (highlighted in yellow) with the parallel vertical lines referring to the planes shown in the display (−4 to +4). Interplane distance and total number of planes are chosen by the examiner. The −4 plane is hidden behind the orientation plane A.

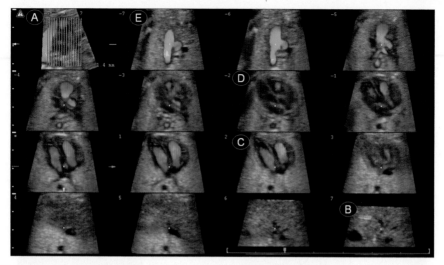

Figure 9-9. Tomographic ultrasound imaging of spatio-temporal image correlation (STIC) volume of the fetal heart in color Doppler demonstrating the orientation plane in **A** with 15 parallel vertical lines corresponding to 15 planes that span the abdomen inferiorly to the upper chest superiorly. The upper abdomen is shown in **B,** the four-chamber-view in **C,** the five chamber view in **D,** and the three-vessel-trachea view in **E.**

There are different rendering modes that are based on varying thresholds resulting in various displays that have been shown to be clinically relevant.

Surface Mode Display

In its classic form, surface rendering has been synonymous with 3-D ultrasound in the lay population by its ability to display near-perfect images of the fetal face. In 3-D or STIC the surface of the cardiac cavities with their interface with the blood can be easily demonstrated. This display allows the *en face* view of several regions of interest within the fetal heart. The correct anatomic placement of the rendered box and the rendering direction required for the surface-rendering display of clinically relevant regions of the fetal heart are described in Figures 9-10 and 9-11. The impact of these rendered views in the demonstration of abnormalities involving the atrioventricular valves (valve dysplasia or atrioventricular septal defects) and the great vessels (transposed great arteries) has been analyzed (25). New planes in the surface-rendering mode could facilitate understanding of the spatial relationship of cardiac structures, and clinically appropriate views remain to be investigated (25).

Application in Fetal Cardiac Anomalies Surface mode can be used to demonstrate the typical fetal cardiac planes providing a three-dimensional impression as shown in Figure 9-10. This can be used in anomalies that are present in the four-chamber view or that can be summarized in one 3-D view. Three-dimensional surface mode of cardiac anomalies is shown in this book for critical aortic stenosis (Fig. 11-13A), hypoplastic left heart syndrome (Fig. 11-24), atrioventricular septal defect (Fig. 15-31), Ebstein anomaly (Fig. 14-8), double inlet ventricle (Fig. 16-6), and tricuspid atresia with ventricular septal defect (Fig. 16-14).

Transparent Minimum Mode

Transparent minimum mode can be added to a static or STIC acquisition and displays structures in similar appearance to x-ray and magnetic resonance projection by accentuating anechoic structures (dark colors) and blurring the surrounding echogenic structures (26) (Fig. 9-12). In this mode the spatial anatomic details of structures are limited, but the projection of anechoic structures such as the cardiac chambers and great vessels allows for a useful display of cardiac anatomy.

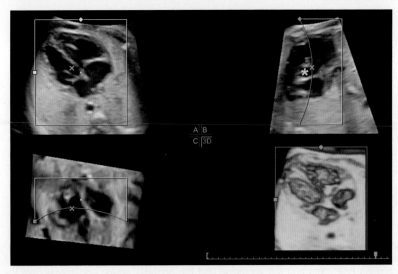

Figure 9-10. Surface-rendering mode of a spatio-temporal image correlation (STIC) volume in gray scale demonstrating the four-chamber view (three-dimensional [3-D], **right lower image**). In order to obtain the view of the four chambers as seen in 3-D right lower image, the 3-D–rendering box is placed over the heart as demonstrated in **plane B** with the rendering line from cranial to caudal (*asterisk*) placed just under the ascending aorta. The reference plane **(A)** is obtained at the level of the four-chamber view.

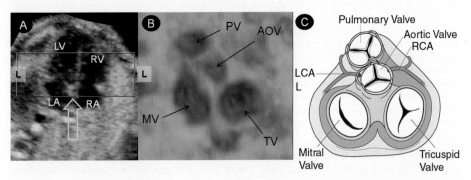

Figure 9-11. Surface-rendering mode of a spatio-temporal image correlation (STIC) volume in gray scale demonstrating the basic cardiac view of the atrioventricular and semilunar valves in **plane B.** In order to obtain this view the three-dimensional (3-D)–rendering box is placed over the four-chamber plane with the rendering view (*open arrow*) in the atria **(A).** The reference plane (A) is obtained at the level of the four-chamber view. **Plane C** is a drawing of the anatomic relationship of the cardiac valves. RV, right ventricle; RA, right atrium; LV, left ventricle; LA, left atrium; LCA, left coronary artery; RCA, right coronary artery; TV, tricuspid valve; MV, mitral valve; AOV, aortic valve; PV, pulmonary valve; L, left.

Application in Fetal Cardiac Anomalies Minimum mode can be used to demonstrate a plane represented as a thin slice of cardiac anatomy such as the chambers or the great vessels. Figure 9-12A shows the crossing of the great vessels in a normal heart, and Figure 9-12B shows the parallel course of the great vessels in a fetus with transposition. The use of minimum mode in double outlet right ventricle is shown in Figure 19-9 and in heterotaxy in Figure 22-14B. The clinical utility of this mode is currently limited.

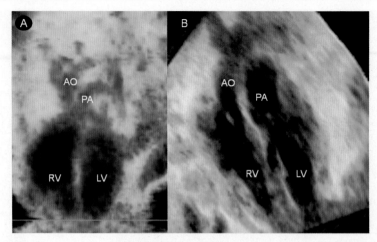

Figure 9-12. Transparent minimum mode display in a normal fetal heart **(A)** and a heart with a complete transposition of the great arteries **(B)**. A: Anterior view with a projection through the heart showing both right and left ventricles and the normally arising and crossing of the aorta and pulmonary artery. B: The same view shows parallel arising great vessels from the discordant ventricles representing a D-transposition of the great vessels. RV, right ventricle; LV, left ventricle; PA, pulmonary artery; AO, aorta.

Inversion Mode

Inversion mode can be added to a static or STIC acquisition in a rendered display. The inversion mode inverts, as the name implies, the echogenicity of volume components. In other words, it is the inversion of the information displayed with the minimum mode. When applied to the fetal heart, fluid-filled spaces, such as cardiac chambers, appear bright, while cardiac and vessel walls or lungs disappear (Fig. 9-13). The amount of echogenicity shown on the screen can be changed by increasing or decreasing the threshold of gray-to-black information (Fig. 9-13). Artifacts, which can be produced by shadowing from the fetal ribs and spine, can be removed by using the electronic scalpel (Fig. 9-13). Display of rendered 3-D volumes using inversion mode provides information similar to volumes acquired with power Doppler or B flow. Advantages of the inversion mode, however, reside within the quality of the image, which is superior to power Doppler given a higher frame rate and resolution. Figure 9-13 shows preferred steps for the anatomic display of a rendered volume of the fetal heart in inversion mode.

Application in Fetal Cardiac Anomalies Inversion mode can be applied to create "digital casts" of the cardiac chambers and great vessels (27), and reports have analyzed the role of inversion mode in visualizing cardiac and extracardiac fluid-filled structures in the fetus (28,29). Inversion mode can also be used in demonstrating the spatial relationship of the great vessels (Fig. 9-14). The use of inversion mode is demonstrated in double outlet right ventricle (Fig. 19-10), common arterial trunk (Fig. 18-11), transposition of the great arteries (Fig. 20-11A), pulmonary atresia with intact septum (Fig. 13-17B), and others. In Figure 9-14A, a frontal view of the fetal heart shows the normal crossing of the great vessels and the right atrial appendage.

Three-dimensional Color Doppler and Glass Body Mode

Color Doppler, power Doppler, and high-definition flow (similar to bidirectional power Doppler) can be combined with 3-D static and STIC acquisitions. Options for rendered display of such volumes include the color information alone, the gray-scale information alone, or a combination of both, termed "glass body" mode (Fig. 9-15).

Application in Fetal Cardiac Anomalies Glass body and color Doppler display is helpful in the demonstration of the relationship of the great vessels in congenital heart disease (2–4,30) and especially the heart cycle–related flow events. Approach to the heart using color

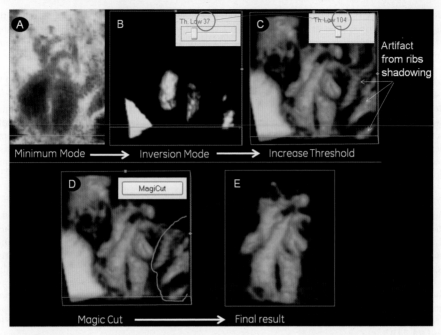

Figure 9-13. Step-by-step demonstration of inversion mode rendering: The volume in Figure 9-12A is used as an example **(A).** First inversion mode is activated **(B)** and hypoechoic information is shown with disappearance of the surrounding structures. The minimum threshold is then increased until the targeted anatomic details are seen **(C).** Artifact from rib shadowing is seen in **plane C** (*arrows*). The electronic scalpel is activated and the artifact is digitally removed **(D),** leading to the final result displayed in **plane E.**

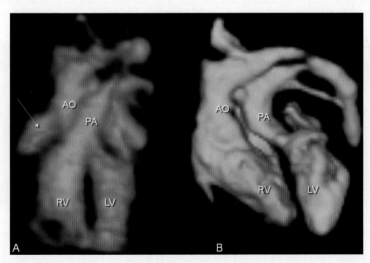

Figure 9-14. Inversion mode showing an anterior view of a normal heart (rendered in Fig. 9-13) with the normal crossing of the great arteries **(A)** and a heart **(B)** with parallel course of the great vessels in transposition of the great arteries. The right atrial appendage is shown in plane A (*arrow*). RV, right ventricle; LV, left ventricle; PA, pulmonary artery; AO, aorta.

Doppler in glass body mode includes the four-chamber view showing abnormal flow events during diastole or systole. It can also include a cranial view of the great vessels demonstrating their spatial relationship (see normal finding in Figure 17-11A) and a lateral view of the heart and upper abdomen showing the great and abdominal vessels (Fig. 9-15). Later in this book 3-D color, power Doppler, and high-definition color rendering are demonstrated in critical aortic stenosis (Fig. 11-13B), interrupted inferior vena cava with azygos continuation (Fig. 22-14A), tetralogy of Fallot (Fig. 17-11B), right aortic arch (Fig. 21-10), ductal and aortic arch flow events in hypoplastic left heart syndrome (Fig. 11-21B), anomalous pulmonary venous drainage (Fig. 23-20 and 23-21A), aortic coarctation (Fig. 12-12), major aortopulmonary collateral arteries in pulmonary atresia (Fig. 17-20), and an *en face* view of a ventricular septal defect in systole and diastole (Fig. 15-19). It has to be emphasized that many figures of glass body mode shown in this book do not reveal the complete information since a still image cannot display changes in flow events between systole and diastole.

Three-dimensional B-flow Rendering

B flow is a Doppler-independent approach to imaging of vascular flow. This technique allows the direct visualization of blood cell reflectors and as such is angle independent, which makes it appealing for vascular structures at a perpendicular angle to the direction of ultrasound beam. Only flow events are visualized, and any other information from neighboring structures is not seen. A 3-D volume acquired in B-flow mode allows for vascular imaging within the volume in a nongated angle-independent approach (Fig. 9-16) (31). The image is similar to the inversion mode display, but it shows flow patterns and is best suited for the demonstration of the relationship of vessels and also small vasculature, such as pulmonary veins and aberrant arising vessels (31). Examples of anomalies are presented in figures 21-11B, 21-15B, and 23-21B.

 CONCLUSION

Three-dimensional ultrasound has been a valuable addition to fetal echocardiography with a multitude of options in acquisition and display, which has undoubtedly helped in the understanding of normal and abnormal cardiac anatomy. In this book the reader will find in the chapters on cardiac anomalies a short description of the application of 3-D ultrasound with characteristic figures.

Application of 3-D ultrasound has also extended into the ability to provide sophisticated fetal echocardiography to underserved areas by sending 3-D volume sets for remote review by

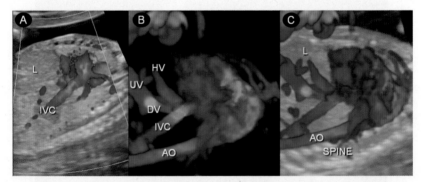

Figure 9-15. A: Color Doppler demonstration of the longitudinal view of the inferior vena cava (IVC) in two-dimensional ultrasound. **B:** A three-dimensional (3-D) volume acquisition in color Doppler displayed as "3-D color Doppler mode," which shows the vasculature without any surrounding tissue. The projection shows the descending aorta, the heart, and the liver vasculature in addition to the vascularity displayed in A. **C:** The 3-D volume is rendered in glass body mode, which shows the combination of 3-D color Doppler and 3-D gray-scale information with the spine, liver (L), and neighboring structures. AO, aorta; DV, ductus venosus; UV, umbilical vein; HV, hepatic vein.

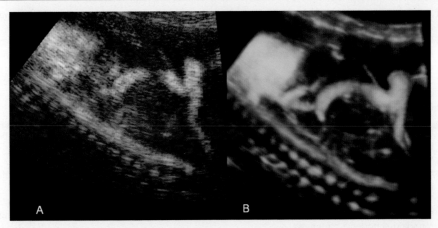

Figure 9-16. B flow demonstrates vasculature in an angle-independent approach. **Plane A** shows B flow applied to a sagittal view of the abdomen and chest. In **plane B,** three-dimensional rendering of an acquired spatio-temporal image correlation (STIC) volume with B flow permits the demonstration of small vessels and their spatial relationship. These figures show views in similar anatomic orientation to those in Figure 9-15.

experienced operators (32,33). New modalities are allowing the calculation of cardiac chamber volumes and the attainment of data on stroke volume and ejection fraction in the fetus (34–36). Future advances will include matrix transducers more suitable for obstetric scanning, which will open the door for real-time 3-D ultrasound. Combining automation software with a real-time 3-D ultrasound examination holds great promise for simplifying the fetal cardiac examination, which may translate into increased prenatal detection of congenital heart disease.

▦ KEY POINTS: THREE-DIMENSIONAL FETAL ECHOCARDIOGRAPHY

- ■ Three-dimensional ultrasound provides a volume of a target anatomic region that contains an infinite number of 2-D planes.
- ■ The first step in 3-D volume acquisition is the optimization of the 2-D ultrasound examination, because the quality of the 3-D volume is dependent on the quality of the 2-D ultrasound examination.
- ■ The term *reference plane* is used to designate the starting 2-D plane for a 3-D acquisition.
- ■ The ROI determines two parameters of a 3-D volume, the height and width, corresponding to the x and y axis.
- ■ The smallest ROI size that contains all the anatomic components of the fetal heart and its vascular connections will ensure the fastest acquisition while minimizing artifact within the volume.
- ■ The angle of acquisition refers to the depth of a volume, corresponding to the z axis.
- ■ Ensuring the smallest angle of acquisition of a 3-D volume will enhance the speed of acquisition, reduce artifact, and optimize the quality of the 3-D volume.
- ■ Plane A (left upper) in a multiplanar display corresponds to the reference plane, which is the starting anatomic 2-D plane of a 3-D volume and thus displays the respective size of the ROI in that volume.
- ■ Plane B (right upper) in a multiplanar display is a reconstructed orthogonal plane to plane A and shows the respective angle of acquisition of that volume.
- ■ Static 3-D acquisition refers to the acquisition of a 3-D volume in a nongated static mode.
- ■ Advantages of static 3-D acquisition of the fetal heart include its speed of acquisition (0.5 to 2 seconds) and the ease of volume manipulation.
- ■ STIC acquisition is an indirect, motion-gated, offline mode based on the concept of using tissue excursion concurrent with cardiac motion to extract the temporal information regarding the cardiac cycle.

- Advantages of STIC volume acquisition include the ability to assess atrial and ventricular wall motion and valve excursion.
- Disadvantages of STIC acquisition include a fairly delayed acquisition time, which can be hampered by fetal movements or maternal breathing movements, thus introducing artifact into the volume.
- Real-time 3-D acquisition of cardiac volumes is best obtained with matrix 3-D transducers allowing real-time dynamic 3-D evaluation.
- Multiplanar display is commonly used for 3-D static and STIC acquisitions.
- TUI, or multislice analysis, is a modification to multiplanar imaging, where numerous parallel 2-D planes are simultaneously displayed, giving a sequential anatomic view of a region within the acquired volume.
- Volume rendering describes the display of external or internal surfaces of acquired volumes.
- Surface mode display allows the *en face* view of several regions of interest within the fetal heart.
- Transparent minimum mode displays structures in similar appearance to x-ray and magnetic resonance projection by accentuating anechoic structures (dark colors) and blurring the surrounding echogenic structures.
- The inversion mode inverts, as the name implies, the echogenicity of volume components.
- B flow is a Doppler-independent approach to imaging of vascular flow; it allows the direct visualization of blood cell reflectors and as such is angle independent.

References

1. Deng J. Terminology of three-dimensional and four-dimensional ultrasound imaging of the fetal heart and other moving body parts. *Ultrasound Obstet Gynecol* 2003;22:336–344.
2. Chaoui R, Kalache KD, Hartung J. Application of three dimensional power Doppler ultrasound in prenatal diagnosis. *Ultrasound Obstet Gynecol* 2001;17:22–29.
3. Chaoui R, Kalache KD. Three-dimensional power Doppler ultrasound of the fetal great vessels. *Ultrasound Obstet Gynecol* 2001;17:455–456.
4. Chaoui R, Schneider MBE, Kalache KD. Right aortic arch with vascular ring and aberrant left subclavian artery: prenatal diagnosis assisted by three-dimensional power Doppler ultrasound. *Ultrasound Obstet Gynecol* 2003;22:661–663.
5. Chaoui R, Kalache KD. Three-dimensional color power imaging: principles and first experience in prenatal diagnosis. In: Merz E, ed. *3D ultrasonography in obstetrics and gynecology*. Philadelphia: Lippincott Williams & Wilkins, 1998;135–142.
6. Nelson TR, Pretorius DH, Sklansky M, et al. Three-dimensional echocardiographic evaluation of fetal heart anatomy and function: acquisition, analysis, and display. *J Ultrasound Med* 1996;15:1–9.
7. Falkensammer P. *Spatio-temporal image correlation for volume ultrasound. Studies of the fetal heart.* Zipf, Austria: GE Healthcare, 2005.
8. DeVore GR, Falkensammer P, Sklansky MS, et al. Spatiotemporal image correlation (STIC): new technology for evaluation of the fetal heart. *Ultrasound Obstet Gynecol* 2003;22:380–387.
9. Goncalves LF, Lee W, Chaiworapongsa T, et al. Four-dimensional ultrasonography of the fetal heart with spatiotemporal image correlation. *Am J Obstet Gynecol* 2003;189:1792–1802.
10. Arzt W, Tulzer G, Aigner M. Real time 3D sonography of the normal fetal heart–clinical evaluation. *Ultraschall Med* 2002;23(6):388–391.
11. Acar P, Laskari C, Rhodes J, et al. Determinants of mitral regurgitation after atrioventricular septal defect surgery: a three-dimensional echocardiographic study. *Am J Cardiol* 1999;83:745–749.
12. Acar P, Dulac Y, Roux D, et al. Comparison of transthoracic and transesophageal three-dimensional echocardiography for assessment of atrial septal defect diameter in children. *Am J Cardiol* 2003;91:500–502.
13. Acar P, Saliba Z, Bonhoeffer P, et al. Influence of atrial septal defect anatomy in patient selection and assessment of closure by the CardioSEAL device: a three-dimensional transesophageal echocardiography. *Eur Heart J* 2000;21:573–581.
14. Marx GR, Fulton DR, Pandian NG, et al. Delineation of site, relative size and dynamic geometry of atrial septal defect by real-time three-dimensional echocardiography. *J Am Coll Cardiol* 1995;25:482–490.
15. Hata T, Shu-Yan D, Eisuke I, et al. Real-time three-dimensional color Doppler fetal echocardiographic features of congenital heart disease. *J Obstet Gynecol Res* 2008;34:670–673.
16. Marx GR. The real deal: real-time 3-D echocardiography in congenital heart diseases. *Pediatr Cardiol Today* 2003;1:9–11.
17. Acar P, Dulac Y, Taktak A, et al. Real-time three-dimensional fetal echocardiography using matrix probe. *Prenat Diagn* 2005;25:370–375.
18. Abuhamad A. Standardization of 3-dimensional volumes in obstetric sonography: a required step for training and automation. *J Ultrasound Med* 2005;24:397–401.
19. Abuhamad A, Falkensammer P, Reichartseder F, et al. Automated retrieval of standard diagnostic fetal cardiac planes in the second trimester of pregnancy: a prospective evaluation of software. *Ultrasound Obstet Gynecol* 2008;31:30–36.
20. Devore GR, Polanco B, Sklansky MS, et al. The 'spin' technique: a new method for examination of the fetal outflow tracts using three-dimensional ultrasound. *Ultrasound Obstet Gynecol* 2004;24:72–82.

21. Chaoui R, Hoffmann J, Heling KS. Three-dimensional (3D) and 4D color Doppler fetal echocardiography using spatiotemporal image correlation (STIC). *Ultrasound Obstet Gynecol* 2004;23:535–545.

22. Paladini D, Vassallo M, Sglavo G, et al. The role of spatio-temporal image correlation (STIC) with tomographic ultrasound imaging (TUI) in the sequential analysis of fetal congenital heart disease. *Ultrasound Obstet Gynecol* 2006;27(5):555–561.

23. Abuhamad A, Falkensammer P, Zhao Y. Automated sonography: defining the spatial relationship of standard diagnostic fetal cardiac planes in the second trimester of pregnancy. *J Ultrasound Med* 2007;26:501–507.

24. Rizzo G, Capponi A, Cavicchioni O, et al. Application of automated sonography on 4-dimensional volumes of fetuses with transposition of the great arteries. *J Ultrasound Med* 2008;27:771–776.

25. Chaoui R, Hoffmann J, Heling KS. Basal cardiac view on 3D/4D fetal echocardiography for the assessment of AV valves and great vessels arrangement. *Ultrasound Obstet Gynecol* 2004;22:228.

26. Espinoza J, Goncalves LF, Lee W, et al. The use of the minimum projection mode in 4-dimensional examination of the fetal heart with spatio-temporal image correlation. *J Ultrasound Med* 2004;23:1337–1348.

27. Goncalves LF, Espinoza J, Lee W, et al. A new approach to fetal echocardiography: digital casts of the fetal cardiac chambers and great vessels for detection of congenital heart disease. *J Ultrasound Med* 2005;24:415–424.

28. Goncalves LF, Espinoza J, Lee W, et al. Three- and four-dimensional reconstruction of the aortic and ductal arches using inversion mode: a new rendering algorithm for visualization of fluid-filled anatomical structures. *Ultrasound Obstet Gynecol* 2004;24:696–698.

29. Lee W, Goncalves LF, Espinoza J, et al. Inversion mode: a new volume analysis tool for 3-dimensional ultrasonography. *J Ultrasound Med* 2005;24:201–207.

30. Goncalves LF, Espinoza J, Romero R, et al. A systematic approach to prenatal diagnosis of transposition of the great arteries using 4-dimensional ultrasonography with spatiotemporal image correlation. *J Ultrasound Med* 2004;23:1225–1231.

31. Volpe P, Campobasso G, Stanziano A, et al. Novel application of 4D sonography with B-flow imaging and spatio-temporal image correlation (STIC) in the assessment of the anatomy of pulmonary arteries in fetuses with pulmonary atresia and ventricular septal defect. *Ultrasound Obstet Gynecol* 2006;28:40–46.

32. Vinals F, Poblete P, Giuliano A. Spatio-temporal image correlation (STIC): a new tool for the prenatal screening of congenital heart defects. *Ultrasound Obstet Gynecol* 2003;22:388–394.

33. Vinals F, Mandujano L, Vargas G, et al. Prenatal diagnosis of congenital heart disease using four-dimensional spatiotemporal image correlation (STIC) telemedicine via an Internet link: a pilot study. *Ultrasound Obstet Gynecol* 2005;25:25–31.

34. Meyer-Wittkopf M, Cole A, Cooper SG, et al. Three-dimensional quantitative echocardiographic assessment of ventricular volume in healthy human fetuses and in fetuses with congenital heart disease. *J Ultrasound Med* 2001;20:317–327.

35. Esh-Broder E, Ushakov FB, Imbar T, et al. Application of free-hand three-dimensional echocardiography in the evaluation of fetal cardiac ejection fraction: a preliminary study. *Ultrasound Obstet Gynecol* 2004;23:546–551.

36. Messing B, Rosenak D, Valsky DV, et al. 3D inversion mode combined with spatiotemporal image correlation (STIC): a novel technique for fetal heart ventricle volume quantification [Abstract]. *Ultrasound Obstet Gynecol* 2006;28:397.

FETAL ECHOCARDIOGRAPHY IN EARLY GESTATION

 ## INTRODUCTION

The prenatal diagnosis of cardiac malformations has been traditionally limited to the mid-second and third trimesters of pregnancy. The first description of a fetal cardiac anomaly at 11 weeks' gestation occurred 20 years ago (1) and since then several studies reported on the detection of cardiac anomalies in the late first and early second trimesters of pregnancy by the transvaginal and the transabdominal ultrasound approach (2–6). The ability to image the fetal heart in early gestation with sufficient clarity to make a diagnosis of a cardiac malformation was made possible by the advent of high-resolution transvaginal and transabdominal probes (Figs. 10-1 and 10-2). The widespread adoption of first trimester risk assessment with nuchal translucency and other first trimester ultrasound markers increased interest in early fetal echocardiography. Nuchal translucency screening allowed for the detection of fetuses with chromosomal abnormalities in the first trimester with associated cardiac defects (7). Furthermore, an enlarged nuchal translucency is a risk factor for cardiac malformations (7–10).

Discrepancy exists in the literature with regard to the gestational age window, which warrants the term *early fetal echocardiography*. Some authors consider a targeted cardiac examination prior to 16 weeks' gestation as early echocardiography (2), whereas others have established the nuchal translucency gestational age window of 11 to 13^{+6} weeks for early echocardiography (3). Nevertheless, most practitioners consider a targeted cardiac examination performed in the first and early second trimester window (10 to 16 weeks) as early fetal echocardiography (4).

Sufficient data on the efficacy of early fetal echocardiography have been mounting, and this examination is now considered an integral part of fetal cardiology in several centers with expertise in this area. In this book, we have integrated in each chapter discussing specific cardiac malformation a separate section on the detection of the abnormality in early gestation. In this chapter, we discuss basic and technical aspects related to the early fetal cardiac examination in addition to common indications and potential limitations of early fetal echocardiography.

 ## TRANSVAGINAL VERSUS TRANSABDOMINAL ROUTE

It is widely accepted that the transvaginal ultrasound (TVUS) examination of the fetus is superior to the transabdominal approach in early gestation as the former provides enhanced image resolution and quality. Disadvantages of the TVUS cardiac examination include the inconvenience involved in the preparation of the vaginal probe and its sterilization after the examination is completed and the added skills required by the operator (4). The tilting range of the probe is limited in TVUS and the operator should be familiar with manipulating the probe in one hand and the uterus in the other hand in order to optimize the approach to the fetal chest if needed. The most optimum fetal position is the low transverse position, which explains why the best TVUS examination is achieved before 13 weeks' gestation (crown-rump length <70 mm), when the uterine size is still small and the fetus often lies in a transverse position. Beyond 13 weeks, the fetus commonly assumes a longitudinal position, and the approach to the heart is thus limited by the reduced depth of the high-resolution transvaginal probe. In our experience, fetal cardiac imaging performed by the TVUS approach is achievable and reliable in most cases between 12 and 13 weeks (crown-rump length 60 to 70 mm). After 13 weeks, the transabdominal route provides excellent quality with the latest transducers, assuming the fetus is examined in a dorsoposterior position.

We recommend an approach that is targeted to the gestational age, maternal body habitus, and the position of the fetus in utero. A combined transvaginal and transabdominal approach may be required in some cases.

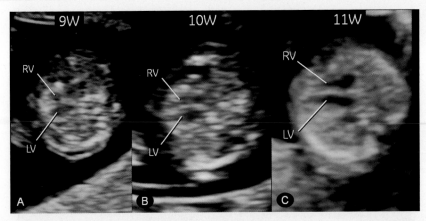

Figure 10-1. Transverse four-chamber views in three normal fetuses at 9+4 **(A)**; 10+3 **(B)**; and 11+2 **(C)** weeks' gestation as demonstrated by transvaginal ultrasound. The lumen of right (RV) and left (LV) ventricle separated by the interventricular septum can be clearly identified by the lateral insonation. From 11 weeks' gestation and beyond (C), the image quality under optimum conditions becomes of such clarity that reliable diagnoses can be expected.

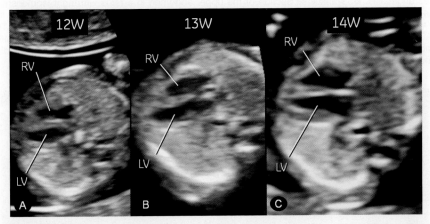

Figure 10-2. Transverse four-chamber views in three normal fetuses at 12+4 **(A)**; 13 **(B)**; and 14+4 **(C)** weeks' gestation. Fetus at 12 (A) weeks' gestation was examined transvaginally, while both fetuses at 13 (B) and 14 (C) weeks' gestation were examined by high-resolution transabdominal probe (4 to 8 MHz). The switch from a transvaginal to a transabdominal approach can be achieved between 12 and 13 weeks' gestation in most cases. LV, left ventricle; RV, right ventricle.

CARDIAC PLANES IN GRAY SCALE AND COLOR DOPPLER

A transverse view of the fetal abdomen (Fig. 10-3) and the four-chamber view (Fig. 10-4) are reliably achieved with two-dimensional gray scale in early gestation. Abnormal cardiac anatomy at the level of the four-chamber view can be clearly demonstrated as early as 12 weeks' gestation under optimal scanning conditions (Fig. 10-5). In many cases, the anatomic orientation of the right and left ventricular outflow tracts are not reliably seen due to their small size. By changing the insonation angle and aligning the great vessels in a transverse position, the lumen of the vessel can be better delineated (Fig. 10-6).

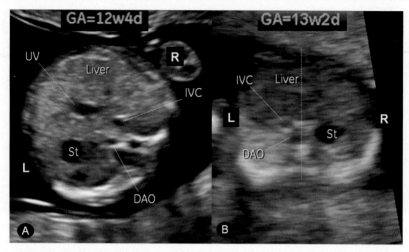

Figure 10-3. A: Transverse section of the upper abdomen in a normal fetus at 12+4 weeks' gestation imaged by high-resolution transvaginal ultrasound. The stomach (St) and the descending aorta (DAO) are left-sided, while the inferior vena cava (IVC) and liver are right sided. The umbilical vein (UV) can also be identified. This plane is visualized routinely in order to exclude situs anomalies. **B:** Transverse section of the upper abdomen in a fetus with right isomerism at 13+2 weeks' gestation imaged with high-resolution transabdominal scanning. The stomach (St) is right-sided, whereas the aorta (DAO), inferior vena cava (IVC), and liver are left-sided. The DAO and IVC are on the same side (called juxtaposition), suggesting the presence of situs ambiguous with right isomerism (see also Chapter 22). This fetus also had a complex cardiac defect, L, left; R, right.

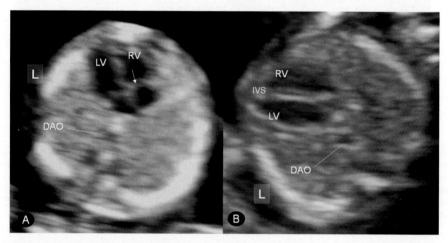

Figure 10-4. Apical **(A)** and axial **(B)** planes of the four-chamber view at 13 weeks' gestation in two normal fetuses imaged transabdominally. Note the more apical insertion of the septal leaflet of the tricuspid valve (*arrow*) in A. Descending aorta (DAO) is seen in both planes and the interventricular spetum (IVS) is most optimally seen in the axial or transverse plane (B). LV, left ventricle; RV, right ventricle; L, left.

Color or high-definition power Doppler provides significant advantages in cardiac imaging in early gestation by demonstrating blood flow events in addition to flow direction. The color or high-definition power Doppler filling of an apical or basal four-chamber view separated by the septum is a good adjunct to the gray scale image. We feel that color Doppler at

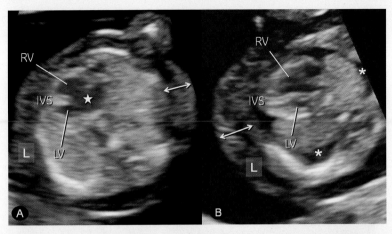

Figure 10-5. Transverse four-chamber views of two fetuses at 12 weeks' gestation with abnormal cardiac anatomy. In fetus **A,** a large atrioventricular septal defect (*star*) is demonstrated in the center of the heart between the right (RV) and left (LV) ventricle. In fetus **B,** ventricular discrepancy is seen with a diminutive left ventricle (LV) in hypoplastic left heart syndrome. Note the presence of skin edema (*double-sided arrow*) in both fetuses and pleural effusion (*asterisk*) in fetus B. Fetus A had trisomy 21 and fetus B had trisomy 13. IVS, interventricular septum; L, left.

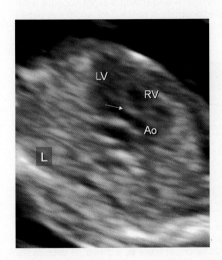

Figure 10-6. Left ventricular outflow tract in a normal fetus at 13 weeks' gestation. Note the continuity of the medial wall of the aorta (Ao) with the ventricular septum (*arrow*). The lumen of the ascending aorta is best demonstrated in an insonating angle that is almost perpendicular to its course. LV, left ventricle; RV, right ventricle; L, left.

the level of the four-chamber view in early fetal echocardiography is essential in identifying normal and abnormal cardiac anatomy (Figs. 10-7 and 10-8). Color or high-definition power Doppler demonstration of the upper transverse views in the chest including the three-vessel-trachea and the transverse ductal views is, however, superior to what can be provided by the two-dimensional evaluation alone (Fig. 10-9). Aortic and ductal arches are more easily recognized in their anatomic location, size, patency, and blood flow direction. Several cardiac abnormalities involving the outflow tracts can be recognized in the three-vessel-trachea view, and a right aortic arch can also be clearly identified. Color or high-definition power Doppler is also superior to gray-scale imaging in the demonstration of aortic and ductal arches in early gestation (Fig. 10-10) and the right and left pulmonary veins draining into the left atrium (Fig. 10-11).

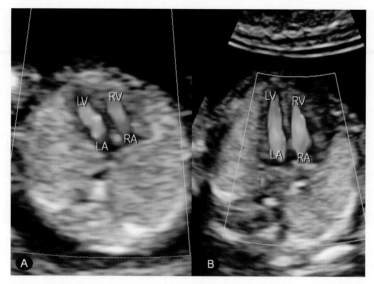

Figure 10-7. Color Doppler of an apical four-chamber view at 12 weeks' gestation by transabdominal **(A)** and transvaginal **(B)** ultrasound examination demonstrating diastolic flow from both right (RA) and left (LA) atrium into right (RV) and left (LV) ventricle, respectively. Note that the information provided by color Doppler is very similar in both A and B with a slight superior resolution by the transvaginal approach (B). When a cardiac anomaly is suspected, additional details may be provided by the transvaginal approach.

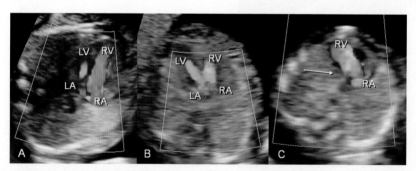

Figure 10-8. Abnormal apical four-chamber views in color Doppler in three fetuses with cardiac anomalies at 12 to 13 weeks' gestation. In fetus **A,** discrepant ventricular chamber size is seen with a diminutive left ventricle in a case of aortic coarctation. In fetus **B,** a defect is seen in the center of the heart (single color channel) in a case of atrioventricular septal defect. In fetus **C,** a single chamber (right ventricle) is perfused on color Doppler in a case of hypoplastic left heart syndrome (*arrow* points to the hypoplastic left ventricle). RV, right ventricle; LV, left ventricle; RA, right atrium; LA, left atrium.

 CARDIAC AXIS IN EARLY GESTATION

Evaluation of the fetal cardiac axis is part of the fetal cardiac examination in the mid-second and third trimesters of pregnancy. In this gestational age window, the normal cardiac axis is defined at a 45-degree angle to the left of the midline with a range of plus or minus 20 degrees (11). Several studies have established an association between an abnormal cardiac axis and congenital heart disease in mid-second and third trimesters of pregnancy (12,13). The specific embryologic event that results in an abnormal cardiac axis in some fetuses with

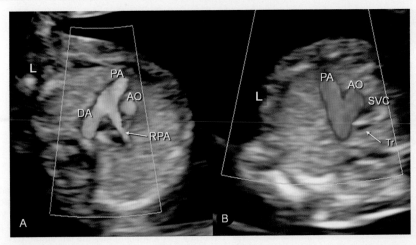

Figure 10-9. Transverse section of the ductal arch **(A)** and the three-vessel-trachea transverse view **(B)** in high-definition power and color Doppler in two normal fetuses at 13 weeks' gestation. These transverse views, which are especially helpful in early gestation, provide critical information on the anatomic relationship of the great vessels and the direction of blood flow. PA, pulmonary artery; AO, aorta; SVC, superior vena cava; DA, ductal arch; RPA, right pulmonary artery; Tr, trachea; L, left.

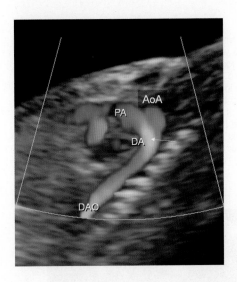

Figure 10-10. Ductal (DA) and aortic arch (AoA) view in color Doppler in a normal fetus at 13 weeks' gestation. Note the presence of high velocities (*arrow*) at the junction of the DA with descending aorta (DAO). PA, pulmonary artery.

cardiac abnormalities is not currently known, however an over-rotation of the bulboventricular loop in early embryogenesis has been proposed as the underlying mechanism (11,12).

Defining the cardiac axis in early gestation may be particularly helpful in identifying congenital heart disease given the limitations involved in fetal cardiac imaging in this gestational window. Based on a prospective study of cardiac axis measurement between 11 and 15 weeks' gestation on 100 fetuses, we have found the cardiac axis to be between 40 and 60 degrees (14) (Fig. 10-12). The cardiac axis tends to be higher (levorotation) at 11 to 12 weeks' compared to 14 to 15 weeks' gestation in normal fetuses (14). The use of color or power Doppler is helpful in the technical measurement of the cardiac axis in early gestation by identifying the interventricular septum, which can then guide the accurate placement of the intersecting angle line (Fig. 10-13). In our study, 4 of 100 fetuses had abnormal cardiac axis

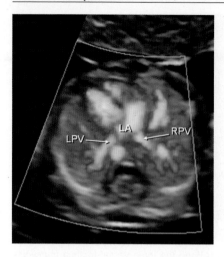

Figure 10-11. Transverse view in high-definition power Doppler in a normal fetus at 12 weeks' gestation at the level of the four-chamber view demonstrating the left (LPV) and right (RPV) pulmonary veins draining into the left atrium (LA).

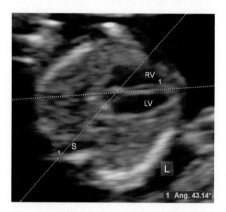

Figure 10-12. Normal cardiac axis in a fetus at 13 weeks' gestation. Cardiac axis is measured in a four-chamber view of the heart by the angle of two lines; the first line starts at the spine (S) posteriorly and ends in mid-chest anteriorly, bisecting the chest into two equal halves (*long dashed line*), the second line runs through the ventricular septum (*short dashed line*). The angle shown in this case is 43 degrees (normal). RV, right ventricle; LV, left ventricle; L, left.

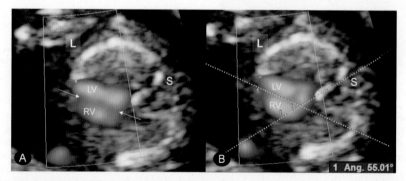

Figure 10-13. Power Doppler at the four-chamber view in a normal fetus at 12 weeks' gestation showing in **plane A** the right (RV) and left (LV) ventricles in bright color separated by a dark line, which represents the interventricular septum (*arrows*). Applying power (or color) Doppler in early gestation helps in the identification of the interventricular septum which aids in cardiac axis measurements as shown in **plane B**. S, spine; L, left.

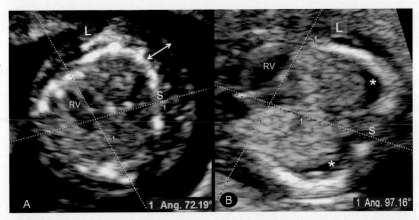

Figure 10-14. Cardiac axis measurements in two fetuses with congenital heart disease and left axis deviations at 13 weeks' gestation. The fetus in **plane A** has tetralogy of Fallot, and the fetus in **plane B** has hypoplastic left heart syndrome. Cardiac axes measurements, which are abnormal in both fetuses, are 72 and 97 degrees in A and B, respectively. Note the presence of hydrops (*double-sided arrow*) in A and bilateral pleural effusion (*asterisk*) in B. RV, right ventricle; S, spine; L, left.

measurements; one with dextrocardia in a fetus with single ventricle and heterotaxy syndrome and three with left axis deviations (>60 degrees). All three fetuses with left axis deviations had congenital heart disease including hypoplastic left heart syndrome, tetralogy of Fallot, and atrioventricular canal defect. Figure 10-14 shows cardiac axis measurements in two fetuses with left axis deviations in early gestation.

BENEFITS AND DISADVANTAGES OF EARLY FETAL ECHOCARDIOGRAPHY

The spectrum of cardiac defects encountered in early gestation differs from that in the second and third trimesters. Some cardiac defects diagnosed in early gestation are associated with hydrops or chromosomal abnormalities, which may result in fetal demise before reaching the second trimester. It is generally believed that cardiac defects that are diagnosed in early gestation are more complex and have a higher association with chromosomal abnormalities than those seen in the second and third trimesters of pregnancy. Early fetal echocardiography provides some benefit to patients such as an early reassurance of a normal heart in patients with a high risk for cardiac defects, and when a major cardiac malformation is diagnosed, the option for first trimester termination is thus available, which carries a significantly lower risk of morbidity than second trimester termination.

Disadvantages of early fetal echocardiography include the need for a repeat targeted cardiac examination in the second trimester when normal cardiac anatomy is seen in early gestation, as several cardiac malformations are more visible at a later gestation such as ventricular septal defects, valve stenosis, and lung vein anomalies, among others. Another disadvantage of early fetal echocardiography is that it requires a skilled and experienced operator who is well versed in early fetal echocardiography. Furthermore, completion of early fetal echocardiography may require a combined transabdominal and a transvaginal approach, which may be time-consuming.

In the absence of associated fetal hydrops, an enlarged nuchal translucency, or extracardiac abnormalities, the authors recommend confirming the diagnosis of a cardiac malformation during serial examinations in order to reduce possible false-positive and false-negative diagnoses. False-positive diagnoses in early fetal echocardiography include ventricular septal defect due to gray-scale echo dropout or color Doppler artifacts, atrioventricular septal defect suspected in a fetus with left superior vena cava and dilated coronary sinus, or discrepant ventricular size in a fetus with tricuspid regurgitation, which may resolve in the second trimester. Furthermore, the wrong orientation in the transvaginal probe may result in the erroneous assumption of abnormal situs in a fetus. False-negative diagnoses include tetralogy of Fallot where pulmonary stenosis is mild, transposition of the great arteries, atrioventricular septal defect, ventricular septal defect, hypoplastic left or right heart syndrome, or anomalies of aortic arch including coarctation and interruption. Detection of abnormal flow patterns over the great vessels is almost always associated with cardiac abnormalities.

 ## INDICATIONS FOR EARLY FETAL ECHOCARDIOGRAPHY

Almost all known indications for fetal echocardiography can be applied for a cardiac examination in early gestation. Based on our experience however, indications for patient referral for early fetal echocardiography are limited and primarily include an enlarged nuchal translucency, a positive family history of a previous child with severe cardiac malformation, or the presence of a major extracardiac malformation detected in the first trimester. With wide application of first trimester screening in recent years, an enlarged nuchal translucency became the most common indication for early fetal echocardiography (see Chapter 3's section on nuchal translucency). When an enlarged nuchal translucency is encountered, we prefer to perform an early fetal echocardiography during the same examination rather than rescheduling the patient at 15 to 16 weeks for a fetal cardiac evaluation. The presence of reverse flow in the ductus venosus or the detection or tricuspid or mitral regurgitation in early gestation are other indications for early fetal echocardiography (15).

 ## SAFETY ASPECTS

Ultrasonography is safe for the fetus when used appropriately and when medical information about a pregnancy is needed; however, ultrasound energy delivered to the fetus cannot be assumed to be completely innocuous, and the possibility exists that such biological effects may be identified in the future (16). Early fetal echocardiography should therefore be performed only when there is a valid medical indication, and the lowest possible ultrasound exposure setting should be used to gain the necessary diagnostic information under the as-low-as-reasonably achievable principle (ALARA) (17,18). Doppler ultrasound, especially pulsed Doppler, is associated with a higher energy than gray-scale or color Doppler imaging and thus its use in the first trimester should be limited to specific indications guided by an abnormal gray-scale or color Doppler evaluation. Furthermore, limiting the duration of the examination and abiding by the safety principles of ultrasound should be established. The authors recommend a cineloop sweep acquisition in color Doppler and after the image is frozen, single images can be retrieved from the cineloop and stored in the image archives. This technique limits the color Doppler time exposure of the fetus. The potential risk should be balanced to the benefit of diagnosis when a complex cardiac malformation is suspected.

■ KEY POINTS: FETAL ECHOCARDIOGRAPHY IN EARLY GESTATION

- ■ Most practitioners consider a targeted cardiac examination performed in the first and early second trimester window (10 to 16 weeks) as early fetal echocardiography.
- ■ The most optimum fetal position for a transvaginal examination of the fetal heart in early gestation is the low transverse position.
- ■ In our experience, fetal cardiac imaging performed by the transvaginal approach is achievable and reliable in most cases between 12 and 13 weeks (crown-rump length 60 to 70 mm).
- ■ The cardiac outflow tracts are best imaged in early gestation when the insonation angle is almost perpendicular to their course.
- ■ Color or high-definition power Doppler provides significant advantages in cardiac imaging in early gestation by demonstrating blood flow events in addition to flow direction.
- ■ Color or high-definition power Doppler demonstration of the upper transverse views in the chest including the three-vessel-trachea and the transverse ductal views is superior to what can be provided by the two-dimensional evaluation alone.

■ We have found the cardiac axis to be between 40 and 60 degrees between 11 and 15 weeks' gestation.

■ It is generally believed that cardiac defects that are diagnosed in early gestation are more complex and have a higher association with chromosomal abnormalities than those seen in the second and third trimesters of pregnancy.

■ Disadvantages of early fetal echocardiography include the need for a repeat targeted cardiac examination in the second trimester when normal cardiac anatomy is seen in early gestation.

■ Early fetal echocardiography should therefore be performed only when there is a valid medical indication, and the lowest possible ultrasound exposure setting should be used.

References

1. Gembruch U, Knopfle G, Chatterjee M, et al. First-trimester diagnosis of fetal congenital heart disease by transvaginal two-dimensional and Doppler echocardiography. *Obstet Gynecol* 1990;75:496–498.
2. Bronshtein M, Zimmer EZ, Milo S, et al. Fetal cardiac abnormalities detected by transvaginal sonography at 12–16 weeks gestation. *Obstet Gynecol* 1991;78:374–378.
3. Becker R, Wegner RD. Detailed screening for fetal anomalies and cardiac defects at the 11–13-week scan. *Ultrasound Obstet Gynecol* 2006;27:613–618.
4. Yagel S, Achiron R. First and early second trimester fetal heart screening. In: Yagel S, Silvermann N, Gembruch U, eds. *Fetal cardiology*. London: Martin Dunitz, 2003;160–168.
5. Achiron R, Weissman A, Rotstein Z, et al. Transvaginal echocardiographic examination of the fetal heart between 13 and 15 weeks' gestation in a low-risk population. *J Ultrasound Med* 1994;13:783–789.
6. Simpson JM, Jones A, Callaghan N, et al. Accuracy and limitations of transabdominal fetal echocardiography at 12–15 weeks of gestation in a population at high risk for congenital heart disease. *BJOG* 2000;107:1492–1497.
7. Hyett J, Perdu M, Sharland G, et al. Using fetal nuchal translucency to screen for major congenital cardiac defects at 10–14 weeks of gestation: population based cohort study. *BMJ* 1999;318:81–85.
8. Makrydimas G, Sotiriadis A, Huggon IC, et al. Nuchal translucency and fetal cardiac defects:a pooled analysis of major fetal echocardiography centers. *Am J Obstet Gynecol* 2005;192:89–95.
9. Huggon IC, Ghi T, Cook AC, et al. Fetal cardiac abnormalities identified prior to 14 weeks' gestation. *Ultrasound Obstet Gynecol* 2002;20:22–29.
10. Lynn S, Malone F, Bianchi D, et al.; for the First and Second Trimester Evaluation of Risk Research Consortium. Nuchal translucency and the risk of congenital heart disease. *Obset Gynecol* 2007(109, Pt 1):376–383.
11. Comstock CH. Normal fetal heart axis and position. *Obstet Gynecol* 1987;70:255.
12. Crane JM, Ash K, Fink N, et al. Abnormal fetal cardiac axis in the detection of intrathoracic anomalies and congenital heart disease. *Ultrasound Obstet Gynecol* 1997;10:90–93.
13. Smith RS, Comstock CH, Kirk JS, et al. Ultrasonographic left cardiac axis deviation: a marker for fetal anomalies. *Obstet Gynecol* 1995;85:187–191.
14. Sinkovskaya ES, Horton S, Berkley EMF, et al. Fetal cardiac axis in the first and early second trimester of pregnancy. Paper presented at: 19th World Congress on Ultrasound in Obstetrics and Gynecology, September 2009, Hamburg.
15. Matias A, Huggon I, Areias JC, et al. Cardiac defects in chromosomally normal fetuses with abnormal ductus venosus blood flow at 10–14 weeks. *Ultrasound Obstet Gynecol* 1999;14:307–310.
16. Abramowicz JS, Fowlkes JB, Skelly AC, et al. Conclusions regarding epidemiology for obstetric ultrasound. *J Ultrasound Med* 2008;27:637–644.
17. American Institute of Ultrasound in Medicine. *Medical ultrasound safety*. Laurel, MD: AIUM, 1994; reapproved 2002.
18. Duck FA. Is it safe to use diagnostic ultrasound during the first trimester? *Ultrasound Obstet Gynecol* 1999;13:385–388.

AORTIC STENOSIS AND CRITICAL AORTIC STENOSIS

Definition, Spectrum of Disease, and Incidence

Aortic stenosis is defined as narrowing at the level of the aortic valve leading to an obstruction of left ventricular outflow (Fig. 11-1). The stenosis is classified as valvular, subvalvular, or supravalvular according to the anatomic location of the obstruction in relation to the aortic valve. Valvular aortic stenosis is the most common type diagnosed prenatally; the other two are rarely encountered on prenatal ultrasound, especially in an isolated form.

In valvular aortic stenosis, the valve leaflets are dysplastic and are either tricuspid with fused commissures, bicuspid, unicuspid, or noncommissural. The spectrum of aortic stenosis varies from an isolated mild lesion, *mild aortic stenosis* (Fig. 11-1A), to a severe lesion, *critical aortic stenosis*, which may lead to a secondary dysfunction of the left ventricle, signs of endocardial fibroelastosis, and hypoplastic left heart syndrome (Fig. 11-1B). Figure 11-2 demonstrates an anatomic specimen of critical aortic stenosis with endocardial fibroelastosis, and Table 11-1 lists differentiating characteristics of mild and critical aortic stenosis.

Aortic stenosis occurs in 3% to 6% of structural heart defects and is more common in boys, with a ratio of 3:1 to 5:1 (1–3). Isolated mild aortic stenosis is rare in fetal series, whereas critical aortic stenosis is more common and easily detectable due to the abnormal four-chamber anatomy (4) (Figs. 11-1B and 11-2). Bicuspid aortic valve, which occurs in about 1% of the population and represents one of the most common congenital heart malformations, can be detected prenatally and is not associated with hemodynamic abnormalities in the absence of aortic stenosis (5).

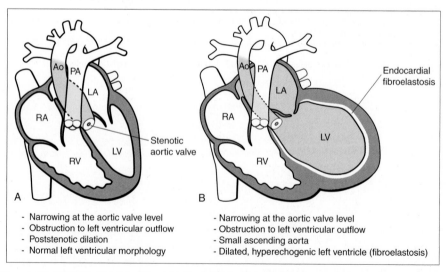

- Narrowing at the aortic valve level
- Obstruction to left ventricular outflow
- Poststenotic dilation
- Normal left ventricular morphology

- Narrowing at the aortic valve level
- Obstruction to left ventricular outflow
- Small ascending aorta
- Dilated, hyperechogenic left ventricle (fibroelastosis)

Figure 11-1. Aortic stenosis **(A)** and critical aortic stenosis **(B)**. RV, right ventricle; LV, left ventricle; RA, right atrium; LA, left atrium; PA, pulmonary artery; Ao, aorta.

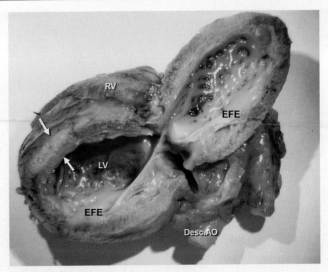

Figure 11-2. Anatomic specimen of a fetal heart with critical aortic stenosis. The lateral left ventricular (LV) wall is open, demonstrating the thickened and echogenic endocardium (*arrows*). Desc AO, descending aorta; RV, right ventricle; EFE, endocardial fibroelastosis.

Ultrasound Findings

Gray Scale (Mild Aortic Stenosis)
Mild aortic stenosis is difficult to detect prenatally due to a normal four-chamber anatomy in the majority of cases (Fig. 11-3). The typical left ventricular myocardial hypertrophy found postnatally is occasionally noted in late gestation. The five-chamber view may show a poststenotic dilation of the ascending aorta (Fig. 11-4). At the level of the aortic valve, thickened valve leaflets, doming of the cusps, and lack of complete valve opening during systole may be observed (Fig. 11-4). A cross section at the level of the aortic valve (short axis of right ventricle) may show the number of cusps and the presence of any thickening of the commissures (5) (Fig. 11-5).

Color Doppler (Mild Aortic Stenosis)
The detection of mild aortic stenosis is mainly achieved by the routine use of color Doppler with the detection of turbulent flow across the aortic valve (Fig. 11-6). Pulsed Doppler reveals high peak systolic velocities of greater than 200 cm/sec (Fig. 11-7). The three-vessel view on color Doppler shows a turbulent antegrade flow through a normal-size aortic arch (Fig. 11-8).

TABLE 11-1	Differentiating Characteristics of Mild and Critical Aortic Stenosis	
	Mild aortic stenosis	**Critical aortic stenosis**
Aortic valve	Thickened	Thickened
Systolic aortic flow	Antegrade turbulent	Antegrade turbulent
LV size	Normal	Dilated
LV contractility	Normal	Reduced
LV wall echogenicity	Normal	Hyperechogenic (fibroelastosis)
Mitral flow	Antegrade	Short diastole and mitral regurgitation
Aortic isthmus flow	Antegrade flow	Partially reverse flow
Foramen ovale	Right-to-left shunt	Left-to-right shunt when mitral regurgitation
LV, left ventricle.		

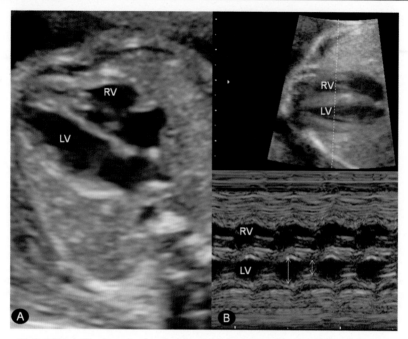

Figure 11-3. Mild aortic stenosis showing a normal four-chamber view **(A)** and normal contractility of the left and right ventricle (LV, RV) on M-mode tracing **(B).**

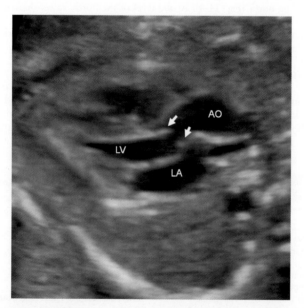

Figure 11-4. Parasagittal long-axis view of the ascending aorta in a fetus with mild (simple) aortic stenosis. Poststenotic dilation of the ascending aorta (AO) is noted. The incomplete opening of the aortic valve in systole with doming is recognized (*arrows*). The four-chamber view of this fetus is shown in Figure 11-3. LA, left atrium; LV, left ventricle.

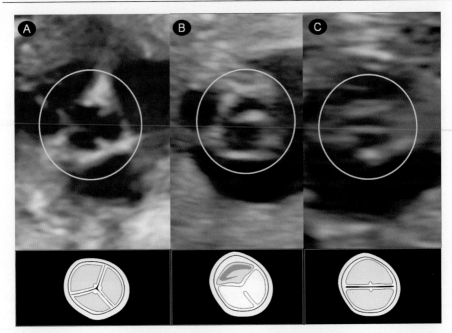

Figure 11-5. Short-axis view at the level of the aortic root. **A:** The three leaflets in a normal aortic valve. **B:** Thickened and fused valve leaflets in a fetus with mild aortic stenosis. **C:** A bicuspid aortic valve in a fetus with a ventricular septal defect and coarctation of the aorta.

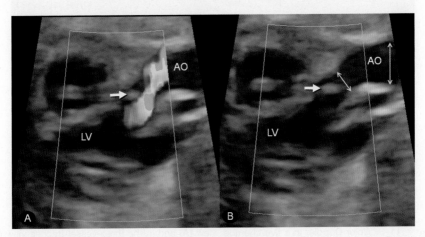

Figure 11-6. Parasagittal long-axis view of the left ventricular outflow tract in color Doppler **(A)** and two-dimensional image **(B)** in a fetus with mild aortic stenosis. A demonstrates color Doppler turbulence in the ascending aorta (AO) during systole (*white arrow*). B shows the corresponding two-dimensional image, which demonstrates limited excursion of the thickened aortic valve (*white arrow*) with poststenotic dilation (*yellow arrows*). Cross section of the thickened aortic root is shown in Figure 11-5B. LV, left ventricle.

Gray Scale (Critical Aortic Stenosis)

Critical aortic stenosis is typically associated with an abnormal four-chamber view where the left ventricle is dilated and more circular with reduced contractility (Fig. 11-9). Commonly, the left ventricular wall is echogenic, a sign of endocardial fibroelastosis (Fig. 11-9). The left atrium may be dilated due to mitral valve regurgitation. The five-chamber view shows a

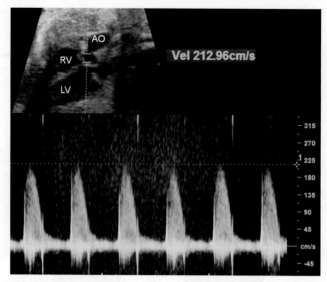

Figure 11-7. Pulsed Doppler interrogation of the aortic valve in a fetus with mild aortic stenosis showing high peak velocities (212 cm/sec). LV, left ventricle; RV, right ventricle; AO, aorta.

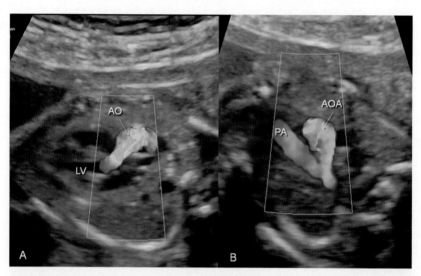

Figure 11-8. Color Doppler in a five-chamber view **(A)** and in the three-vessel-trachea view **(B)** in a fetus with mild aortic stenosis showing typical turbulent flow. Cross section of the aortic valve and parasagittal long axis of the aorta in the same fetus are shown in Figures 11.5B and 11.6. LV, left ventricle; AO, aorta; AOA, aortic arch; PA, pulmonary artery.

narrow aortic root (Fig. 11-10) with reduced movement of valve leaflets. The ascending aorta may show poststenotic dilation or narrowing (Fig. 11-10).

Color Doppler (Critical Aortic Stenosis)
Color Doppler at the level of the four-chamber view shows right and left ventricular filling during diastole with mitral valve regurgitation in systole (Fig. 11-11). In severe cases, reduced filling of the left ventricle is seen with left-to-right shunting at the level of the foramen ovale.

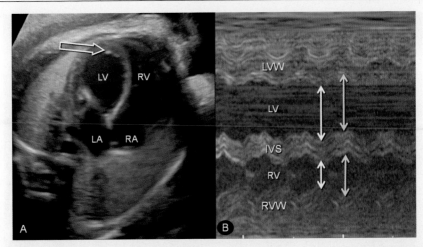

Figure 11-9. Four-chamber view **(A)** and M-mode display **(B)** in a fetus with critical aortic stenosis. A shows the left ventricle (LV) dilated and globular in shape, with echogenic dots in its wall (*arrow*) representing initial stages of endocardial fibroelastosis. M-mode tracing is shown in B demonstrating hypocontractile LV in comparison to the right ventricle (RV). Ventricular width is nearly identical in the LV in systole (*white arrow*) and diastole (*yellow arrow*) in contrast to that of the RV. IVS, interventricular septum; LVW, left ventricular wall; RVW, right ventricular wall; RA, right atrium; LA, left atrium.

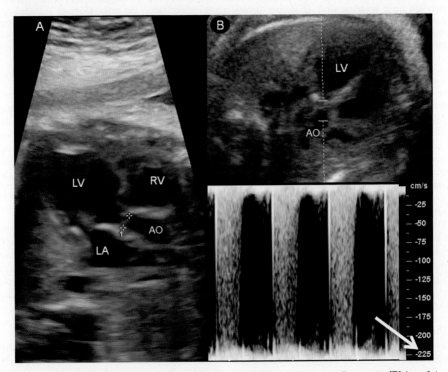

Figure 11-10. Five-chamber view **(A)** and pulsed Doppler of the ascending aorta **(B)** in a fetus with critical aortic stenosis, demonstrating dilated dysfunctional left ventricle (LV), narrow aortic root, and poststenotic dilation of the ascending aorta (AO). Pulsed Doppler interrogation (B) shows antegrade turbulent blood flow with high velocities (>225 cm/sec) (*arrow*). Unlike hypoplastic left heart syndrome, forward flow in the aorta is commonly present in critical aortic stenosis. LA, left atrium; RV, right ventricle.

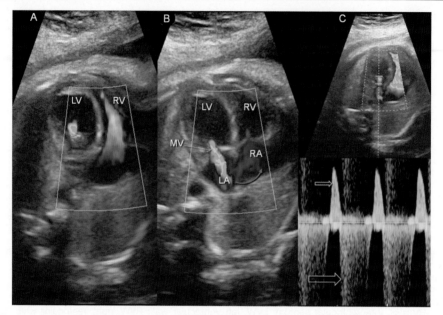

Figure 11-11. Color **(A,B)** and pulsed Doppler **(C)** across the mitral valve (MV) in a fetus with critical aortic stenosis. A shows reduced diastolic filling into the left ventricle (LV) in comparison with the right ventricle (RV). B shows severe mitral regurgitation on color Doppler with left-to-right shunting across the foramen ovale (*curved arrow*). C demonstrates monophasic mitral inflow in diastole (*small arrow*) and severe holosystolic mitral regurgitation (*large arrow*). LA, left atrium; RA, right atrium.

In the five-chamber view turbulent antegrade flow is found in the ascending aorta with reverse flow in late systole and diastole in severe cases. Pulsed Doppler interrogation of the mitral valve shows, in severe cases, an abnormal monophasic mitral flow pattern with short diastolic filling (Fig. 11-11). Peak velocities across the aortic valve in the second half of gestation are generally high (>200 cm/sec) but may also be reduced (between 80 and 200 cm/sec). Reduction in systolic peak velocities on follow-up examination may be considered a sign of left ventricular dysfunction (6). Color Doppler at the three-vessel view may show reverse flow in the aortic isthmus in late systole and diastole in severe cases.

Early Gestation
The diagnosis of mild aortic stenosis has been reported in early gestation (7). The authors have also diagnosed two fetuses with mild aortic stenosis by demonstrating elevated peak systolic velocities across the aortic valves (>100 cm/sec) as compared to normal velocities across the pulmonary valves (30 cm/sec) (Fig. 11-12). Poststenotic dilation of the aortic root was already noted in one of the cases (Fig. 11-12). Critical aortic stenosis with a dilated echogenic hypocontractile left ventricle can be easily recognized in early gestation during targeted cardiac evaluation.

Three-dimensional Ultrasound
Tomographic ultrasound imaging of a three-dimensional (3-D) volume can demonstrate various features of aortic stenosis by displaying multiple planes at different anatomic levels. Application of spatio-temporal image correlation (STIC) allows for evaluation of ventricular anatomy and contractility and can be used to monitor progress of disease. Surface-rendering mode combined with STIC can be used to obtain an *en face* plane of the stenotic aortic valve. This is better achieved in the third trimester, but shadowing from the ribs can be a limiting factor. Rendering of the ventricular volume using inversion mode can also be of help in the

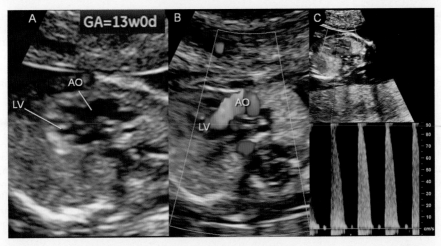

Figure 11-12. Transvaginal ultrasound at 13 weeks' gestation in a fetus with mild aortic stenosis. Note the dilated ascending aorta (AO) **(A)** with turbulent flow on color Doppler **(B)** and high aortic flow velocities on pulsed Doppler **(C)**. Ultrasound findings in this fetus at 25 weeks' gestation are shown in Figures 11.5B and 11.6. LV, left ventricle.

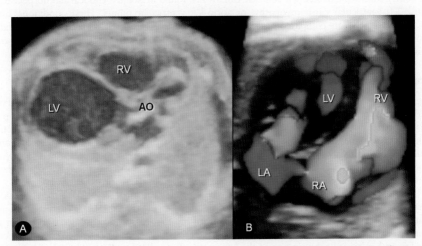

Figure 11-13. Three-dimensional ultrasound of two fetuses with critical aortic stenosis. **A:** A dilated left ventricle (LV) in surface mode with a narrow aortic root (AO). **B:** A glass body mode in a spatio-temporal image correlation (STIC) volume showing limited filling of the dilated left ventricle in diastole in comparison to the right ventricle (RV). LA, left atrium; RA, right atrium.

differentiation of the contractility between the right and left ventricles. Figure 11-13 demonstrates rendering of three-dimensional ultrasound volumes in two fetuses with critical aortic stenosis.

Associated Cardiac and Extracardiac Findings

Associated cardiac malformations occur in about 20% of patients with aortic stenosis including ventricular septal defect, coarctation of the aorta, and patent ductus arteriosus (postnatally) (8). In some cases, aortic stenosis progresses toward hypoplastic left heart syndrome. A rare subgroup of aortic stenosis is the Shone complex, which is a combination of left ventricular inflow and outflow obstruction with a normally contractile left ventricle. In the prenatal cases of Shone complex, there is a narrowing of the mitral valve orifice with a regular filling of the small, normally contractile left ventricle. Occasionally, the presence of a ventricular septal defect and a narrow aortic valve combined with a narrow aortic arch are suggestive of aortic coarctation.

Extracardiac malformations are uncommon in aortic stenosis and the association with chromosomal abnormalities is rare. If karyotyping is offered, consider screening for Williams-Beuren syndrome (deletion 7q11.23, see Table 2-6) given its association with aortic stenosis. The combination of aortic stenosis with extracardiac findings such as renal anomalies, nuchal thickening, or hydrops may suggest the presence of Turner syndrome (see Table 2-4).

Differential Diagnosis

Mild Aortic Stenosis

High velocities or turbulent flow across the aortic valve may be present in other cardiac anomalies such as tetralogy of Fallot, pulmonary atresia with ventricular septal defect, and common arterial trunk. A dilated root of a vessel (pulmonary artery) in the five-chamber view in complete transposition of the great arteries may mimic the poststenotic dilation occasionally noted in aortic stenosis. Aortic stenosis can also be present in fetuses with a congenital heart block due to maternal autoantibodies. Normal aortic flow on color and Doppler evaluation does not rule out mild aortic stenosis in midgestation.

Critical Aortic Stenosis

Critical aortic stenosis and some forms of hypoplastic left heart syndrome constitute a continuum and thus, hypoplastic left heart syndrome should be considered in the differential diagnosis (9). The poorly contractile dilated left ventricle can also be found in isolated endocardial fibroelastosis, dilative left ventricular cardiomyopathy, or aorto-left ventricular tunnel. These conditions, however, are extremely rare compared to critical aortic stenosis. A short left ventricle is also found in atrioventricular discordance in corrected transposition of the great arteries. Conversely to the critical stenosis, the atrioventricular valves and ventricular filling are normal in these conditions.

Prognosis and Outcome

Prognosis of mild aortic stenosis is generally good, provided it remains mild until birth. Postnatal therapy may include medical management consisting of bacterial endocarditis prophylaxis, exercise restrictions, and close follow-up to monitor progression of valve dysfunction (10). Surgical management includes balloon valvuloplasty. Some cases cannot be adequately treated by balloon valvuloplasty and a surgical commissurotomy is then performed (11). Aortic valve replacement is also required in some cases. Options for aortic valve replacement include the pulmonary valve (Ross-Kono operation), homograft, or prosthetic valve.

In utero follow-up of aortic stenosis is recommended, at an interval of 2 to 4 weeks, in order to identify progression and worsening of the disease (11) (Fig. 11-14). Progression of aortic stenosis to hypoplastic left heart syndrome from the first to second trimesters and from the second to third trimesters has been reported on numerous occasions (6,7,9,12,13). Reduced contractility and increased echogenicity of the left ventricular wall, as well as a decrease in the peak systolic aortic velocity, can be considered as signs of progression and worsening prognosis.

Recently, the option of catheter intervention in utero to alter the natural course of aortic stenosis has been offered at several institutions (14–17). Investigators have noted that the anatomic characteristics of severe aortic stenosis are not predictive of growth failure of left heart structures, whereas the direction of blood flow across the foramen ovale (left-to-right shunt) and left ventricular diastolic filling (monophasic mitral valve flow) are sensitive parameters for prediction of growth failure of left heart function during later pregnancy (17,18). The authors suggest that these parameters may be used in patient selection for fetal intervention (18). An excellent editorial on this subject is presented elsewhere (19).

■ KEY POINTS: AORTIC STENOSIS

■ Aortic stenosis is defined as narrowing at the level of the aortic valve leading to an obstruction of left ventricular outflow.

■ The stenosis is classified as valvular, subvalvular, or supravalvular according to the anatomic location of the obstruction.

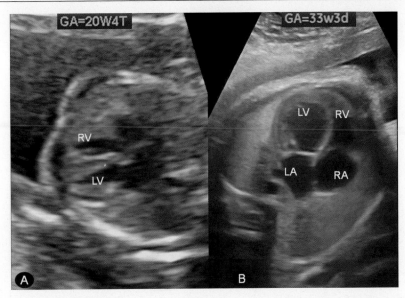

Figure 11-14. Progression of mild aortic stenosis to critical aortic stenosis. **A:** Mild aortic stenosis at 20 weeks' gestation with mitral insufficiency and normal ventricular anatomy and contractility. Follow-up at 33 weeks' gestation **(B)** shows dilated hypocontractile left ventricle (LV) with early-stage endocardial fibroelastosis. RV, right ventricle; LA, left atrium; RA, right atrium.

- Valvular aortic stenosis is the most common type diagnosed prenatally.
- Bicuspid aortic valve, which occurs in about 1% of the population, represents one of the most common congenital heart malformations.
- The five-chamber view may show a poststenotic dilation of the ascending aorta.
- Aortic valve peak systolic velocities are generally more than 200 cm/sec.
- Mild aortic stenosis is associated with a normal four-chamber anatomy in most cases.
- Critical aortic stenosis is typically associated with an abnormal four-chamber view with left ventricular dilation.
- In severe cases, reduced filling of the left ventricle is seen with left-to-right shunting at the level of the foramen ovale.
- Reduction in aortic systolic peak velocities on follow-up examination may be considered a sign of left ventricular dysfunction.
- Associated cardiac malformations occur in about 20% of patients including ventricular septal defect, coarctation of the aorta, and patent ductus arteriosus.
- Extracardiac malformations and chromosomal abnormalities are rare.
- Aortic stenosis is associated with Williams-Beuren syndrome.
- Normal aortic flow on color and Doppler evaluation does not rule out mild aortic stenosis in midgestation.
- Prognosis of mild aortic stenosis is generally good.
- The direction of blood flow across the foramen ovale (left-to-right shunt) and left ventricular diastolic filling (monophasic mitral valve flow) are sensitive parameters for left heart function in late gestation.

HYPOPLASTIC LEFT HEART SYNDROME

Definition, Spectrum of Disease, and Incidence

Hypoplastic left heart syndrome (HLHS) is a spectrum of complex cardiac malformations involving significant underdevelopment of the left ventricle and the left ventricular outflow tract (Fig 11.15), resulting in an obstruction to systemic cardiac output. Two classic forms of HLHS

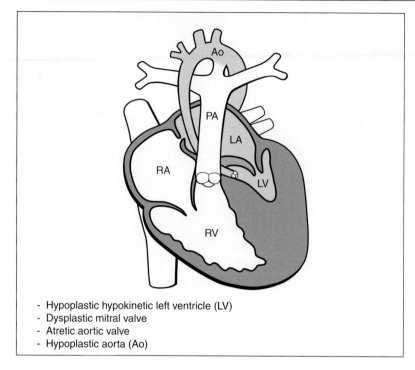

- Hypoplastic hypokinetic left ventricle (LV)
- Dysplastic mitral valve
- Atretic aortic valve
- Hypoplastic aorta (Ao)

Figure 11-15. Hypoplastic left heart syndrome. RA, right atrium; RV, right ventricle; PA, pulmonary artery; LA, left atrium.

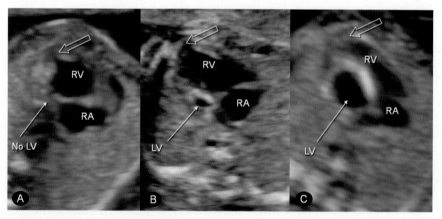

Figure 11-16. Spectrum of hypoplastic left heart syndrome (HLHS) showing absent or hypoplastic left ventricle (LV) **(A,B)** or dilated/normal-size left ventricle **(C).** The cardiac apex is formed by the right ventricle (RV) (*open arrows*) in all cases. RA, right atrium.

exist. One form involves atresia of both the mitral and aortic valves, with no communication between the left atrium and left ventricle and a severely, to nearly absent, hypoplastic left ventricle (Fig. 11-16A,B). The other form involves a patent, often dysplastic, mitral valve with aortic atresia, and a hyperechoic, globular, and poorly contractile left ventricle (Fig. 11-16C). Figure 11-17 shows an anatomic specimen of hypoplastic left heart syndrome.

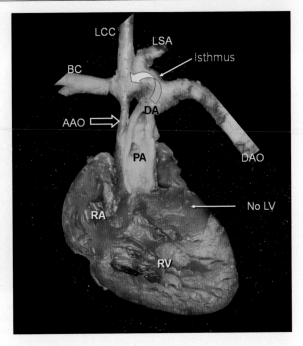

Figure 11-17. Anatomic specimen of a hypoplastic left heart in a fetus. The heart is opened at the level of the four-chamber view, demonstrating the absence of the left ventricle (LV). The ascending aorta (AAO) is hypoplastic in comparison to the dilated main pulmonary artery (PA). Retrograde flow through the ductus arteriosus (DA) provides blood to the aortic arch (*curved arrow*). RA, right atrium; RV, right ventricle; DAO, descending aorta; BC, brachiocephalic; LCC, left common carotid artery; LSA, left subclavian artery.

The reported birth incidence of HLHS is 0.1 to 0.25 per 1000 live births (20). HLHS accounts for 3.8% of all congenital cardiac abnormalities, and up to seven-tenths of cases occur in boys (1,21). Although HLHS is one of the most commonly diagnosed congenital heart abnormalities in utero (4), it is still missed in a significant proportion of fetuses. Recurrence of left-sided congenital heart disease has been reported in the range of 2% to 13% (22).

Ultrasound Findings

Gray Scale

In HLHS the four-chamber view is markedly abnormal with a small, hypokinetic left ventricle (Fig. 11-18). The apex of the heart is therefore predominantly formed by the right ventricle (Fig. 11-18). The size of the left ventricle, however, can vary and can be absent, small, of normal size, or even dilated (Fig. 11-16), but in all cases this ventricle is hypocontractile with absent function. In most cases the aortic valve is atretic, the mitral valve is patent but dysplastic, and the left ventricle is typically globular in shape and hypokinetic, with a bright echogenic inner wall due to the associated endocardial fibroelastosis (Fig. 11-16C). The left atrium is small relative to the right atrial size with a paradoxical movement of the leaflet of the foramen ovale from the left to right atrium. In the five-chamber view, the aortic outflow is difficult to visualize due to its hypoplastic size (<3 mm). At the level of the three-vessel view, the compensatory dilated pulmonary trunk is seen adjacent to the superior vena cava with a nonvisible or hypoplastic transverse aortic arch (Fig. 11-19).

Color Doppler

Color Doppler evaluation demonstrates minimal to absent filling of the left ventricle (Fig. 11-18B). In cases with a patent mitral valve, mitral regurgitation can be found. Typically a left-to-right shunting across the foramen ovale is found, owing to the increased pressure in the left atrium (Fig. 11-20). In the five-chamber view, color Doppler confirms lack of forward flow across the atretic aortic valve. Color Doppler at the level of the three-vessel view shows

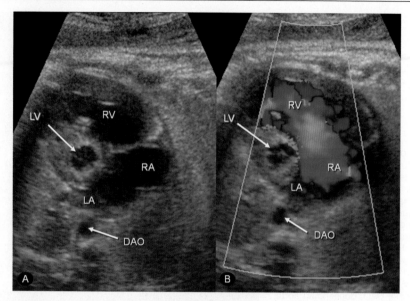

Figure 11-18. Four-chamber view of a hypoplastic left heart syndrome at 22 weeks' gestation in two-dimensional **(A)** and color Doppler **(B)** imaging. Note the diminutive left ventricle (LV) with wall hypertrophy (A) and without blood filling on color Doppler in diastole (B). DAO, descending aorta; RV, right ventricle; RA, right atrium; LA, left atrium.

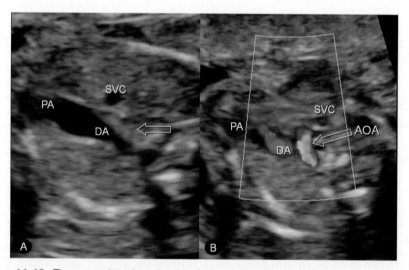

Figure 11-19. Three-vessel-trachea view in a fetus with hypoplastic left heart syndrome in two-dimensional **(A)** and color Doppler **(B)** imaging. In A, the ascending aorta is not visible on two-dimensional ultrasound (*open arrow*). Color Doppler as seen in B aids in the visualization of the aortic arch (AOA) (*open arrow*) with reverse blood flow to that of the ductal arch (DA). PA, pulmonary artery; SVC, superior vena cava.

the reversal of flow across the aortic isthmus and transverse aortic arch, a typical finding in HLHS (Fig. 11-19B). Longitudinal view of the aortic arch with color Doppler confirms the retrograde flow to the aortic root supplied by the pulmonary artery though the ductus arteriosus (Fig. 11-21B).

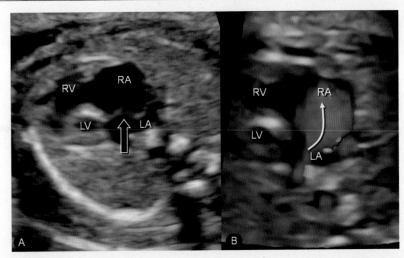

Figure 11-20. Four-chamber view in two-dimensional **(A)** and color Doppler **(B)** imaging in a fetus with hypoplastic left heart syndrome at 21 weeks' gestation. The atrial septum bulges into the right atrium (RA) (*black open arrow*) due to left-to-right shunting at the foramen ovale. B demonstrates left-to-right blood shunting at the foramen ovale on color Doppler (*white curved arrow*). LA, left atrium; LV, left ventricle; RV, right ventricle.

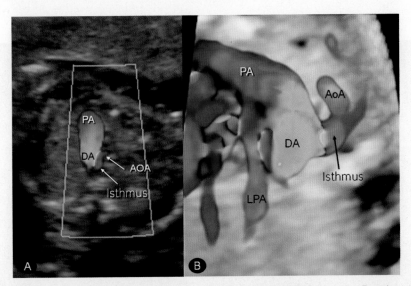

Figure 11-21. A: Reverse flow in the transverse aortic arch (AOA) on color Doppler at the three-vessel-trachea view. **B:** A three-dimensional-rendered image in glass body mode showing a sagittal view of the ductal arch (DA) with retrograde flow across the aortic isthmus (*arrow*) into the aortic arch. LPA, left pulmonary artery; PA, pulmonary artery.

Early Gestation

HLHS is detectable in early gestation at 11 to 14 weeks, primarily in cases with a combined mitral and aortic atresia, showing an absence or severely hypoplastic left ventricle (Fig. 11-22). It has also been shown that HLHS can develop between the first and second trimesters, emphasizing that a normal-appearing four-chamber view at the time of nuchal translucency measurement does not rule out the development of HLHS in later gestation. With this caveat,

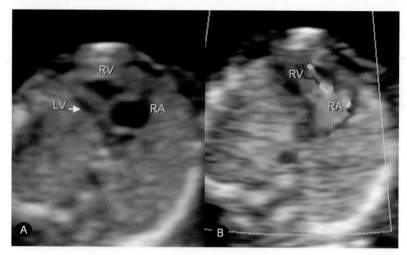

Figure 11-22. Four-chamber view in a fetus with hypoplastic left heart syndrome at 13 weeks' gestation with two-dimensional **(A)** and color Doppler **(B)** imaging. A small left ventricular cavity is seen on two-dimensional ultrasound (A) and absence of mitral inflow is noted on color Doppler during diastole (B). RA, right atrium; RV, right ventricle; LV, left ventricle.

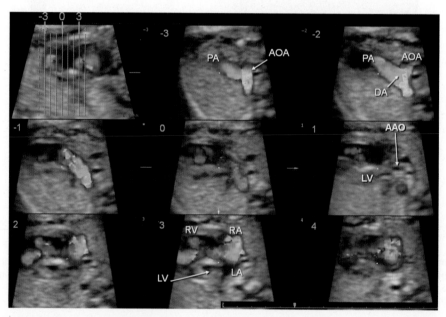

Figure 11-23. Tomographic ultrasound display of a three-dimensional color Doppler spatio-temporal image correlation (STIC) volume in a fetus at 22 weeks' gestation with hypoplastic left heart syndrome (HLHS). Several ultrasound features of HLHS can be demonstrated in this display, including absence of perfusion of the small echogenic left ventricle (LV) (**planes 2, 3**), left-to-right shunting across the interatrial septum (**plane 3**), absence of flow into the ascending aorta (AAO) (**plane 1**), and antegrade flow into the pulmonary artery (PA) and ductus arteriosus (DA) with reverse flow into the isthmus and transverse aortic arch (AOA) (**planes −2, −3**). RA, right atrium; LA, left atrium; RV, right ventricle; LV, left ventricle.

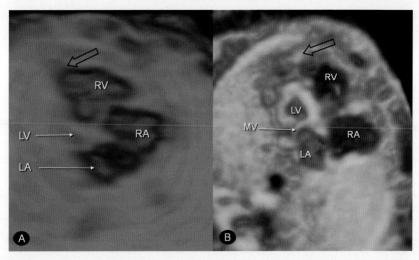

Figure 11-24. Three-dimensional ultrasound in surface mode rendering in two fetuses with hypoplastic left heart syndrome. **A:** A left ventricle (LV) that is nearly absent and a hypoplastic left atrium (LA). **B:** A hypoplastic and hyperechogenic LV with a thickened mitral valve (MV). In both cases the apex of the heart is formed by the right ventricle (*open arrow*). RA, right atrium; RV, right ventricle.

it has been the authors' experience that the diagnosis of HLHS is possible in early gestation. In one case, however, the presence of a stenotic aortic valve with a normal-looking left ventricle at 12 weeks' gestation progressed into HLHS at 19 weeks' gestation. This observation has also been reported by other authors (7).

Three-dimensional Ultrasound
Three-dimensional tomographic imaging combined with color Doppler can demonstrate various anatomic abnormalities of HLHS (23,24) (Fig. 11-23). In addition, 3-D volume rendering of the four-chamber view can emphasize the size of the hypoplastic left chamber, and in the basic cardiac view the hypoplastic aortic root and mitral valve annulus can be better assessed (Fig. 11-24).

Associated Cardiac and Extracardiac Findings

HLHS is associated with a 4% to 5% incidence of chromosomal abnormalities (4,25) such as Turner syndrome, trisomies 13, 18, and others. Extracardiac malformations have been reported in 10% to 25% of infants with HLHS (26,27) with associated genetic syndromes such as Turner syndrome, Noonan syndrome, Smith-Lemli-Opitz syndrome, and Holt-Oram syndrome (26,28). Growth restriction may be seen in fetuses with HLHS probably due to a 20% reduction in combined cardiac output (29).

Differential Diagnosis

Differential diagnosis typically includes cardiac malformations that result in a diminutive left ventricle. The most common cardiac abnormality in this differential diagnosis is coarctation of the aorta, when it is suspected due to a narrow and small left ventricle. Table 11-2 highlights the differentiation between HLHS and coarctation of the aorta. The most challenging differential diagnosis, however, is critical aortic stenosis, which can develop in utero to HLHS (see first section of this chapter). Other abnormalities that should be considered include mitral atresia with a ventricular septal defect, an unbalanced atrioventricular septal defect, double outlet right ventricle, and corrected transposition of great vessels. Detailed discussion on the ultrasound findings associated with these malformations will be presented in their corresponding chapters.

TABLE 11-2	Differentiating Anatomic Characteristics of Hypoplastic Left Heart Syndrome and Coarctation of the Aorta	
Cardiac anatomy	Hypoplastic left heart syndrome	Coarctation of the aorta
LV size	Small	Narrow but normal length
Apex of the heart	Built by right ventricle	Built by left ventricle
LV contractility	Reduced	Normal
LV wall echogenicity	Hyperechogenic (fibroelastosis)	Normal
Mitral flow	Absent or reduced	Normal
Ventricular septal defect	Absent	Occasional
Aortic valve	Atretic	Patent
Aortic arch	Tubular, hypoplastic, tortuous	Narrow either at the isthmus region or tubular hypoplastic
Systolic aortic flow	Absent	Antegrade
Aortic isthmus flow	Reverse flow	Antegrade or partially reverse flow
Foramen ovale	Left-to-right shunt	Right-to-left shunt

LV, left ventricle.

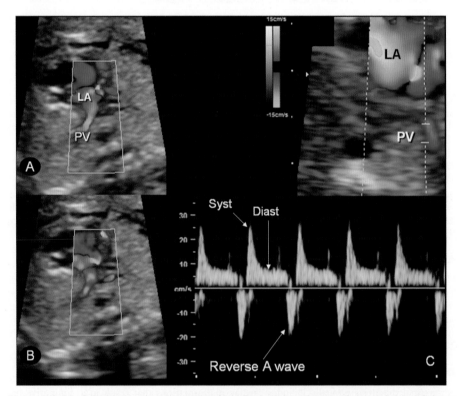

Figure 11-25. Pulmonary vein color and pulsed Doppler in a fetus with hypoplastic left heart syndrome and restrictive foramen ovale. Color Doppler shows bidirectional flow in the pulmonary vein (PV) (**A:** red; **B:** blue). Pulsed Doppler **(C)** shows high systolic velocity (Syst), low diastolic velocity (Diast), and reverse flow during the atrial contraction (reverse A-wave). LA, left atrium.

Prognosis and Outcome

Serial prenatal ultrasound evaluation every 4 to 6 weeks is recommended to assess for fetal growth, tricuspid valve function, and flow across the foramen ovale. The presence of tricuspid

TABLE 11-3	Reconstructive Strategy for Hypoplastic Left Heart Syndrome		
Operation	**Age**	**Procedure**	**Physiologic impact**
Stage I (Norwood operation)	Newborn	• Atrial septectomy • Proximal pulmonary artery to aorta anastomosis • Reconstruction of the aortic arch arising from the right ventricle • Creation of a reliable source for pulmonary blood flow (aorto-pulmonary shunt or right ventri-cle–to–pulmonary artery conduit)	• Right ventricle as the systematic and pulmonic ventricle • Right ventricle volume overload • Peripheral oxygen saturation 75%–85%
Stage II (superior cavopulmonary connection)	4 to 6 mo	• Elimination of shunt or conduit • Anastomosis of superior vena cava to the branch pulmonary arteries (bidirectional Glenn, or hemi-Fontan) • Augmentation of branch pulmo-nary arteries as necessary	• Volume unloading of the right ventricle • Peripheral oxygen saturation 80%–85%
Stage III (Fontan operation)	18 mo to 3 y	• Inferior vena cava flow chan-neled to the pulmonary arteries (Fontan operation, many modifications)	• Increased pulmonary blood flow • Peripheral oxygen saturation >90%

Modified from Rychik J. Hypoplastic left heart syndrome: from in-utero diagnosis to school age. *Semin Fetal Neonatal Med* 2005;10:553–566, with permission.

TABLE 11-4	Morbidities in Children with Hypoplastic Left Heart Syndrome after Fontan Operation	
Morbidity		**Frequency**
Exercise intolerance (varying degrees)		Majority
Arrhythmia (varying degrees)		25%–50%
Thromboembolic disease (e.g., pulmonary embolism, stroke)		Approximately 10%
Protein-losing enteropathy		<5%
Neurocognitive disabilities (e.g., learning differences, attention deficit/hyperactivity disorder) (varying degrees)		10%–70%

(Modified from Rychik J. Hypoplastic left heart syndrome: from in-utero diagnosis to school age. *Semin Fetal Neonatal Med* 2005;10:553–566, with permission.)

valve dysfunction (regurgitation) and/or restriction of flow across the foramen ovale cast a poor prognostic outlook (30). Doppler evaluation of flow pattern in the pulmonary veins is helpful in indirectly assessing the patency of the foramen ovale (31,32) in fetuses with HLHS. The presence of restricted flow across the foramen ovale also casts a poor postnatal prognostic outlook (33), since it reflects a high pressure in the left atrium and is associated with severe pulmonary vascular disease (Fig. 11-25).

Surgical outcome of HLHS has improved in the past 10 years, but this cardiac abnormality is still considered one of the most complex heart malformations, leading to a palliative correction with at least three or more operations. The goal of postnatal palliative treatment of HLHS includes the establishment of an unobstructed systemic cardiac output, a controlled source of pulmonary flow, a reliable source of coronary blood flow, and an unobstructed egress of pulmonary flow across the atrial septum (34). Current modes of therapy include the

Norwood protocol and cardiac transplantation. Given the scarcity of donors and an overall improved outcome of the Norwood protocol reported in several centers, cardiac transplantation, as a treatment option, is offered less commonly to neonates with HLHS. Overall reported infant mortality, while awaiting transplantation, is in the range of 21% to 37% (35). Long-term problems associated with cardiac transplantation include rejection, accelerated atherosclerosis, and chronic infection (36). The Norwood protocol involves three stages, which are described in Table 11-3. Stage 1 survival has been reported to range from 46% to 76%, with some centers reporting a 90% survival (34,36). Survival of stages 2 and 3 are in the range of 95% (34,36). Long-term morbidity in children following a successful Norwood protocol is listed in Table 11-4. Etiology of the neurocognitive disabilities is unclear at this time (37). Possibilities include an association of central nervous system abnormalities with HLHS, hemodynamic instability in the preoperative period, and the effect of the intraoperative perfusion techniques (37,38). Prenatal diagnosis of HLHS has been associated with a lower incidence of perioperative neurologic events in some series (39). Risk factors for increased operative mortality for the Norwood protocol include low birth weight, prematurity, significant extracardiac malformations, severe preoperative obstruction to pulmonary venous return, right ventricular dysfunction, and a small ascending aorta (40–43).

■ KEY POINTS: HYPOPLASTIC LEFT HEART SYNDROME

■ HLHS is a spectrum of complex cardiac malformations involving significant underdevelopment of the left ventricle and the left ventricular outflow tract.

■ HLHS is one of the most commonly diagnosed congenital heart abnormalities in utero.

■ The left ventricle is hypocontractile, small, or absent but can also be of normal size or dilated with no filling on color Doppler.

■ The aortic root is rudimentary and difficult to image on ultrasound.

■ The apex of the heart is predominantly formed by the right ventricle.

■ The foramen ovale bulges into the right atrium with left-to-right shunting on color Doppler.

■ Pulmonary trunk and ductus arteriosus are compensatory dilated.

■ There is reverse flow into the aortic arch in the three-vessel-trachea view or in a longitudinal ductal arch view.

■ HLHS is associated with a 4% to 5% incidence of chromosomal abnormalities such as Turner syndrome, among others.

■ Extracardiac malformations have been reported in 10% to 25% of infants.

■ The presence of tricuspid valve dysfunction (regurgitation) and/or restriction of flow across the foramen ovale cast a poor prognostic outlook.

■ Current modes of therapy include the Norwood protocol and cardiac transplantation.

■ Prenatal diagnosis of HLHS has been associated with a lower incidence of perioperative neurologic events in some series.

References

1. Ferencz C, Rubin JD, Loffredo CA, et al. *Epidemiology of congenital heart disease: the Baltimore-Washington infant study 1981–1989.* Austin, TX: Futura Publishing, 1993;38.
2. Campbell M. The natural history of congenital aortic stenosis. *Br Heart J* 1968;30:514–526.
3. Frank S, Johnson A, Ross J. Natural history of valvular aortic stenosis. *Br Heart J* 1973;35:41–46.
4. Allan LD, Sharland GK, Milburn A, et al. Prospective diagnosis of 1,006 consecutive cases of congenital heart disease in the fetus. *J Am Coll Cardiol* 1994;23:1452–1458.
5. Paladini D, Russo MG, Vassallo M, et al. Ultrasound evaluation of aortic valve anatomy in the fetus. *Ultrasound Obstet Gynecol* 2002;20(1):30–34.
6. Hornberger LK, Sanders SP, Rein AJ, et al. Left heart obstructive lesions and left ventricular growth in the midtrimester fetus. A longitudinal study. *Circulation* 1995;92(6):1531–1538.
7. Axt-Fliedner R, Kreiselmaier P, Schwarze A, et al. Development of hypoplastic left heart syndrome after diagnosis of aortic stenosis in the first trimester by early echocardiography. *Ultrasound Obstet Gynecol* 2006;28(1):106–109.
8. Braunwald E, Goldblatt A, Aygen MM, et al. Congenital aortic stenosis. I. Clinical and hemodynamic findings in 100 patients. II. Surgical and the results of operation. *Circulation* 1963;27:426–462.
9. Sharland GK, Chita SK, Fagg NL, et al. Left ventricular dysfunction in the fetus: relation to aortic valve anomalies and endocardial fibroelastosis. *Br Heart J* 1991;66(6):419–424.
10. Maron BJ, Zipes DP. 36th Bethesda Conference: eligibility recommendations for competitive athletes with cardiovascular abnormalities. *J Am Coll Cardiol* 2005;45:1313–1375.
11. Drury NE, Veldtman GR, Benson LN. Neonatal aortic stenosis. *Expert Rev Cardiovasc Ther* 2005;3(5):831–843.

12. Allan LD, Sharland G, Tynan MJ. The natural history of the hypoplastic left heart syndrome. *Int J Cardiol* 1989;25(3):341–343.

13. Simpson JM, Sharland GK. Natural history and outcome of aortic stenosis diagnosed prenatally. *Heart* 1997;77(3):205–210.

14. Maxwell D, Allan LD, Tynan MJ. Balloon dilatation of the aortic valve in the fetus: a report of two cases. *Br Heart J* 1991;65:256–258.

15. Kohl T, Sharland G, Allan LD, et al. World experience of percutaneous ultrasound-guided balloon valvuloplasty in human fetuses with severe aortic valve obstruction. *Am J Cardiol* 2000;85(10):1230–1233.

16. Gardiner HM. Progression of fetal heart disease and rationale for fetal intracardiac interventions. *Semin Fetal Neonatal Med* 2005;10(6):578–585.

17. Tworetzky W, Wilkins-Haug L, Jennings RW, et al. Balloon dilation of severe aortic stenosis in the fetus: potential for prevention of hypoplastic left heart syndrome: candidate selection, technique, and results of successful intervention. *Circulation* 2004;110(15):2125–2131.

18. Makikallio K, McElhinney DB, Levine JC, et al. Fetal aortic valve stenosis and the evolution of hypoplastic left heart syndrome: patient selection for fetal intervention. *Circulation* 2006;113(11):1401–1405.

19. Kleinman CS. Fetal cardiac intervention Innovative therapy or a technique in search of an indication? *Circulation* 2006;113:1378–1381.

20. Ferencz C, Rubin JD, McCarter RJ, et al. Congenital heart disease: prevalence at livebirth: the Baltimore-Washington infant study. *Am J Epidemiol* 1985;121:31–36.

21. Morris CD, Outcalt J, Menashe VD. Hypoplastic left heart syndrome: natural history in a geographically defined population. *Pediatrics* 1990;85:977–983.

22. Boughman JA, Berg KA, Astemborski JA, et al. Familial risks of congenital heart defects assessed in a population based epidemiologic study. *Am J Med Genet* 1987;26:839–849.

23. Chaoui R, Hoffmann J, Heling KS. Three-dimensional (3D) and 4D color Doppler fetal echocardiography using spatio-temporal image correlation (STIC). *Ultrasound Obstet Gynecol* 2004;23(6):535–545.

24. Paladini D, Vassallo M, Sglavo G, et al. The role of spatio-temporal image correlation (STIC) with tomographic ultrasound imaging (TUI) in the sequential analysis of fetal congenital heart disease. *Ultrasound Obstet Gynecol* 2006;27(5):555–561.

25. Raymond FL, Simpson JM, Sharland GK, et al. Fetal echocardiography as a predictor of chromosomal abnormality. *Lancet* 1997;360:930.

26. Natowicz M, Chatten J, Clancy R, et al. Genetic disorders and major extra-cardiac anomalies associated with the hypoplastic left heart syndrome. *Pediatrics* 1988;82:698–706.

27. Callow LB. Current strategies in the nursing care of infants with hypoplastic left heart syndrome undergoing first-stage palliation by the Norwood operation. *Heart Lung* 1992;21(5):463–470.

28. Connor JA, Thiagarajan R. Hypoplastic left heart syndrome. *Orphanet J Rare Dis* 2007;2:23.

29. Rosenthal GL. Patterns of prenatal growth among infants with cardiovascular malformations: possible fetal hemodynamic effects. *Am J Epidemiol* 1996;143:505–513.

30. Rychik J. Hypoplastic left heart syndrome: from in-utero diagnosis to school age. *Semin Fetal Neonatal Med* 2005;10:553–566.

31. Lenz F, Machlitt A, Hartung J, et al. Fetal pulmonary venous flow pattern is determined by left atrial pressure: report of two cases of left heart hypoplasia, one with patent and the other with closed interatrial communication. *Ultrasound Obstet Gynecol* 2002;19:392–395.

32. Lenz F, Chaoui R. Changes in pulmonary venous Doppler parameters in fetal cardiac defects. *Ultrasound Obstet Gynecol* 2006;28:63–70.

33. Michelfelder E, Gomez C, Border W, et al. Predictive value of fetal pulmonary venous flow patterns in identifying the need for atrial septoplasty in the newborn with hypoplastic left ventricle. *Circulation* 2005;112:2974–2979.

34. Alsoufi B, Bennetts J, Verma S, et al. New developments in the treatment of hypoplastic left heart syndrome. *Pediatrics* 2007;119(1):109–117.

35. Jenkins PC, Flanagan MF, Jenkins KJ, et al. Survival analysis and risk factors for mortality in transplantation and staged surgery for hypoplastic left heart syndrome. *J Am Coll Cardiol* 2000;36:1178–1185.

36. Simpson JM. Hypoplastic left heart syndrome. *Ultrasound Obstet Gynecol* 2000;15:271–278.

37. Goldberg CA, Gomez CA. Hypoplastic left heart syndrome: new developments and current controversies. *Semin Neonatol* 2003;8:461–468.

38. Glauser TA, Zackie E, Weinberg P, et al. Congenital brain anomalies associated with the hypoplastic left heart syndrome. *Pediatrics* 1990;85:984–989.

39. Mahle WT, Clancy RR, McGaurn SP, et al. Impact of prenatal diagnosis on survival and early neurologic morbidity in neonates with the hypoplastic left heart syndrome. *Pediatrics* 2001;107:1277–1282.

40. Daebritz SH, Nollert GD, Zurakowski D, et al. Results of Norwood stage I operation: comparison of hypoplastic left heart syndrome with other malformations. *J Thorac Cardiovasc Surg* 2000;119:358–367.

41. Mahle WT, Spray TL, Wernovsky G, et al. Survival after reconstructive surgery for hypoplastic left heart syndrome: a 15-year experience from a single institution. *Circulation* 2000;102(19 suppl 3):III136–III141.

42. Azakie T, Merklinger SL, McCrindle BW, et al. Evolving strategies and improving outcomes of the modified Norwood procedure: a 10-year single-institution experience. *Ann Thorac Surg* 2001;72:1349–1353.

43. Gaynor JW, Mahle WT, Cohen MI, et al. Risk factors for mortality after the Norwood procedure. *Eur J Cardiothorac Surg* 2002;22:82–89.

COARCTATION OF THE AORTA

Definition, Spectrum of Disease, and Incidence

Coarctation of the aorta involves narrowing of the aortic arch, typically located at the isthmic region, between the left subclavian artery and the ductus arteriosus (Fig. 12-1). Alternatively, coarctation of the aorta may involve a long segment of the aortic arch, termed *tubular hypoplasia of the aortic arch*. Coarctation of the aorta is a common anomaly, found in about 5% of newborns with congenital heart disease (1). It occurs more commonly in boys, with a male-to-female ratio of 1.27 to 1.74 (2,3). Coarctation of the aorta has a fairly high recurrence risk, between 2% and 6% for a previously affected child and 4% for an affected mother (4,5). Chromosomal and extracardiac abnormalities are common associations with coarctation of the aorta (6). The embryologic origin of coarctation of the aorta is complex and not well understood, with two proposed concepts; the ductus tissue theory proposes that aortic constriction is due to migration of ductal smooth muscle cell into the aorta (7), whereas the hemodynamic theory proposes that coarctation results from reduced flow through the aortic arch in fetal life (8). Coarctation of the aorta can be classified as simple when it occurs without important intracardiac lesions and complex when it occurs in association with significant intracardiac pathology. When associated with hypoplastic left heart syndrome and aortic atresia, hypoplastic aortic arch should not be classified as coarctation of the aorta but rather as part of the main cardiac anomaly. Table 12-1 lists cardiac malformations that may include

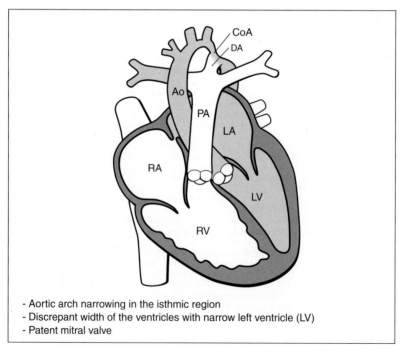

- Aortic arch narrowing in the isthmic region
- Discrepant width of the ventricles with narrow left ventricle (LV)
- Patent mitral valve

Figure 12-1. Coarctation of the aorta. RA, right atrium; RV, right ventricle; LA, left atrium; PA, pulmonary artery; Ao, aorta; DA, ductus arteriosus; CoA, coarctation of the aorta.

TABLE 12-1	Cardiac Anomalies That May Include Coarctation of the Aorta or Tubular Aortic Hypoplasia as Part of the Abnormalities

Unbalanced atrioventricular defect with a narrow left ventricle
Hypoplastic left heart syndrome
Double outlet right ventricle
Tricuspid atresia with ventricular septal defect and malposition of great vessels (type II)
Corrected transposition of the great arteries
Double inlet ventricle (single ventricle)

aortic coarctation or tubular aortic hypoplasia as part of the main cardiac anomaly. Figure 12-2 demonstrates coarctation of the aorta in an anatomic specimen of a fetal heart.

Ultrasound Findings

Gray Scale

Coarctation of the aorta is often associated with an abnormal four-chamber view, where the left ventricle appears narrow when compared to the right ventricle (9–11) (Fig. 12-3). The right ventricular–to–left ventricular width ratio, reported as 1.19 in normal fetuses, is 1.69 in fetuses with coarctation of the aorta (12). Conversely to hypoplastic left heart syndrome, in coarctation of the aorta the contractility of the left ventricle is normal and the mitral valve is patent. The five-chamber view shows the arising aorta with a generally normal diameter. The aortic root can be narrow on occasions, especially when a perimembranous ventricular septal defect and/or aortic stenosis are present. In the three-vessel-trachea view, the diameter of the transverse aortic arch is narrow when compared to the main pulmonary artery (12), and this narrowing of the transverse aortic arch is most impressive in the isthmus region (Fig. 12-4). In the diagnosis of aortic coarctation, the three-vessel-trachea view, depicting the great vessel disproportion, is more specific than ventricular disproportion alone noted on a four-chamber view. Once coarctation of the aorta is suspected in the transverse planes (four-chamber and three-vessel-trachea views), a longitudinal view of the aortic arch should be attempted. In this

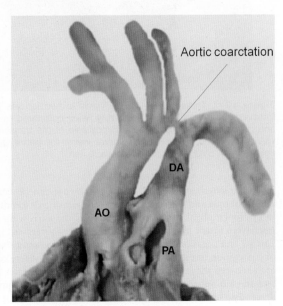

Figure 12-2. Anatomic specimen of coarctation of the aorta in a fetal heart showing aortic narrowing at the aortic isthmus (labeled *aortic coarctation*). AO, aorta; PA, pulmonary artery; DA, ductus arteriosus.

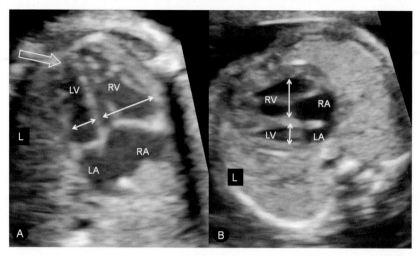

Figure 12-3. Four-chamber view in two fetuses **(A,B)** with coarctation of the aorta showing typical ventricular disproportions. The left ventricle (LV) is small in width when compared to the width of the right ventricle (RV). Cardiac apex is still formed by the left ventricle in both fetuses (*open arrow* in A). RA, right atrium; LA, left atrium; L, left.

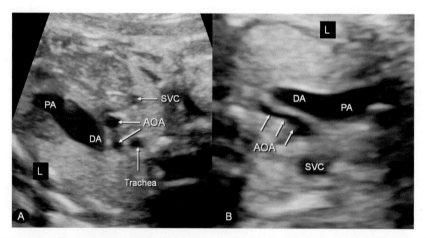

Figure 12-4. Three-vessel-trachea views in two fetuses with coarctation of the aorta. **A:** The transverse aortic arch (AOA) is narrow when compared to the size of the pulmonary artery (PA) and ductal arch (DA). **B:** Tubular hypoplasia of the transverse AOA is demonstrated in a lateral view. The authors recommend lateral views for better demonstration of small vessels in the upper chest. SVC, superior vena cava; L, left.

plane the length and degree of the narrowing can be better assessed and the junction of the aortic isthmus and the ductus arteriosus with the descending aorta better evaluated (Fig. 12-5). In this longitudinal view of the aortic arch, the narrowing is commonly located between the left subclavian artery and the origin of the ductus arteriosus (Fig. 12-5A). The aortic arch appears narrow and occasionally tortuous, termed *contraductal shelf*, an important hint for the presence of coarctation of the aorta (13). In the presence of severe coarctation of the aorta, the transverse arch between the left common and left subclavian arteries (Fig. 12-5B) is elongated and narrow, and the left subclavian artery appears to arise at the junction of ductus arteriosus with the descending aorta. Z-scores for the measurements of the size of the aortic isthmus, the transverse

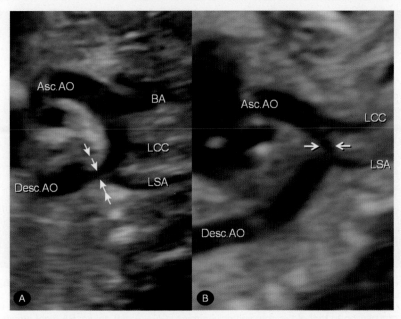

Figure 12-5. Sagittal views of the aortic arches in two fetuses **(A,B)** with coarctation of the aorta. A: The narrowing is mainly in the aortic isthmic region (*arrows*) after the origin of the left subclavian artery (LSA). B: The narrowing is in the middle portion of the transverse aortic arch (*arrows*) between the origins of the LSA and the left common carotid artery (LCC). Asc.O, ascending aorta; Desc. AO, descending aorta; BA, brachiocephalic artery.

arch, and the angle between the aortic isthmus and the ductus arteriosus were proposed to improve the accurate description of this cardiac anomaly (14–16).

Color Doppler
Color Doppler helps in differentiating coarctation of the aorta from other cardiac abnormalities and in occasionally demonstrating the narrow isthmic region. Applied to the four-chamber view, color Doppler confirms normal left ventricular filling in diastole and thus differentiates aortic coarctation from hypoplastic left heart syndrome (Fig. 12-6). At the level of the five-chamber view, color Doppler demonstrates forward flow across the aortic valve and a perimembranous ventricular septal defect when present in association with coarctation of the aorta. In the three-vessel-trachea view or the transverse aortic arch view, a narrow transverse aortic arch can be recognized, which progressively becomes smaller in diameter as it approaches the aortic isthmus (Fig. 12-7). The aortic arch can also be visualized in a longitudinal plane. The use of power Doppler in this plane is preferred for a better definition of the aortic coarctation (Fig. 12-8), where a typical "shelf sign" is seen at the junction between the ductus arteriosus and the descending aorta (Fig. 12-9). Pulsed Doppler evaluation of the atrioventricular valves may show an increase in right heart flow and a decrease in left ventricular flow (9).

Early Gestation
Coarctation of the aorta can be suspected in early pregnancy at the 11- to 14-week scan by demonstrating ventricular discrepancy as well as narrowing of the aortic arch in the three-vessel-trachea view (Fig. 12-10). Color Doppler may be helpful in early gestation in identifying the vessels in the three-vessel-trachea view (Fig. 12-10). The longitudinal view of the aortic arch may be helpful in early gestation in the diagnosis of coarctation of the aorta (17). Confirming the presence of coarctation of the aorta in the second trimester is critical because ventricular discrepancies found in early pregnancy may resolve with advancing gestation. An accurate differentiation between a normal finding and a true coarctation is difficult in

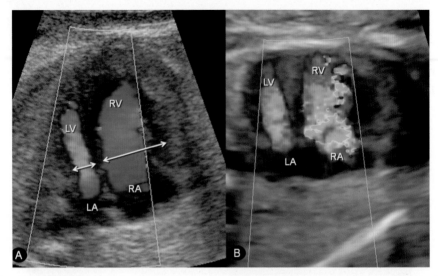

Figure 12-6. Color Doppler at the level of the four-chamber view in two fetuses **(A,B)** with coarctation of the aorta, demonstrating filling of both the left (LV) and right ventricles (RV) during diastole confirming patency of the atrioventricular valves. Note the narrow width of the left ventricle in comparison to that of the right ventricle (*arrows* in A). LA, left atrium; RA, right atrium.

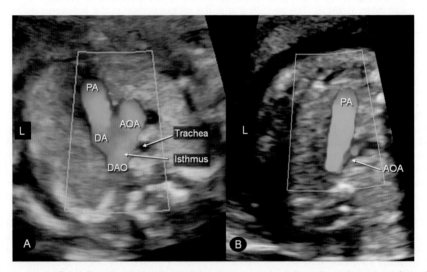

Figure 12-7. Color Doppler at the level of the three-vessel-trachea view in a normal fetus **(A)** and in a fetus with coarctation of the aorta **(B)**. In the normal fetus (A), the aortic arch (AOA) and ductal arch (DA) have nearly the same size and merge together toward the descending aorta (DAO). The aortic isthmus is well developed. In the fetus with coarctation of the aorta (B), forward flow is noted in the AOA, which progressively narrows as it approaches the aortic isthmus. PA, pulmonary artery; L, left.

early gestation, making such false-positive diagnoses unavoidable. If, however, coarctation of the aorta is suspected in the presence of other findings such as cystic hygroma and/or early fetal hydrops, Turner syndrome is a likely diagnosis (18), or, when combined with impaired fetal growth and multiple structural anomalies, trisomy 13 is a likely diagnosis, since both are commonly associated with coarctation of the aorta.

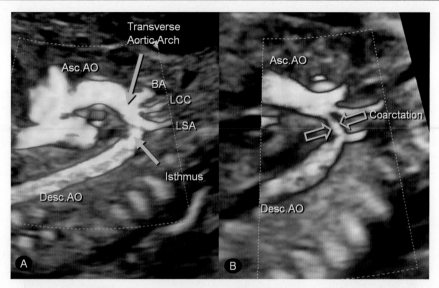

Figure 12-8. Power Doppler in a sagittal view of the aortic arch in a normal fetus **(A)** and in a fetus with coarctation of the aorta **(B).** In the normal fetus (A), power Doppler displays the ascending aorta (Asc.AO), the transverse aortic arch, the aortic isthmus, and the descending aorta (Desc.AO). A also shows the three arteries that arise from the transverse arch: the brachio-cephalic artery (BA), the left common carotid artery (LCC), and the left subclavian artery (LSA). In the fetus with coarctation of the aorta (B), the narrowing in the transverse aortic arch (*open arrows*) is shown between the left common carotid and the left subclavian artery.

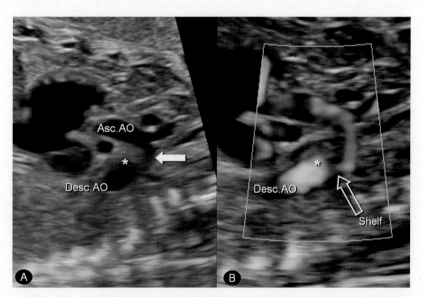

Figure 12-9. Gray scale **(A)** and color Doppler **(B)** in a sagittal view of the aortic arch in a fetus with coarctation of the aorta showing the typical shelf (*open arrow* in B) in the region of the junction of the aortic arch with the ductus arteriosus. The *asterisk* marks the location where the ductus arteriosus enters the descending aorta (Desc.AO); the *solid arrow* in A shows the region of coarctation. Asc.AO, ascending aorta.

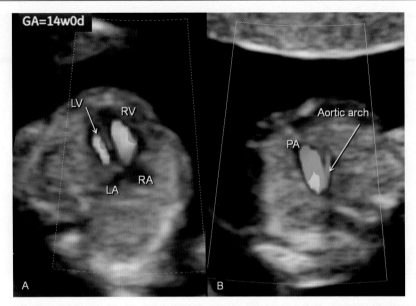

Figure 12-10. Color Doppler at the level of the four-chamber view **(A)** and three-vessel-trachea view **(B)** in a fetus with coarctation of the aorta at 14 weeks' gestation. A diminutive left ventricle (LV) is noted in the four-chamber view (A) and a small aortic arch is noted in the three-vessel-trachea view (B). Figure 12-8B shows the longitudinal view of the aortic arch in this fetus at 26 weeks' gestation. RV, right ventricle; RA, right atrium; LA, left atrium; PA, pulmonary artery.

Three-dimensional Ultrasound

The tomographic mode display of three-dimensional ultrasound can be used for the demonstration of coarctation of the aorta at different planes (Fig. 12-11) (19). The additional use of color Doppler, high-definition flow Doppler, or power Doppler to a three-dimensional (3-D) volume may improve visualization of the coarctation segment (Fig. 12-12). Inversion mode can also be applied to demonstrate narrowing at the aortic isthmic region. By acquiring a 3-D volume of a fetal chest, a longitudinal axis of the aortic arch with the shelf sign may be retrieved even under suboptimal volume acquisition (20,21). We recommend volume acquisition to commence from a sagittal or parasagittal two-dimensional (2-D) reference plane in order to minimize shadowing and optimize imaging of the aortic arch.

Associated Cardiac and Extracardiac Findings

Associated cardiac abnormalities are common in complex coarctation of the aorta, with a large ventricular septal defect representing the most common associated lesion. Various left-sided lesions are also commonly associated with coarctation, including bicuspid aortic valve, aortic stenosis at the valvular and subvalvar levels, and mitral stenosis (22–24). The presence of multiple left-sided obstructive cardiac lesions with coarctation of the aorta has been referred to as Shone syndrome (13,25). The presence of a persistent left superior vena cava has also been associated with coarctation of the aorta (Fig. 12-12) (26,27). The presence of a persistent left superior vena cava with a slight discrepancy of ventricular dimensions should alert the examiner for its association with aortic coarctation, and follow-up examinations looking for signs of coarctation should be performed (26,27).

Associated extracardiac malformations are common in fetuses with coarctation of the aorta and include vascular and nonvascular anomalies (28). Vascular anomalies primarily involve variations in brachiocephalic anatomy and in berry aneurysms of the circle of Willis, which may lead to intracerebral bleeding. Berry aneurysms of the cerebral circulation have been reported in up to 3% to 5% of patients with coarctation. Non–vascular-associated

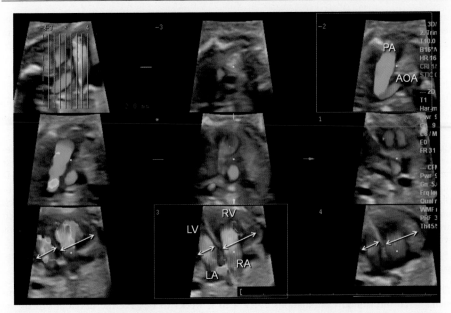

Figure 12-11. Three-dimensional ultrasound volume obtained in color spatio-temporal image correlation (STIC) of a fetus with coarctation of the aorta. The three-dimensional volume is displayed in tomographic mode showing the typical signs of aortic coarctation: narrow left ventricle (LV) in the four-chamber view (*lower box*) and narrow aortic arch (AOA) in the three-vessel-trachea view (*upper box*). LA, left atrium; PA, pulmonary artery; RA, right atrium; RV, right ventricle.

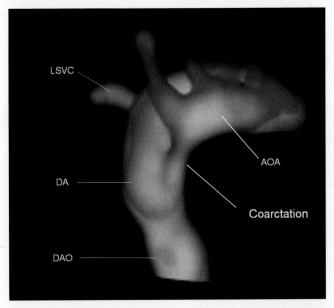

Figure 12-12. Three-dimensional ultrasound volume in power Doppler of a fetus with coarctation of the aorta and persistent left superior vena cava demonstrating a lateral view to the aortic arch with the narrow isthmic region (coarctation). AOA, transverse aortic arch; DAO, descending aorta; DA, ductus arteriosus; LSVC, left superior vena cava.

anomalies involve multiple organ systems such as the genitourinary, musculoskeletal, gastrointestinal, and others, and may be present in up to 30% of children with coarctation of the aorta (2,29). Chromosomal abnormalities are commonly associated with aortic coarctation diagnosed prenatally, with a reported aneuploidy rate up to 35% in a retrospective referral-based review, and Turner syndrome representing the most common abnormality (29). Aortic coarctation can also be found in association with other chromosomal aberrations such as trisomy 13 or 18, especially when coarctation is associated with multiple extracardiac malformations.

Differential Diagnosis

Coarctation of the aorta is difficult to detect prenatally, with a high false-positive and false-negative diagnosis (10,11). The most common differential diagnosis includes hypoplastic left heart syndrome and type A interrupted aortic arch. Assessing ventricular contractility on 2-D ultrasound and flow across the mitral valve on color Doppler can help differentiate hypoplastic ventricle from coarctation (see Table 11-2). Documenting flow across the aortic arch on color Doppler in longitudinal views can help differentiate coarctation from interrupted arch (no flow across). Other conditions associated with discrepant ventricular dimensions with a diminutive-appearing left ventricle are listed in Table 12-2.

Prognosis and Outcome

The in utero course of a fetus with coarctation of the aorta is generally uneventful. We recommend serial ultrasound examinations every 4 to 6 weeks to observe the development of the transverse arch and the progression of the coarctation. When a ventricular septal defect is present, the growth of the ascending aorta is also controlled. Prenatal diagnosis of aortic coarctation should lead to the delivery of the neonate at a tertiary center with immediate availability of pediatric cardiology services. Prostaglandin infusion should be commenced immediately after delivery to maintain ductal patency. Prenatal diagnosis of coarctation of the aorta has been shown to improve neonatal outcome (30).

Long-term studies of outcome following prenatal diagnosis of coarctation of the aorta and surgical repair in infancy are not currently available. Available data on long-term follow-up, however, show that chronic hypertension, surgery site complications (aneurysm, stricture), and coronary artery disease play a significant role in the long-term outcome (31,32). Long-term follow-up of treated infants with coarctation of the aorta is therefore critical in the early identification of potential comorbidities. The prognosis following successful repair in childhood of simple coarctation, without extracardiac anomalies, should be considered excellent.

TABLE 12-2	Conditions Associated with Ventricular Size Discrepancy with an Increased Right Ventricle–to–left Ventricle Ratio (RV/LV)

Differential diagnosis of RV/LV asymmetry
Aortic coarctation
Hypoplastic left heart syndrome
Physiologic condition in some fetuses in late gestation >32 weeks
Transient RV > LV seen before 18 weeks (i.e., trisomy 21)
Interruption of aortic arch
Atrioventricular septal defect (unbalanced) with small left ventricle
Mitral atresia with ventricular septal defect
Total anomalous pulmonary venous return
Left superior vena cava (with or without coarctation)
Double outlet right ventricle
Absent pulmonary valve syndrome
Ebstein anomaly/tricuspid dysplasia
Left congenital diaphragmatic hernia
Peripheral arteriovenous fistula with RV volume overload (Galen aneurysm and others)
Severe tricuspid insufficiency in different fetal conditions (see also Table 14-2)

Similar to other cardiac lesions, the prognosis of coarctation of the aorta when detected prenatally seems to be worse than reported in postnatal series, probably due to selection bias and associated malformations (29). An overall adjusted survival rate of 79% was reported in a prenatal series after excluding pregnancy terminations and extracardiac and chromosomal abnormalities (29). The presence of fetal growth restriction had a significant negative effect on survival (29). Complex coarctation, with its association with other cardiac anomalies, has a worse prognosis.

▨ KEY POINTS: COARCTATION OF THE AORTA

- ■ Coarctation of the aorta involves narrowing of the aortic arch, typically located at the isthmic region, between the left subclavian artery and the ductus arteriosus.
- ■ When a long segment of the aortic arch is narrowed, the descriptive term is tubular hypoplasia of the aortic arch.
- ■ The four-chamber view is abnormal, where the left ventricle appears narrow when compared to the right ventricle.
- ■ The three-vessel-trachea view, depicting great vessel disproportion, is more specific than ventricular disproportion alone on a four-chamber view in the diagnosis of aortic coarctation.
- ■ Longitudinal view of the aortic arch demonstrates tortuosity and narrowing between the left subclavian artery and the origin of the ductus arteriosus (coarctation shelf).
- ■ Associated cardiac abnormalities are common, with a large ventricular septal defect representing the most common associated lesion.
- ■ Various left-sided lesions are commonly associated including bicuspid aortic valve, aortic stenosis at the valvular and subvalvar levels, and mitral stenosis.
- ■ The presence of multiple left-sided obstructive cardiac lesions with coarctation of the aorta has been referred to as Shone syndrome.
- ■ The presence of a persistent left superior vena cava has been associated with coarctation of the aorta.
- ■ Associated extracardiac malformations are common.
- ■ Berry aneurysms of the cerebral circulation have been reported in up to 3% to 5% of patients with coarctation.
- ■ Chromosomal abnormalities are common, with Turner syndrome representing the most common abnormality.
- ■ Chronic hypertension, surgery site complications (aneurysm, stricture), and coronary artery disease play a significant role in the long-term outcome.

▨ INTERRUPTION OF THE AORTIC ARCH

Definition, Spectrum of Disease, and Incidence

Interruption of the aortic arch (IAA) is characterized by complete separation of the ascending and descending aorta. IAA is classified as type A, B, or C based on the anatomic location of the interruption in relation to the brachiocephalic vessels (Fig. 12-13). IAA is a rare cardiac malformation occurring in about 1% of congenital heart disease and is rarely encountered in fetal series. Of the three types, type B is the most common and is noted in about 55% of IAA cases. Type B cases are also associated with a large malalignment-type ventricular septal defect with posterior displacement of the infundibular septum in 90% of cases. IAA type A has similar hemodynamic characteristics as coarctation of the aorta (13), and type C is very rare. Therefore, this chapter will provide a detailed discussion on IAA type B. Figure 12-14 demonstrates IAA type B in an anatomic specimen of a fetal heart.

Ultrasound Findings

Gray Scale

Conversely to coarctation of the aorta where ventricular size disproportion is evident on the four-chamber view, the size of the left ventricle is generally normal in IAA type B (Fig. 12-15A), especially when the ventricular septal defect (VSD) is large (Fig. 12-15B) (13). Thus, IAA type B is generally not suspected in the four-chamber view unless the ventricular septal defect is apparent in this plane. The five-chamber view reveals the VSD and a rather small

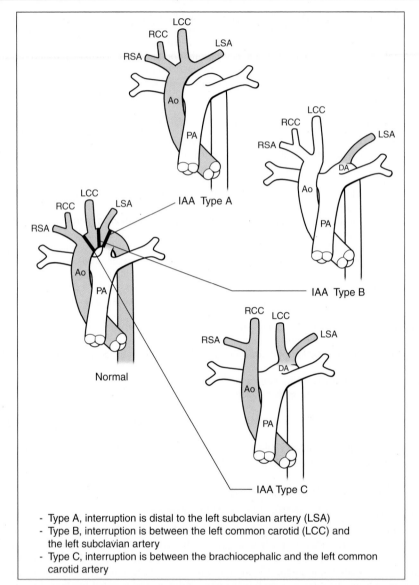

- Type A, interruption is distal to the left subclavian artery (LSA)
- Type B, interruption is between the left common carotid (LCC) and the left subclavian artery
- Type C, interruption is between the brachiocephalic and the left common carotid artery

Figure 12-13. Interruption of the aortic arch (IAA). Ao, aorta; DA, ductus arteriosus; RCC, right common carotid artery; RSA, right subclavian artery; PA, pulmonary artery.

aortic root (Fig. 12-15B). In IAA, the continuity of the aortic arch in the three-vessel-trachea view cannot be demonstrated (Fig. 12-16). Longitudinal view of the aortic arch fails to show the typical "candy cane" curvature of the aortic arch, but rather a straight course of the aorta with two branching vessels: the brachiocephalic and left common carotid arteries (Fig. 12-17). The short-axis and three-vessel-trachea view reveals a slightly dilated pulmonary trunk.

Color Doppler
Color Doppler confirms the presence of ventricular septal defect in the four- and five-chamber view, with nonturbulent flow across the aortic valve in the five-chamber view and the absence

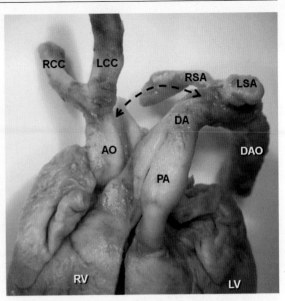

Figure 12-14. Anatomic specimen of a fetal heart with interrupted aortic arch (type B). There is no connection between the ascending (AO) and descending aorta (DAO) (*broken arrow*). The right common carotid artery (RCC) and the left common carotid artery (LCC) are seen to arise from the AO. The left subclavian artery (LSA) arises from the ductus arteriosus (DA). The right subclavian artery (RSA) arises as an aberrant vessel from the DA in this fetus. LV, left ventricle; RV, right ventricle; PA, pulmonary artery.

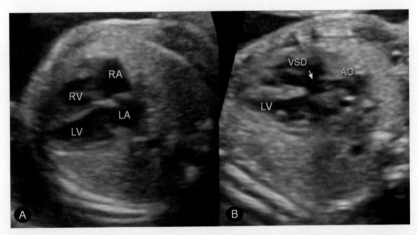

Figure 12-15. Four-chamber view **(A)** and longitudinal axis of the left ventricle **(B)** in a fetus with an interrupted aortic arch type B. The four-chamber view (A) appears normal, and the longitudinal axis of the left ventricle (B) demonstrates a ventricular septal defect (*arrow*, VSD) and a small ascending aorta (AO). The interrupted aortic arch is demonstrated in Figures 12-16 and 12-17. RV, right ventricle; LV, left ventricle; RA, right atrium; LA, left atrium.

of the continuity of the aortic arch in the three-vessel-trachea view. In the longitudinal view, color Doppler will show the straight course of the aorta from the heart toward the neck (Fig. 12-18) and a left subclavian artery arising from the ductus arteriosus (in type B) (Figs. 12-18 and 12-19). The three-vessel-trachea view on color Doppler may show on occasion an aberrant right subclavian artery arising from the ductus region with a course behind the trachea and esophagus (as in Fig. 12-14).

Early Gestation

The diagnosis of IAA is very difficult in early gestation, unless the lack of continuity of the aortic arch in the three-vessel-trachea view is noted on color Doppler evaluation. The four-chamber

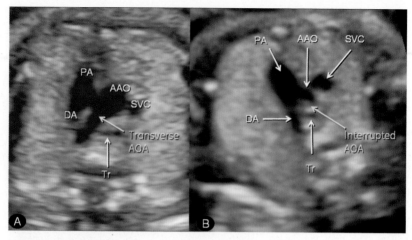

Figure 12-16. Three-vessel-trachea view in a normal fetus **(A)** and in a fetus with interrupted aortic arch (IAA) **(B)**. The continuity of the transverse aortic arch (AOA) toward the descending aorta cannot be demonstrated in IAA, as shown in B. B represents the same fetus as in Figures 12-15 and 12-17B. PA, pulmonary artery; DA, ductus arteriosus; AAO, ascending aorta; SVC, superior vena cava; Tr, trachea.

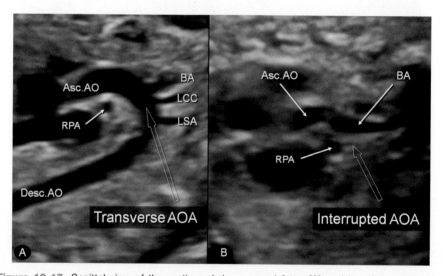

Figure 12-17. Sagittal view of the aortic arch in a normal fetus **(A)** and in a fetus with interrupted aortic arch (IAA type B) **(B)**. In IAA type B (B), the ascending aorta (Asc. AO) is straight and does not show the "candy cane"–shaped curvature as seen in A. Furthermore, a transverse aortic arch (AOA) is not demonstrated in B. BA, brachiocephalic artery; LCC, left common carotid artery; LSA, left subclavian artery; RPA, right pulmonary artery; Desc. AO, descending aorta.

view may appear normal in type B and the ventricular septal defect is not easily detected. A thickened nuchal translucency can lead to suspicion for the presence of cardiac anomaly and the association with microdeletion of 22q11.

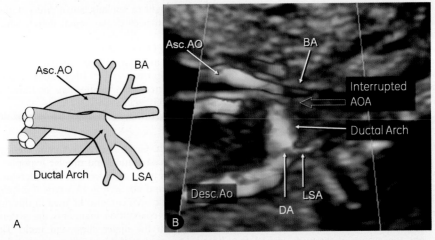

Figure 12-18. Color Doppler of a sagittal view of the chest in a fetus with interrupted aortic arch type B **(B)** showing the straight course of the ascending aorta (Asc.AO) toward the head with a missing transverse aortic arch (AOA). Anatomic details of the ultrasound image (B) are highlighted in the drawing in **A,** which shows a straight course of the ascending aorta and the left subclavian artery (LSA) arising from the ductus arteriosus (DA). Desc.AO, descending aorta; BA, brachiocephalic artery.

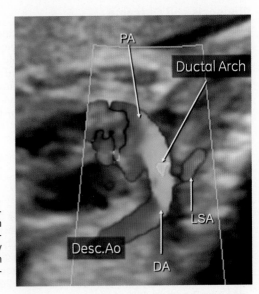

Figure 12-19. Color Doppler of the sagittal view of the ductal arch in a fetus with interrupted aortic arch type B demonstrating the origin of the left subclavian artery (LSA) from the ductus arteriosus region (DA). Desc. AO, descending aorta; PA, pulmonary artery.

Three-dimensional Ultrasound

Three-dimensional ultrasound in combination with color Doppler, B-flow, or inversion flow in the volume-rendered mode can demonstrate the straight course of the interrupted arch in IAA type B.

Associated Cardiac and Extracardiac Findings

IAA type B is considered as a conotruncal anomaly with normally aligned great arteries, a large malalignment-type ventricular septal defect associated with posterior displacement of the infundibular septum, a right aortic arch, and an aberrant right or left subclavian artery. Other associated cardiac anomalies may also coexist, such as atrioventricular septal defect, single ventricle, and double outlet right ventricle.

Extracardiac malformations primarily involve the 22q11 microdeletion, which is associated with IAA type B in about 50% of cases (33,34). In a large series of patients with DiGeorge syndrome, IAA type B was found in 43% of cases (35). Other chromosomal anomalies can also be found, such as Turner syndrome. Extracardiac malformations found in IAA either are related to the 22q11 microdeletion or are nonspecific.

Differential Diagnosis

Differentiating between the three subtypes of IAA is difficult. Given the very common association of IAA type B with a ventricular septal defect, aortic coarctation and tubular hypoplasia with a ventricular septal defect are major cardiac anomalies to be considered in the differential diagnosis. Ventricular size discrepancy seen in coarctation and not seen in IAA type B is helpful in differentiating these anomalies. The shape of the aortic arch can also be used in this differentiation; in the authors' experience the aortic arch in coarctation maintains the normal curvature, whereas in IAA, the aorta remains straight in the upper chest and neck. The straight appearance of the aorta in IAA may be misdiagnosed as the superior vena cava, but the origin of the aorta from the middle of the heart and color Doppler showing forward flow from the heart to the neck vessels helps in differentiating these vessels. The examiner should also be very careful in the assessment of longitudinal views, since the ductal arch, which may give rise to a brachiocephalic artery in IAA (e.g., the left subclavian), may be misinterpreted as a "normal aortic arch."

Prognosis and Outcome

Prenatal diagnosis of IAA, similar to aortic coarctation, should lead to the delivery of the neonate at a tertiary center with immediate availability of pediatric cardiology services. Prostaglandin infusion should be commenced immediately after delivery to maintain ductal patency. Treatment is surgical, involving aortic reconstruction using the main pulmonary artery and homograft augmentation when appropriate. Prognosis is related to the very common association of IAA with 22q11 microdeletion. Overall, short-term and long-term outcome is fair, but may worsen depending on additional cardiac and extracardiac anomalies. Type B has an overall worse prognosis than type A.

▓ KEY POINTS: INTERRUPTION OF THE AORTIC ARCH

- Interruption of the aortic arch (IAA) is characterized by complete separation of the ascending and descending aorta.
- IAA is classified as types A, B, and C.
- Type B is the most common and is noted in about 55% of cases.
- Type B is associated with a ventricular septal defect in 90% of cases.
- The four-chamber view is generally normal in IAA type B.
- Longitudinal view of the aortic arch shows a straight course into the neck with two branching vessels: the brachiocephalic and left common carotid arteries.
- Extracardiac malformations primarily involve the 22q11 microdeletion, which is associated with IAA type B in about 50% of cases.

References

1. Ferencz C, Rubin JD, Loffredo CA, et al., eds. *Perspectives in pediatric cardiology. Epidemiology of congenital heart disease: the Baltimore-Washington Infant Study 1981–1989.* Armonk, NY: Futura Publishing, 1993.
2. Fyler DC, Buckley LP, Hellenbrand WE, et al. Report of the New England regional infant cardiac program. *Pediatrics* 1980;65:432–436.
3. Campbell M, Polani PE. The aetiology of coarctation of the aorta. *Lancet* 1961;1:463–468.
4. Nora JJ, Berg K, Nora AH. *Cardiovascular diseases: genetics, epidemiology and prevention.* New York: Oxford University Press, 1991;53–80.
5. Allan LD, Crawford DC, Chita SK, et al. Familial recurrence of congenital heart disease in a prospective series of mothers referred for fetal echocardiography. *Am J Cardiol* 1986;58(3):334–337.

6. Allan LD, Sharland GK, Milburn A, et al. Prospective diagnosis of 1,006 consecutive cases of congenital heart disease in the fetus. *J Am Coll Cardiol* 1994;23(6):1452–1458.

7. Ho SY, Anderson RH. Coarctation, tubular hypoplasia and the ductus arteriosus. *Br Heart J* 1979;41:268–270.

8. Rudolph AM, Heymann MA, Spitznas U. Hemodynamic considerations in the development of narrowing of the aorta. *Am J Cardiol* 1972;30:514–525.

9. Allan LD, Chita SK, Anderson RH, et al. Coarctation of the aorta in prenatal life: an echocardiographic, anatomical, and functional study. *Br Heart J* 1988;59(3):356–360.

10. Sharland GK, Chan KY, Allan LD. Coarctation of the aorta: difficulties in prenatal diagnosis. *Br Heart J* 1994;71(1):70–75.

11. Brown DL, Durfee SM, Hornberger LK. Ventricular discrepancy as a sonographic sign of coarctation of the fetal aorta: how reliable is it? *J Ultrasound Med* 1997;16(2):95–99.

12. Hornberger LK, Sahn DJ, Kleinman CS, et al. Antenatal diagnosis of coarctation of the aorta: a multicenter experience. *J Am Coll Cardiol* 1994;23(2):417–423.

13. Hornberger LK. Aortic arch anomalies, In: L Allan, L Hornberger, G Sharland, eds. *Textbook of fetal cardiology.* London: Greenwich Medical Media, 2000;305–322.

14. Hornberger LK, Weintraub RG, Pesonen E, et al. Echocardiographic study of the morphology and growth of the aortic arch in the human fetus. Observations related to the prenatal diagnosis of coarctation. *Circulation* 1992;86(3):741–747.

15. Achiron R, Zimand S, Hegesh J, et al. Fetal aortic arch measurements between 14 and 38 weeks' gestation: in-utero ultrasonographic study. *Ultrasound Obstet Gynecol* 2000;15(3):226–230.

16. Pasquini L, Mellander M, Seale A, et al. Z-scores of the fetal aortic isthmus and duct: an aid to assessing arch hypoplasia. *Ultrasound Obstet Gynecol* 2007;29(6):628–633.

17. Bronshtein M, Zimmer EZ. Sonographic diagnosis of fetal coarctation of the aorta at 14–16 weeks of gestation. *Ultrasound Obstet Gynecol* 1998;11(4):254–257.

18. Bronshtein M, Zimmer EZ, Blazer S. A characteristic cluster of fetal sonographic markers that are predictive of fetal Turner syndrome in early pregnancy. *Am J Obstet Gynecol* 2003;188(4):1016–1020.

19. Paladini D, Vassallo M, Sglavo G, et al. The role of spatio-temporal image correlation (STIC) with tomographic ultrasound imaging (TUI) in the sequential analysis of fetal congenital heart disease. *Ultrasound Obstet Gynecol* 2006;27(5):555–561.

20. Quarello E, Trabbia A. The additional value of high definition flow combined with STIC in the diagnosis of fetal coarctation of the aorta. *Ultrasound Obstet Gynecol* 2009;33:365–367.

21. Molina FS, Nicolaides KH, Carvalho JS. Two- and three-dimensional imaging of coarctation shelf in the human fetus. *Heart* 2008;94(5):584.

22. Anderson RH, Lenox CC, Zuberbuhler JR. Morphology of ventricular septal defect associated with coarctation of aorta. *Br Heart J* 1983;50:176–181.

23. Moene RJ, Gittenberger-de Groot AC, Oppenheimer-Dekker A, et al. Anatomic characteristics of ventricular septal defect associated with coarctation of the aorta. *Am J Cardiol* 1987;59:952–955.

24. Rosenquist GC. Congenital mitral valve disease associated with coarctation of the aorta. *Circulation* 1974;49:985–989.

25. Shone JD, Sellers RD, Anderson RC, et al. The development complex of "parachute mitral valve," supravalvar ring of left atrium, subaortic stenosis and coarctation of the aorta. *Am J Cardiol* 1963;11:714–725.

26. Pasquini L, Fichera A, Tan T, et al. Left superior caval vein: a powerful indicator of fetal coarctation. *Heart* 2005;91(4):539–540.

27. Berg C, Knuppel M, Geipel A, et al. Prenatal diagnosis of persistent left superior vena cava and its associated congenital anomalies. *Ultrasound Obstet Gynecol* 2006;27(3):274–280.

28. Greenwood RD, Rosenthal A, Parisi L, et al. Extracardiac abnormalities in infants with congenital heart disease. *Pediatrics* 1975;55:485–492.

29. Paladini D, Volpe P, Russo MG, et al. Aortic coarctation: prognostic indicators of survival in the fetus. *Heart* 2004;90(11):1348–1349.

30. Franklin O, Burch M, Manning N, et al. Prenatal diagnosis of coarctation of the aorta improves survival and reduces morbidity. *Heart* 2002;87(1):67–69.

31. Rosenthal E. Coarctation of the aorta from fetus to adult: curable condition or life long disease process? *Heart* 2005;91(11):1495–1502.

32. Taro-Salazar OH, Steinberger J, Thomas W, et al. Long-term follow-up of patients after coarctation of the aorta repair. *Am J Cardiol* 2002;89:541–547.

33. Chaoui R, Kalache KD, Heling KS, et al. Absent or hypoplastic thymus on ultrasound: a marker for deletion 22q11.2 in fetal cardiac defects. *Ultrasound Obstet Gynecol* 2002;20(6):546–552.

34. Volpe P, Marasini M, Caruso G, et al. Prenatal diagnosis of interruption of the aortic arch and its association with deletion of chromosome 22q11. *Ultrasound Obstet Gynecol* 2002;20(4):327–331.

35. Van Mierop LH, Kutsche LM. Cardiovascular anomalies in DiGeorge syndrome and importance of neural crest as a possible pathogenetic factor. *Am J Cardiol* 1986;58:133–137.

PULMONARY STENOSIS, PULMONARY ATRESIA, AND DUCTUS ARTERIOSUS CONSTRICTION

PULMONARY STENOSIS

Definition, Spectrum of Disease, and Incidence

Pulmonary stenosis is defined as obstruction to right ventricular outflow due to pulmonary valve abnormalities, infravalvular (infundibulum) narrowing, or rarely supravalvular narrowing involving the main pulmonary artery or its branches. Valvular pulmonary stenosis, primarily due to fusion of the valve commissures, is the most common cause of pulmonary stenosis (Fig. 13-1). On occasion, pulmonary stenosis is due to unfused thickened dysplastic valve leaflets with associated pulmonary regurgitation. Unfused and dysplastic valve leaflets are seen in cases of pulmonary stenosis with Noonan syndrome (1). Infundibular thickening due to right ventricular wall hypertrophy is a common cause of pulmonary stenosis in the recipient twin of twin-to-twin transfusion syndrome. The severity of stenosis varies from mild lesions, typically missed prenatally, to severe lesions with associated hypertrophy of the right ventricle (Fig. 13-1) and tricuspid regurgitation. Pulmonary stenosis can progressively worsen in utero, resulting in critical pulmonary stenosis and atresia. Pulmonary stenosis can be associated with other cardiac anomalies such as tetralogy of Fallot. Isolated pulmonary stenosis, which occurs with an incidence of 0.73 per 1000 live births, is the second most common cardiac anomaly to ventricular septal defect and accounts for 9% of live births with congenital heart disease (2,3). Most cases of pulmonary stenosis are first diagnosed beyond the neonatal period probably due to the difficulty in the prenatal diagnosis of this lesion and its progressive

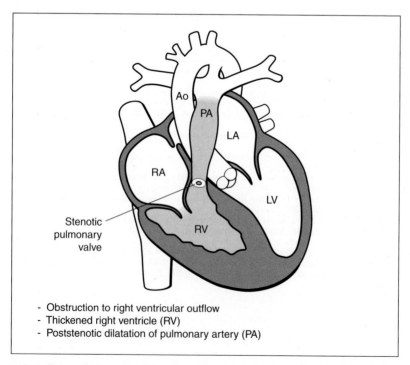

- Obstruction to right ventricular outflow
- Thickened right ventricle (RV)
- Poststenotic dilatation of pulmonary artery (PA)

Figure 13-1. Pulmonary stenosis. LV, left ventricle; LA, left atrium; RA, right atrium; Ao, aorta.

nature in some cases (4). Recurrence of pulmonary stenosis is estimated at 2% for one affected sibling and 6% when two siblings are affected (5).

Ultrasound Findings

Gray Scale

The four-chamber view in pulmonary stenosis shows right ventricular hypertrophy (Fig. 13-2) with bulging of the interventricular septum to the left ventricle. The right ventricular lumen may appear small due to the hypertrophied myocardium, and the tricuspid valve shows normal leaflet excursion with occasional tricuspid regurgitation, which may lead to right atrial dilation. Right ventricular wall hypertrophy is more commonly seen in the third trimester of pregnancy. Confirming the diagnosis of pulmonary stenosis is best performed by direct visualization of the pulmonary valve in the right ventricular outflow view, which shows abnormal excursion and thickening and doming of valve leaflets during systole (Fig. 13-3). Valve leaflets are visible within the pulmonary artery throughout the cardiac cycle in pulmonary stenosis as opposed to a normal pulmonary valve, where the leaflets abut the arterial walls during systole. The three-vessel view and the three-vessel-trachea view will also show poststenotic dilation of the pulmonary artery in many cases (Fig. 13-3). In mild to moderate pulmonary stenosis, ultrasound diagnostic signs are more subtle and primary detection is best achieved by the additional use of color Doppler.

Color Doppler

Color and pulsed Doppler are essential in confirming the diagnosis and in assessing the severity of pulmonary stenosis. Color Doppler of the pulmonary valve in the right ventricular outflow view typically shows turbulent antegrade flow with color aliasing (Fig. 13-4). Pulsed Doppler across the pulmonary valve demonstrates high-flow velocities exceeding 200 cm/sec (Figs. 13-5 and 13-6). Ductus arteriosus flow is antegrade in the majority of cases of pulmonary stenosis. The presence of retrograde flow across the ductus arteriosus, however, is a worsening sign associated with the development of pulmonary atresia and poor outcome (6). Tricuspid regurgitation, which may be absent in mild pulmonary stenosis and holosystolic in moderate or severe cases (Fig. 13-7), can be demonstrated using color Doppler in the four-chamber view. When the valve leaflets are dysplastic, pulmonary regurgitation is demonstrated on color Doppler and flow across the ductus arteriosus may be bidirectional in these conditions. Color and pulsed Doppler of the ductus venosus may show reverse flow during the atrial contraction phase of diastole (7).

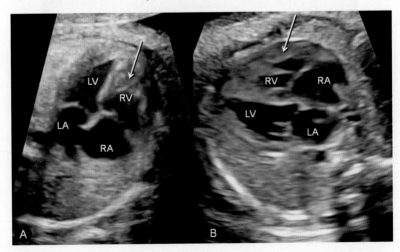

Figure 13-2. Apical **(A)** and lateral **(B)** four-chamber planes in two fetuses with pulmonary stenosis, showing hypertrophy of the right ventricular wall (*arrows*). LA, left atrium; RA, right atrium; RV, right ventricle; LV, left ventricle.

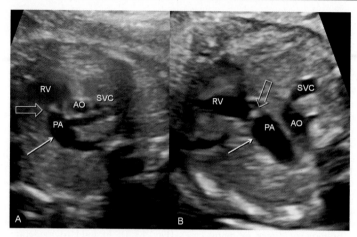

Figure 13-3. Thickened and echogenic pulmonary valve (*open arrows*) in two fetuses with pulmonary stenosis demonstrated at 28 weeks in the three-vessel view **(A)** and at 33 weeks in the three-vessel-trachea view **(B)**. Note the postvalvular dilation of the pulmonary artery (PA) in both cases (*solid arrows*). AO, aorta; SVC, superior vena cava; RV, right ventricle.

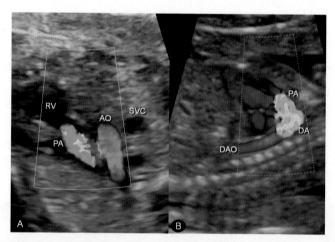

Figure 13-4. Turbulence and aliasing in color Doppler in two fetuses with pulmonary stenosis demonstrated in the three-vessel-trachea view **(A)** and in the ductal arch **(B)**. A shows the same fetus as in Figure 13-3B. AO, aorta; SVC, superior vena cava; PA, pulmonary artery; RV, right ventricle; DAO, descending aorta; DA, ductus arteriosus.

Early Gestation

Pulmonary stenosis is difficult to diagnose in early gestation as the ultrasound findings may be subtle or absent. The presence of tricuspid regurgitation in early gestation should result in targeted examination of the fetal heart including color and pulsed Doppler of the pulmonary artery. The presence of pulmonary stenosis with a thickened nuchal translucency or a hygroma should alert for the association with Noonan syndrome.

Three-dimensional Ultrasound

Three-dimensional (3-D) ultrasound with tomographic imaging in gray scale and color Doppler can demonstrate in one view various ultrasound findings in pulmonary stenosis such as the hypertrophied right ventricle, the dilated pulmonary trunk, the tricuspid regurgitation, and color aliasing across the pulmonary valve during systole (Fig. 13-8). Surface rendering of a 3-D volume may show the stenotic valve with lack of complete excursion in systole (Fig. 13-9).

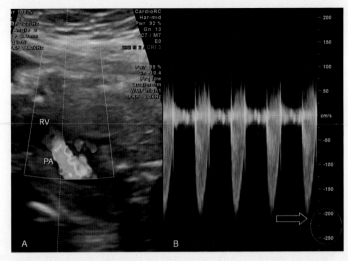

Figure 13-5. Color **(A)** and pulsed **(B)** Doppler of the pulmonary artery in a fetus with pulmonary stenosis. Note the presence of color aliasing across the pulmonary valve on color Doppler (A) and peak systolic velocities at around 210 cm/sec on the spectral Doppler (B) *(open arrow)*, both of which are signs of pulmonary stenosis. PA, pulmonary artery; RV, right ventricle.

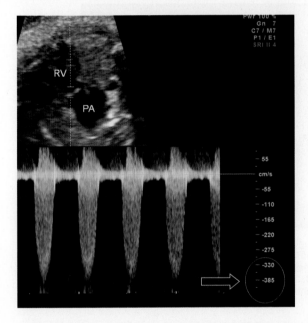

Figure 13-6. Pulsed Doppler in a fetus with pulmonary stenosis demonstrating peak velocities reaching 390 cm/sec *(open arrow)*. PA, pulmonary artery; RV, right ventricle.

Future applications of ventricular volume measurements may be of help in assessing fetuses at risk of developing critical stenosis and right ventricular dysfunction.

Associated Cardiac and Extracardiac Findings

Associated cardiac lesions include right ventricular hypertrophy and tricuspid regurgitation, which are resultant from the hemodynamic changes of pulmonary stenosis. Other associated cardiac abnormalities include atrial septal defect, aortic or tricuspid stenosis, and total anomalous pulmonary venous connection. Table 13-1 lists cardiac malformations having pulmonary stenosis as an associated malformation.

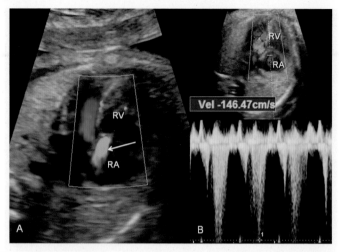

Figure 13-7. Tricuspid regurgitation demonstrated on color **(A)** (*arrow*) and pulsed **(B)** Doppler in a fetus with valvular pulmonary stenosis. Peak velocities of the tricuspid regurgitant jet are at 146 cm/sec (B). RA, right atrium; RV, right ventricle.

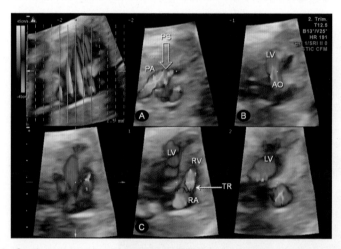

Figure 13-8. Spatio-temporal image correlation (STIC) color Doppler three-dimensional volume in a fetus with pulmonary stenosis (PS) displayed in tomographic mode in systole. Note the presence of turbulent aliased flow across the pulmonary artery (PA) (*open arrow*) in **A** and tricuspid regurgitation (TR) (*solid arrow*) in **C.** The aorta (AO) shows normal laminar flow in **B.** LV, left ventricle; RA, right atrium; RV, right ventricle.

Extracardiac associated findings are rare with the exception of syndromes such as Noonan, Beckwith-Wiedemann, Alagille, and Williams-Beuren, among others. A full listing of genetic associations with cardiac disease is presented in Chapter 2. In Noonan syndrome, approximately 50% of affected infants have congenital heart disease, primarily pulmonary stenosis (8). In twin-to-twin transfusion syndrome, a higher rate of pulmonary stenosis is reported in the recipient twin, possibly related to chronic in utero hemodynamic impairment. Volume overload with chronic tricuspid regurgitation may be associated with reduced antegrade flow across the pulmonary valve and a lack of growth of the valve annulus (9,10). Chromosomal abnormalities are rare associations with cases of pulmonary stenosis. Trisomy 21 may be associated with pulmonary stenosis in rare conditions, especially when additional extracardiac findings are present.

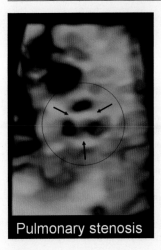

Pulmonary stenosis

Figure 13-9. Three-dimensional volume of the heart in a fetus with pulmonary stenosis, displayed in surface mode in an *en face* view of the stenotic pulmonary valve. Note the three thickened pulmonary artery valve leaflets (*arrows*) with reduced valve aperture.

Differential Diagnosis

Differentiating pulmonary stenosis from pulmonary atresia may be difficult. A false-positive diagnosis of pulmonary stenosis may also occur if color Doppler presets are not adjusted to cardiac flow velocities. Adjusting the velocity scale of the ultrasound machine and confirming the suspicion on pulsed Doppler help in the correct diagnosis.

Prognosis and Outcome

The course of pulmonary stenosis in utero is uneventful except in severe cases where progression may lead to an increase in the severity of tricuspid regurgitation with subsequent dilation of the right atrium, cardiomegaly, and heart failure. Progression may also lead to the development of critical stenosis with progression to pulmonary atresia with intact ventricular septum (6,11). Progression of pulmonary stenosis to atresia, which may alter postnatal surgical management from a biventricular to a univentricular repair, has prompted in utero treatment of critical pulmonary stenosis with balloon valvuloplasty (12). Similar to other cardiac abnormalities, prenatal diagnosis of pulmonary stenosis has a worse outcome than postnatal diagnosis. When diagnosis of pulmonary stenosis was performed before 24 weeks' gestation, a 67% survival rate was reported in one series (6).

We recommend follow-up ultrasound examinations every 2 to 4 weeks on fetuses with pulmonary stenosis in order to assess peak velocities across the stenotic pulmonary valve, the severity of tricuspid regurgitation when present, antegrade or retrograde flow in the ductus arteriosus, and changes in tricuspid valve and right ventricular size. Occurrence of retrograde flow in the ductus arteriosus and a reduction of the right ventricular cavity are signs of worsening disease with poor prognosis. Reverse flow in the ductus venosus is a common finding in right heart obstruction and does not correlate with the prognostic outcome (7).

Prognosis of mild to moderate pulmonary stenosis, if isolated, is excellent, and neonatal management generally depends on the severity of the stenosis assessed postnatally. Mild forms

TABLE 13-1	Cardiac Anomalies with Associated Pulmonary Stenosis
Tetralogy of Fallot	
Absent pulmonary valve syndrome	
Double outlet right ventricle	
Tricuspid atresia with ventricular septal defect	
Ebstein anomaly, tricuspid dysplasia	
D-transposition of the great arteries	
Corrected transposition of the great arteries	
Heterotaxy with cardiac anomaly (right isomerism)	

may only need clinical follow-up with no intervention, whereas moderate to severe forms require treatment primarily with balloon valvuloplasty with excellent results. Children with dysplastic pulmonary valves may require surgical repair.

▓ KEY POINTS: PULMONARY STENOSIS

■ Pulmonary stenosis is an obstruction to right ventricular outflow primarily due to pulmonary valve abnormalities.

■ Fusion of the valve commissures is the most common cause of pulmonary stenosis.

■ Pulmonary stenosis can worsen in utero resulting in critical pulmonary stenosis and atresia.

■ The four-chamber view in pulmonary stenosis shows right ventricular hypertrophy with occasional tricuspid regurgitation, which may lead to right atrial dilation.

■ Direct visualization of the pulmonary valve shows abnormal excursion and thickening and doming of valve leaflets during systole.

■ Valve leaflets are visible within the pulmonary artery throughout the cardiac cycle in pulmonary stenosis.

■ The three-vessel view shows poststenotic dilation of the pulmonary artery in many cases.

■ Color and pulsed Doppler are essential in confirming the diagnosis and in assessing the severity of pulmonary stenosis.

■ Color Doppler shows turbulent antegrade flow with color aliasing and pulsed Doppler demonstrates high-flow velocities.

■ Prognosis of mild to moderate pulmonary stenosis, if isolated, is excellent.

▓ PULMONARY ATRESIA WITH INTACT VENTRICULAR SEPTUM

Definition, Spectrum of Disease, and Incidence

Pulmonary atresia with intact ventricular septum (PA-IVS) is a group of cardiac malformations having in common absent communication between the right ventricle and the pulmonary arterial circulation (pulmonary atresia) in combination with an intact interventricular septum (Fig. 13-10). The pulmonary atresia is usually of the membranous type with complete fusion of the valve commissures and a normally developed infundibulum. On occasion, however, the pulmonary atresia is muscular with a severely distorted right ventricular outflow tract region. The right ventricular cavity is either hypoplastic with thickened right ventricular myocardium (Fig. 13-10) or dilated with significant tricuspid valve regurgitation and a dilated right atrium (see Chapter 14). A hypoplastic right ventricle occurs in the majority of cases (6). The size of the right ventricular cavity correlates with the Z value of the diameter of the tricuspid valve (13,14). One of the major associated findings in hearts with PA-IVS and hypoplastic right ventricles is an anomaly of the coronary circulation, namely, ventriculo-coronary arterial communication (VCAC) (Fig. 13-10B), found in about one third of cases of PA-IVS. Systemic collateral arteries to the lungs, which are typical for pulmonary atresia with ventricular septal defect (see Chapter 17), are not found in pulmonary atresia with intact ventricular septum.

PA-IVS is a rare condition that accounts for approximately 3% of all live births with congenital heart disease and has a prevalence of 0.042 to 0.053 per 1000 live births (15). PA-IVS is more common in fetal series due to the anatomic abnormality seen at the four-chamber view. This chapter will focus on PA-IVS with a hypoplastic right ventricle. The subgroup with a dilated right ventricle and severe tricuspid regurgitation is discussed in Chapter 14.

Ultrasound Findings

Gray Scale

In the four-chamber view PA-IVS is suspected in the presence of a hypoplastic, hypokinetic right ventricle with thickened walls (Fig. 13-11). The anatomic depiction of the right ventricle is similar to the left ventricle in hypoplastic left heart syndrome (see Chapter 11). The degree of "hypoplasia" varies from a nearly absent right ventricle to a normal-sized right ventricle with significantly reduced contractility (Fig. 13-11). The tricuspid valve is often dysplastic with a narrow annulus and abnormal leaflets excursion. The right ventricular wall becomes progressively more hypertrophied with advancing gestation and the hypertrophy of the

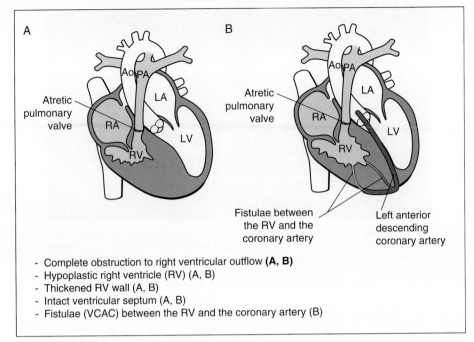

- Complete obstruction to right ventricular outflow **(A, B)**
- Hypoplastic right ventricle (RV) (A, B)
- Thickened RV wall (A, B)
- Intact ventricular septum (A, B)
- Fistulae (VCAC) between the RV and the coronary artery (B)

Figure 13-10. Pulmonary atresia with intact ventricular septum (PA-IVS) **(A)** and PA-IVS with ventriculo-coronary arterial communications (VCAC) **(B)**. RA, right atrium; LV, left ventricle; LA, left atrium; Ao, aorta; PA, pulmonary artery.

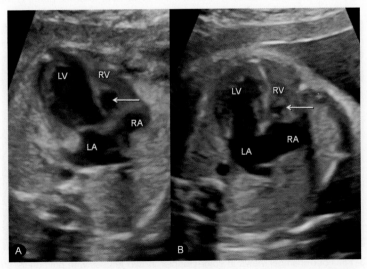

Figure 13-11. Apical four-chamber planes in two fetuses with pulmonary atresia and intact ventricular septum showing varying degrees (*arrows*) of hypoplasia of the right ventricular cavity. The fetus in **A** is at 26 weeks' gestation and the fetus in **B** is at 28 weeks' gestation. RV, right ventricle; LV, left ventricle; RA, right atrium; LA, left atrium.

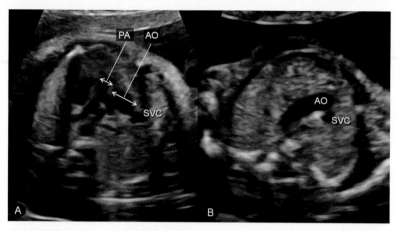

Figure 13-12. Plane A represents the three-vessel view in a fetus with pulmonary atresia. Note the narrow-sized pulmonary artery (PA) in comparison to the size of the aorta (AO). **Plane B** represents the three-vessel-trachea view (more cranial plane than the three-vessel view) in a fetus with pulmonary atresia. Note the presence of the AO and superior vena cava (SVC) with absence of the PA as it is hidden under the AO and can only be demonstrated on color Doppler.

ventricular septum may occasionally lead to a bulge into the left ventricle. The diagnosis of PA-IVS is confirmed by visualizing pulmonary valve and main pulmonary artery: The main pulmonary artery in the right outflow tract view or the three-vessel view is typically small or hypoplastic (Fig. 13-12). In more severe cases the right ventricular outflow tract can be difficult to identify on two-dimensional (2-D) ultrasound and can only be recognized by the additional use of color Doppler.

Color Doppler
Color Doppler is helpful in diagnosing and differentiating between various subgroups of PA-IVS. In most fetuses there is a lack of adequate filling of the right ventricle during diastole (Fig. 13-13). When the right ventricle is near normal or dilated, diastolic filling is followed by

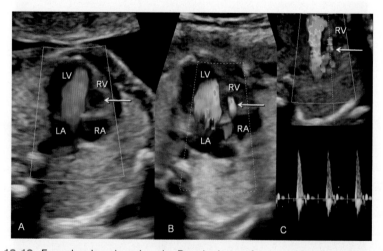

Figure 13-13. Four-chamber views in color Doppler in two fetuses with pulmonary atresia with intact interventricular septum. **Plane A** shows no perfusion across the dysplastic tricuspid valve (*arrow*), whereas in **plane B** minimal perfusion across the tricuspid valve is noted (*arrow*). Pulsed Doppler of the fetus in plane B **(plane C)** shows abnormal monophasic inflow into the hypoplastic right ventricle. RV, right ventricle; LV, left ventricle; RA, right atrium; LA, left atrium.

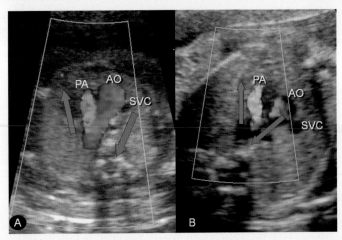

Figure 13-14. Three vessel-trachea views in two fetuses with pulmonary atresia and intact interventricular septum showing the typical antegrade flow (*blue*) across the transverse aortic arch (AO) and the retrograde flow (*red*) into the small pulmonary artery (PA). SVC, superior vena cava.

severe holosystolic tricuspid regurgitation, a condition described in Chapter 14 as tricuspid dysplasia. In the short-axis and three-vessel views, color Doppler shows no antegrade flow across the pulmonary valve and typically reverse flow across the arterial duct (Fig. 13-14). In the three-vessel view the aorta appears dilated with normal antegrade flow, whereas the main pulmonary artery is small and gets reverse flow in late systole via the ductus arteriosus. The diminutive right and left pulmonary arteries are filled retrograde via the ductus arteriosus.

The association of PA-IVS with ventriculo-coronary artery communications can be confirmed or ruled out by color Doppler (16–18). Ventriculo-coronary artery communications, which siphon right ventricular blood during systole, should be sought on color Doppler in the presence of a well-defined right ventricular cavity with diastolic filling and without significant regurgitation. Color Doppler with increased velocity scales may demonstrate these communications at the apex or right ventricular wall as turbulent flow (Fig. 13-15), which

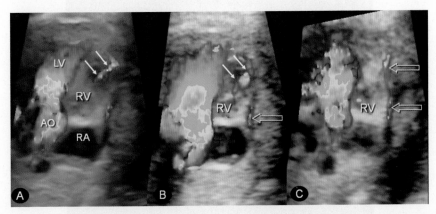

Figure 13-15. Pulmonary atresia with intact interventricular septum and ventriculo-coronary arterial communications (VCAC). Note in systole **(A, B)** drainage of the hypoplastic right ventricle (RV) across a small fistula located at the apex of the heart (*solid arrow*) into a coronary artery. During systole (B) and primarily in diastole **(C),** flow is seen along the pericardium in the coronary artery (*open arrows*). Confirming the presence of VCAC on pulsed Doppler is important in order to avoid its misdiagnosis with pericardial fluid movement. See Figure 13-16. LV, left ventricle; AO, aorta; RA, right atrium.

can be followed along the wall of the right ventricle until the origin of the right or left coronary artery at the aortic root (Figs. 13-10B and 13-15). Care should be taken not to confuse ventriculo-coronary artery communications with movement of pericardial fluid. Pulsed Doppler can be used for confirmation as it shows bidirectional turbulent flow with high velocities (50 to 150 cm/sec) (Fig. 13-16).

Early Gestation

PA-IVS can be present in early gestation and its detection was reported in the late first trimester by color Doppler showing lack of right ventricular filling and reverse flow in the ductus arteriosus (19). Even at this early stage ventriculo-coronary artery communications can be diagnosed (20). Progression of pulmonary stenosis to pulmonary atresia can develop in utero; therefore, the presence of a normal four-chamber view with normal diastolic filling on color Doppler in a fetus with pulmonary stenosis does not exclude progression to atresia.

Three-dimensional Ultrasound

Three-dimensional ultrasound in tomographic ultrasound imaging (TUI) with gray scale and color Doppler can demonstrate in one view anatomic abnormalities associated with PA-IVS such as the hypertrophied, hypoplastic right ventricular cavity and the diminutive pulmonary artery. TUI with color Doppler can demonstrate tricuspid regurgitation, retrograde flow in the ductus arteriosus, and/or right ventricular communication with the coronary arterial system. Surface mode may demonstrate the diminutive right ventricular cavity in comparison to the left ventricle (Fig. 13-17A). Three-dimensional volume measurements of the ventricles or area measurements of the tricuspid and mitral valves may be of help in the future in assessing fetuses at risk for impaired outcome. Inversion mode demonstrates the small cavity and its reduced movements in the 3-D rendering mode (Fig. 13-17B).

Associated Cardiac and Extracardiac Findings

Associated cardiac findings include right ventricular hypoplasia, right atrial dilation, tricuspid valve abnormalities, ventriculo-coronary arterial communications, subvalvular obstruction of the aortic valve due to bulging of the ventricular septum, atrial septal defects, dextrocardia,

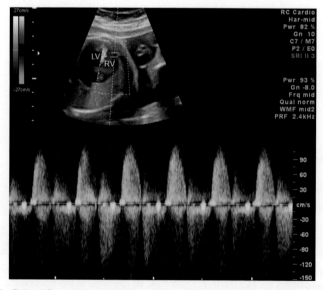

Figure 13-16. Pulsed Doppler in pulmonary atresia with right ventricular-coronary arterial communication. The sample volume is placed at the apex of the heart within the fistula as demonstrated in Figure 13-15B. Pulsed Doppler shows the typical bidirectional flow from the small right ventricle (RV) into the coronary artery in systole and from the coronary artery back into the right ventricle during diastole. LV, left ventricle.

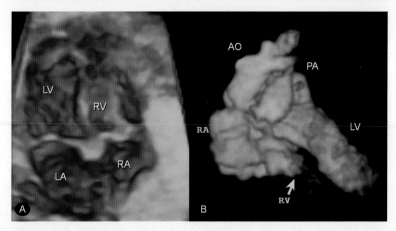

Figure 13-17. Three-dimensional ultrasound in a fetus with pulmonary atresia with intact interventricular septum. In **plane A,** the four-chamber view is shown in surface mode, demonstrating the small right ventricle (RV). In **plane B,** an anterior view of the heart in inversion mode is displayed showing the diminutive size of the hypoplastic right ventricle (*arrow*) when compared to the left ventricle (LV). RA, right atrium; LA, left atrium; AO, aorta; PA, pulmonary artery.

and transposition of great arteries. Sequential evaluation should be performed to rule out the association with heterotaxy, especially with situs abnormalities.

Extracardiac anomalies may be found but without an organ-specific pattern. Chromosomal aberrations such as trisomy 21 or 22q11 microdeletion are rare.

Differential Diagnosis

Differential diagnosis primarily includes pulmonary stenosis, tricuspid atresia with ventricular septal defect, and pulmonary atresia with ventricular septal defect. In pulmonary stenosis, antegrade flow across the pulmonary valve is demonstrated on color Doppler. In tricuspid atresia, color Doppler demonstrates no flow across the tricuspid valve in contrast to PA-IVS, where flow across the tricuspid valve is always demonstrated. Pulmonary atresia with ventricular septal defect is a distinct entity from PA-IVS, both from the embryologic and the hemodynamic points of view. Table 13-2 summarizes the differences between these two conditions.

Prognosis and Outcome

Prognosis of fetuses with PA-IVS is variable and is dependent on the size and function of the right ventricle. The optimum prognosis is noted in cases where biventricular repair is possible

TABLE 13-2	Differentiating Features of Pulmonary Atresia with Intact Ventricular Septum and Pulmonary Atresia with Ventricular Septal Defect	
	Pulmonary atresia with intact ventricular septum	**Pulmonary atresia with ventricular septal defect**
Pulmonary valve	Atretic	Atretic
Four-chamber view	Hypoplastic right ventricle	Normal
Five-chamber view	Normal	Ventricular septal defect with dilated overriding aorta
Main pulmonary artery	Hypoplastic to normal sized	Hypoplastic and may be absent
Ductus arteriosus	Retrograde flow and narrow	Retrograde flow and tortuous
Typical additional cardiac findings	Ventriculo-coronary arterial communications	Major aortopulmonary collateral arteries
Associated chromosomal anomalies	Rare, deletion 22q11	Common, 20% of cases with deletion 22q11

TABLE 13-3	Poor Prognostic Findings in Pulmonary Atresia with Intact Ventricular Septum

Severe tricuspid regurgitation
Small tricuspid valve annulus (Z score <-4)
Small RV/LV length or width (<0.5)
Presence of ventriculo-coronary arterial communications
Associated extracardiac abnormalities
Associated chromosomal abnormalities

RV, right ventricle; LV, left ventricle.

and right ventricular function is preserved. The presence of severe tricuspid regurgitation is associated with a high mortality in utero and in the neonatal period. On the contrary, in the absence of tricuspid regurgitation, the disease is well tolerated in utero. When the right ventricular inlet and outlet are fairly developed, postnatal treatment may include intervention catheterization with pulmonary valve perforation with laser or radiofrequency ablation followed by balloon dilation. In fetal series, PA-IVS is associated with an in utero mortality of 10% and a neonatal survival rate of 63% (21).

Several reports have addressed short- and long-term prognostic indicators for PA-IVS (22–27) and are presented in Table 13-3.

KEY POINTS: PULMONARY ATRESIA WITH INTACT VENTRICULAR SEPTUM

- PA-IVS is a group of cardiac malformations having in common absent communication between the right ventricle and the pulmonary arterial circulation with an intact interventricular septum.
- The right ventricular cavity is either hypoplastic with thickened right ventricular myocardium or dilated with significant tricuspid valve regurgitation.
- Tricuspid valve is usually dysplastic with impaired movements.
- Ventriculo-coronary arterial communications are found in about one third of cases of PA-IVS.
- In the four-chamber view the right ventricle can be hypoplastic, normal in size, or dilated.
- The pulmonary trunk in the right outflow tract view or the three-vessel view is typically small or hypoplastic.
- Color Doppler shows no antegrade flow across the pulmonary valve.
- The three-vessel view shows reversal of blood flow across the ductus arteriosus into the pulmonary trunk.
- Associated chromosomal aberrations are rare.
- Prognosis of fetuses with PA-IVS is variable and is dependent on the size and function of the right ventricle.

 PREMATURE CONSTRICTION OF THE DUCTUS ARTERIOSUS

Introduction

The ductus arteriosus (DA) is a muscular tube that provides a communication between the pulmonary and systemic circulation in fetal life. The DA connects the main pulmonary artery at the anatomic origin of the left pulmonary artery to the descending aorta (Fig. 13-18A) just distal to the left subclavian artery. This communication between the pulmonary and systemic circulation establishes the parallel circulation in the fetus and equalizes pressure in the right and left ventricles. The DA receives the majority of right ventricular output, bypassing the lungs. It is one of the largest vessels in the fetus with a diameter equal to that of the descending aorta. The patency of the ductus arteriosus is an active process maintained during gestation by the anatomic structure of the vessel and by circulating products such as prostaglandins in the fetal circulation. In early gestation, the DA wall is muscular, unlike surrounding vascular structures (28). With advancing gestation, increased deposition of collagen,

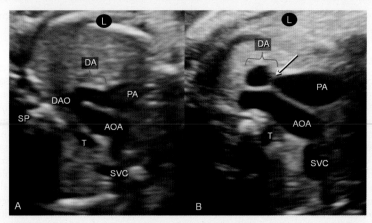

Figure 13-18. Transverse view of the upper fetal thorax showing the three-vessel-trachea view insonated from the left side. **A:** The ductus arteriosus (DA) is shown in a fetus at 29 weeks as a long, well-recognized tube (*brackets*) connecting the main pulmonary artery (PA) and the descending aorta (DAO). **B:** The DA is shown in a fetus at 34 weeks. Note the narrow segment of the DA at this gestation (*arrow*) starting from the pulmonary part toward the DAO in the normal fetus. AOA, aortic arch; SP, spine; SVC, superior vena cava; T, trachea; L, left.

elastin, and glycoproteins occurs, in addition to a proliferation of smooth muscle, to prepare for postnatal closure (28). This narrowing of the DA later in gestation starts at the junction to the pulmonary artery and progresses toward the junction with the descending aorta, a process that can be identified on prenatal ultrasound (Fig. 13-18B). An increase in oxygen tension, which occurs immediately after birth, is thought to be the stimulus for the closure of the DA.

Doppler of the ductus arteriosus can be achieved either in a longitudinal view of the ductal arch or in a cross-sectional plane of the three-vessel-trachea view as shown in Figure 13-19.

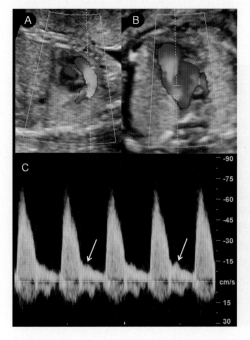

Figure 13-19. The insonation of the ductus arteriosus (DA) is achieved either longitudinally in the ductal arch plane **(A)** or in a transverse plane at the three-vessel-trachea view **(B).** Doppler waveforms **(C)** of the DA show the typical high velocities in systole and a second peak in diastole (*arrows*) with a high pulsatility index.

Doppler velocity waveform of the ductus arteriosus shows a high systolic peak velocity and a prominent diastolic flow as shown in Figure 13-19.

Premature Constriction of the Ductus Arteriosus In Utero

Total occlusion of the DA is extremely rare in fetal life, and most reported conditions addressed a constriction of the DA rather than an occlusion (29,30). Spontaneous constriction of the DA is very rarely seen unless it is part of a complex congenital heart malformation. Most cases of DA constriction, however, are due to maternal drug therapy with prostaglandin synthetase inhibitors such as indomethacin and others. Prostaglandin synthetase inhibitors are used as tocolytic agents for management of polyhydramnios in some cases and for management of degenerating fibroids in pregnancy. The risk for constriction of DA with prostaglandin synthetase inhibitors is increased in late gestation, probably related to the physiologic and anatomic changes of the DA that occur in late pregnancy. Therefore, constriction of the DA is related not only to the dose and duration of maternal drug therapy, but also to the gestational age at treatment. The risk of constriction increases significantly with advancing gestation, and the authors do not advise the use of prostaglandin synthetase inhibitors after 32 weeks' gestation and for a prolonged period. Drug-induced DA constriction is reversible a few days after cessation of treatment. Delivery concomitant with fetal DA constriction is associated with a high risk for the development of pulmonary hypertension in the newborn.

Ultrasound and Doppler Signs

Constriction of the DA is not reliably diagnosed on 2-D ultrasound as color and pulsed Doppler is essential for its diagnosis. The four-chamber view on 2-D ultrasound may show a hypokinetic, dilated right ventricle due to volume overload. Color Doppler reveals tricuspid regurgitation, which is generally holosystolic with maximum velocities at greater than 200 cm/sec. Visualization of the right ventricular outflow tract shows a dilated pulmonary artery with narrow DA. Color and pulsed Doppler, at the level of the constricted DA, shows turbulent high diastolic and systolic velocities with reduced pulsatile flow (Fig. 13-20A). Peak systolic velocities of around 200 to 300 cm/sec are typical (normal levels at 100 to 120 cm/sec), as are high diastolic velocities (greater than 35 cm/sec) with a pulsatility index (PI) less than 1.9 (normal greater than 2). Stopping the drug therapy will lead in most cases to a reversal of the findings (Fig. 13-20B) within 24 to 48 hours, but the tricuspid regurgitation may last longer.

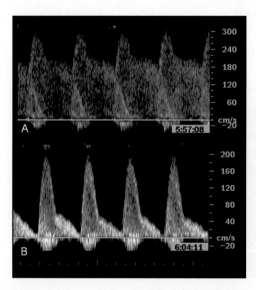

Figure 13-20. Maternal indomethacin therapy and ductus arteriosus (DA) constriction **(A)** in a fetus at 31 weeks with reversal after cessation of therapy **(B).** In A, DA constriction typically shows high systolic and diastolic velocities (systolic peak: 330 cm/sec; diastolic peak: 200 cm/sec) with a low pulsatility index (PI = 0.65). In B, Doppler waveforms are shown in the same fetus 3 days after cessation of indomethacin therapy. Note the near-normal pattern of the DA Doppler spectrum (systolic peak = 197 cm/sec, low diastolic peak = 35 cm/sec, and high PI = 2.57).

■ KEY POINTS: PREMATURE CONSTRICTION OF THE DUCTUS ARTERIOSUS

- The DA connects the main pulmonary artery to the descending aorta.
- The DA receives the majority of the right ventricular output, bypassing the lungs.
- An increase in oxygen tension, which occurs immediately after birth, is thought to be the stimulus for the closure of the DA.
- Most cases of DA constriction, however, are due to maternal drug therapy with prostaglandin synthetase inhibitors (indomethacin).
- DA constriction is related not only to the dose and duration of maternal drug therapy, but also to the gestational age at treatment.
- The authors do not advise the use of prostaglandin synthetase inhibitors after 32 weeks' gestation and for a prolonged period.
- In DA constriction, the four-chamber view shows a hypokinetic, dilated right ventricle with tricuspid regurgitation.
- In DA constriction, peak systolic velocities of around 200 and 300 cm/sec are typical, as are high diastolic velocities with a PI less than 1.9.
- Interruption of indomethacin therapy reverses the constriction and the ductus is patent again.

References

1. Rodriguez-Fernandez HL, Char F, Kelly DT, et al. The dysplastic pulmonic valve and the Noonan syndrome. *Circulation* 1972;46(2 Suppl):98–100.
2. Hoffman JI, Kaplan S. The incidence of congenital heart disease. *Circ Res* 2004;94:1890–1900.
3. Ferencz C, Rubin JD, Loffredo CA, et al. *Epidemiology of congenital heart disease: the Baltimore-Washington Infant Study.* New York: Futura Publishing Company, 1993;38.
4. Ferencz C, Rubin JD, Loffredo CA, et al. *Epidemiology of congenital heart disease: the Baltimore-Washington Infant Study.* New York: Futura Publishing Company, 1993;52.
5. Nora JJ, Fraser FC, Bear J, et al. *Medical genetics: principles and practice,* 4th ed. Philadelphia: Lea & Febiger, 1994;371.
6. Todros T, Paladini D, Chiappa E, et al. Pulmonary stenosis and atresia with intact ventricular septum during prenatal life. *Ultrasound Obstet Gynecol* 2003;21(3):228–233.
7. Berg C, Kremer C, Geipel A, et al. Ductus venosus blood flow alterations in fetuses with obstructive lesions of the right heart. *Ultrasound Obstet Gynecol* 2006;28(2):137–142.
8. Van Der Havwaert LF, Fryns JP, Dumoulin M, et al. Cardiovascular malformations in Turner's and Noonan's syndrome. *Br Heart J* 1978;40:500–505.
9. Zosmer N, Bajoria R, Weiner E, et al. Clinical and echographic features of in utero cardiac dysfunction in the recipient twin in twin-twin transfusion syndrome. *Br Heart J* 1994;72:74–79.
10. Lougheed J, Sinclair B, Fung KFK, et al. Acquired right ventricular outflow tract obstruction in twin-twin transfusion syndrome. *J Am Coll Cardiol* 1999;33:536A.
11. Hornberger LK, Benacerraf BR, Bromley BS, et al. Prenatal detection of severe right ventricular outflow tract obstruction: pulmonary atresia and pulmonary valve. *J Ultrasound Med* 1994;13(10):743–750.
12. Galindo A, Gutierrez-Larraya F, Velasco JM, et al. Pulmonary balloon valvuloplasty in a fetus with critical pulmonary stenosis/atresia with intact ventricular septum and heart failure. *Fetal Diagn Ther* 2006;21(1):100–104.
13. Hanley FL, Sade RM, Blackstone EH, et al. Outcomes in neonatal pulmonary atresia with intact ventricular septum. A multiinstitutional study. *J Thorac Cardiovasc Surg* 1993;105:406–407.
14. Humpl T, Soderberg B, McCrindle BW, et al. Percutaneous balloon valvuloplasty in pulmonary atresia with intact ventricular septum: impact on patient care. *Circulation* 2003;108:826–832.
15. Shinebourne EA, Rigby ML, Carvalho JS. Pulmonary atresia with intact ventricular septum: from fetus to adult: congenital heart disease. *Heart* 2008;94(10):1350–1357.
16. Chaoui R, Tennstedt C, Goldner B, et al. Prenatal diagnosis of ventriculo-coronary communications in a second-trimester fetus using transvaginal and transabdominal color Doppler sonography. *Ultrasound Obstet Gynecol* 1997;9(3):194–197.
17. Taddei F, Signorelli M, Groli C, et al. Prenatal diagnosis of ventriculocoronary arterial communication associated with pulmonary atresia. *Ultrasound Obstet Gynecol* 2003;21(4):413–415.
18. Maeno YV, Boutin C, Hornberger LK, et al. Prenatal diagnosis of right ventricular outflow tract obstruction with intact ventricular septum, and detection of ventriculocoronary connections. *Heart* 1999;81(6):661–668.
19. Paulick J, Tennstedt C, Schwabe M, et al. Prenatal diagnosis of an isochromosome 5p in a fetus with increased nuchal translucency thickness and pulmonary atresia with hypoplastic right heart at 14 weeks. *Prenat Diagn* 2004;24(5):371–374.
20. Chaoui R, Machlitt A, Tennstedt C. Prenatal diagnosis of ventriculo-coronary fistula in a late first-trimester fetus presenting with increased nuchal translucency. *Ultrasound Obstet Gynecol* 2000;15(2):160–162.
21. Daubeney PEF, Sharland GK, Cook AC, et al., for the UK and Eire Collaborative study of Pulmonary Atresia with Intact Ventricular Septum. Pulmonary atresia with intact ventricular septum. Impact of fetal echocardiography on incidence at birth and postnatal outcome. *Circulation* 1998;98:562–566.

22. Roman KS, Fouron JC, Nii M, et al. Determinants of outcome in fetal pulmonary valve stenosis or atresia with intact ventricular septum. *Am J Cardiol* 2007;99(5):699–703.

23. Gardiner HM, Belmar C, Tulzer G, et al. Morphologic and functional predictors of eventual circulation in the fetus with pulmonary atresia or critical pulmonary stenosis with intact septum. *J Am Coll Cardiol* 2008;51(13):1299–1308.

24. Kawazu Y, Inamura N, Kayatani F. Prediction of therapeutic strategy and outcome for antenatally diagnosed pulmonary atresia/stenosis with intact ventricular septum. *Circ J* 2008;72(9):1471–1475.

25. Peterson RE, Levi DS, Williams RJ, et al. Echocardiographic predictors of outcome in fetuses with pulmonary atresia with intact ventricular septum. *J Am Soc Echocardiogr* 2006;19(11):1393–1400.

26. Favilli S, Giusti S, Vangi V, et al. Pulmonary atresia or critical pulmonary stenosis with intact interventricular septum diagnosed in utero: echocardiographic findings and post-natal outcome. *Pediatr Med Chir* 2003;25(4):266–268.

27. Salvin JW, McElhinney DB, Colan SD, et al. Fetal tricuspid valve size and growth as predictors of outcome in pulmonary atresia with intact ventricular septum. *Pediatrics* 2006;118(2):e415–e420.

28. Silver MM, Freedom RM, Silver MD, et al. The morphology of the human newborn ductus arteriosus: a reappraisal of its structure and closure with special reference to prostaglandin E1 therapy. *Hum Pathol* 1981;12:1123–1136.

29. Luchese S, Manica JL, Zielinsky P. Intrauterine ductus arteriosus constriction: analysis of a historic cohort of 20 cases. *Arq Bras Cardiol* 2003;81(4):399–404.

30. Huhta JC, Moise KJ, Fisher DJ, et al. Detection and quantitation of constriction of the fetal ductus arteriosus by Doppler echocardiography. *Circulation* 1987;75:406–412.

EBSTEIN ANOMALY

Definition, Spectrum of Disease, and Incidence

In the normal heart the tricuspid valve inserts more apically on the interventricular septum than the mitral valve (see Chapter 5). In Ebstein anomaly the septal and posterior leaflets of the tricuspid valve are displaced inferiorly from the tricuspid valve annulus, toward the apex, and originate from the right ventricular myocardium (Figs. 14-1 and 14-2). The anterior tricuspid leaflet maintains its normal attachment to the tricuspid valve annulus. The proximal portion of the right ventricle is then continuous with the true right atrium and forms an "atrialized" portion of the right ventricle (Figs. 14-1 and 14-2). The spectrum of Ebstein anomaly is wide and varies from a minor form, with minimal displacement of the tricuspid valves with mild tricuspid regurgitation, to a severe form, with the "atrialization" of the entire right ventricle (Fig. 14-3).

Associated anomalies are not uncommon and include right ventricular outflow tract obstruction, either as pulmonary stenosis (Fig. 14-4) or atresia, and atrial and ventricular septal defects. The pathogenesis of pulmonary stenosis or atresia in association with Ebstein anomaly may be related to a reduction in flow across the pulmonary valve due to severe tricuspid regurgitation. Atrial septal defect may also result from the dilation of the right atrium due to the severe regurgitation noted in utero. Ebstein anomaly is one of the less common cardiac abnormalities occurring in about 0.5% of congenital heart disease in the neonate, with an equal male-to-female distribution (1,2). Ebstein anomaly is more common in prenatal series as it accounts for 3% to 7% of congenital heart disease in fetuses (3,4). This higher prenatal rate is related to an increase in fetal or early neonatal death in severe cases due to severe tricuspid regurgitation and associated pulmonary hypoplasia.

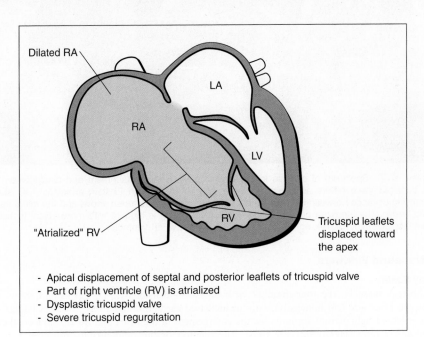

Dilated RA

LA

RA

LV

"Atrialized" RV

RV

Tricuspid leaflets displaced toward the apex

- Apical displacement of septal and posterior leaflets of tricuspid valve
- Part of right ventricle (RV) is atrialized
- Dysplastic tricuspid valve
- Severe tricuspid regurgitation

Figure 14-1. Ebstein anomaly. RA, right atrium; LA, left atrium; LV, left ventricle.

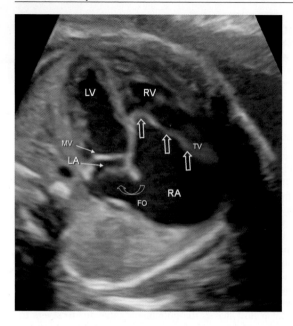

Figure 14-2. Four-chamber view in a fetus with Ebstein anomaly demonstrating the typical apical displacement of the tricuspid valve (TV) (*open straight arrows*) compared to the mitral valve (MV). The right atrium (RA) is dilated due to severe TV regurgitation, and the interatrial communication through the foramen ovale (FO) is wide (*open curved arrow*) due to increased right-to-left shunting of blood. LV, left ventricle; RV, right ventricle; LA, left atrium.

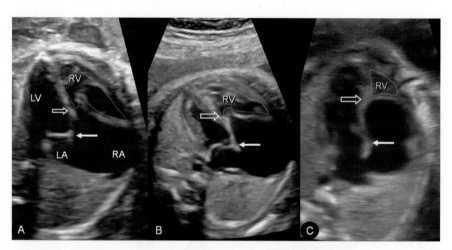

Figure 14-3. Spectrum of disease in Ebstein anomaly. Septal attachment and displacement of the tricuspid valve differs as shown in three fetuses **(A–C)** with Ebstein anomaly. A–C show increasing distance between the attachment of the tricuspid valve (*open arrow*) and the mitral valve (*solid arrow*). The atrialized portion of the right ventricle (RV) is biggest with more apical tricuspid valve displacement (C). RA, right atrium; LA, left atrium; LV, left ventricle.

Ultrasound Findings

Gray Scale

In Ebstein anomaly, the four-chamber view on two-dimensional (2-D) ultrasound shows an enlarged heart size (cardiomegaly) with an increased cardiothoracic ratio (5) (see Chapter 4). The enlarged right atrium accounts for the enlargement of the heart and for the abnormal cardiothoracic ratio (Figs. 14-2 and 14-3). The dilation of the right atrium, however, can be subtle during the second trimester, and a progressive dilation of the right atrium can be

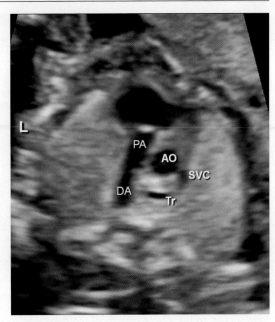

Figure 14-4. Transverse view of the ductal arch (DA) in a fetus with Ebstein anomaly showing right ventricular outflow tract obstruction. Note the narrow pulmonary artery (PA) compared to the size of the ascending aorta (AO). SVC, superior vena cava; Tr, trachea; L, left.

noticed with advancing gestation. The attachment of the septal leaflet of the tricuspid valve to the ventricular wall rather than to the valve annulus can be documented on careful observation of the tricuspid valve anatomy in systole and diastole by using the cine loop technique. This observation is essential for differentiating Ebstein anomaly from tricuspid valve dysplasia (see next section on tricuspid valve dysplasia). In severe Ebstein anomaly, with a large atrialized ventricle, paradoxical movements of the ventricular septum can be observed, with the apical and basal parts of the interventricular septum showing opposite directional movements. When pulmonary stenosis or atresia is present in association with Ebstein anomaly, the pulmonary artery appears smaller than the ascending aorta (Fig. 14-4) and the pulmonary valve may show poor excursion in the short-axis view.

Color Doppler
Color Doppler helps in the detection of severe tricuspid regurgitation even prior to the enlargement of the right atrium (Fig. 14-5). The tricuspid regurgitation occurs during the entire systole (holosystolic), with peak velocities of greater than 200 cm/sec (Fig. 14-6). The systolic regurgitant jet of the tricuspid valve typically arises from the middle of the right ventricle in Ebstein anomaly, in contrast to the regurgitant jet of tricuspid dysplasia, which arises at the level of the tricuspid valve annulus, an important differentiating point (Fig. 14-5). Color Doppler of the right outflow tract shows either a reverse flow in the ductus arteriosus toward the pulmonary valve or an antegrade flow into the often narrow pulmonary trunk when pulmonary atresia and stenosis is present (6).

Early Gestation
The presence of tricuspid regurgitation can be present at 11 to 14 weeks' gestation in fetuses with Ebstein anomaly, but the main findings of cardiomegaly and dilated right atrium are typically seen later in gestation. Early severe cases with cardiomegaly may be associated with a thickened nuchal translucency and fetal hydrops (Fig. 14-7), a sign of impending fetal demise.

Three-dimensional Ultrasound
The display of Ebstein anomaly with three-dimensional ultrasound such as tomographic imaging or orthogonal planes can demonstrate in one view the cardiomegaly, the level of attachment of the tricuspid valve leaflets, and the diminutive pulmonary artery. Surface rendering

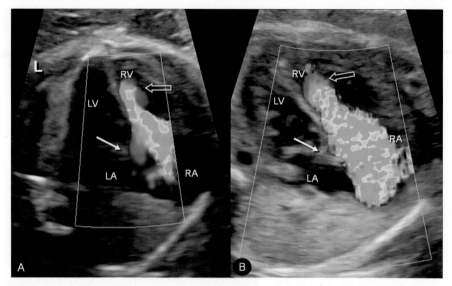

Figure 14-5. Color Doppler during systole at the four-chamber view in two fetuses with Ebstein anomaly demonstrating severe tricuspid regurgitation into the dilated right atrium (RA). Open arrows point to the site of closure of the dysplastic tricuspid valves. Solid arrows point to the attachment of the mitral valves. Note the anatomic origin of the regurgitant jet, deep in the right ventricle (RV), a differentiating point from tricuspid dysplasia (see text for details). LA, left atrium; LV, left ventricle; L, left.

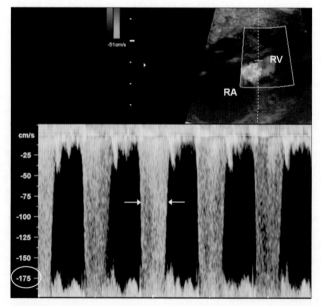

Figure 14-6. Tricuspid regurgitation on color and pulsed Doppler in a fetus with Ebstein anomaly. Note the holosystolic duration of the regurgitant jet (*arrows*) with peak velocities exceeding 175 cm/sec. RA, right atrium; RV, right ventricle.

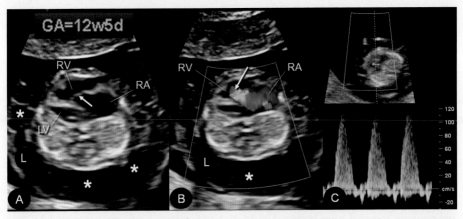

Figure 14-7. Gray scale **(A)**, color **(B)**, and pulsed Doppler **(C)** in a fetus at 12.5 weeks' gestation with Ebstein anomaly. Note the presence of generalized hydrops (*asterisks*) in A and B. The displaced apical attachment of the tricuspid valve in the right ventricle (RV) is shown in A (*arrow*). Severe tricuspid regurgitation originating near the apex of the RV is shown in B (*arrow*). Holosystolic tricuspid regurgitation with peak velocities of 120 cm/sec is demonstrated in C. RA, right atrium; LV, left ventricle; L, left.

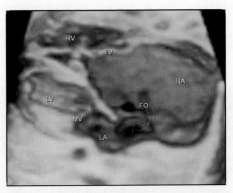

Figure 14-8. Three-dimensional ultrasound in surface mode display in a fetus with Ebstein anomaly showing the four-chamber view. The large right atrium (RA) and the wide foramen ovale (FO) are demonstrated (*open arrow*). Different levels of attachment of the tricuspid (TV) and mitral valves (MV) are noted. LA, left atrium; RV, right ventricle; LV, left ventricle.

(Fig. 14-8) can provide a better assessment of the abnormal valve anatomy (7) and could in the future be of importance in counseling parents for the options of postnatal therapy. Tricuspid regurgitation jets can be displayed in surface rendering and glass body mode (8). Volume measurements of the functional right ventricle may be of help in the future in assessing fetuses at risk for poor prognosis.

Associated Cardiac and Extracardiac Findings

Associated cardiac abnormalities include an obstruction of the right ventricular outflow tract as pulmonary stenosis (Fig. 14-4) or atresia in more than 60% of fetuses diagnosed with Ebstein anomaly prenatally (4). Atrial septal defects represent another common association and have been reported in up to 60% of children with Ebstein anomaly (9). The presence of right atrial enlargement and a high prevalence of accessory pathways increase the risk for supraventricular tachyarrhythmias, primarily seen in postnatal studies (10,11).

Most cases of Ebstein anomaly are isolated findings (12), but an association with chromosomal anomalies such as trisomy 21 or trisomy 13 has been reported in addition to familial cases. Amniocentesis for karyotyping should be offered as part of the workup. Severe tricuspid regurgitation can lead to in utero cardiac failure and development of fetal hydrops, which may be the first sign of the cardiac abnormality. Pulmonary hypoplasia, which increases neonatal morbidity and mortality, can occur when severe cardiomegaly is found. A cardiothoracic area ratio of greater than 0.6 in fetuses with cardiomegaly is associated with the postnatal presence of pulmonary hypoplasia (5).

Differential Diagnosis

On occasion, it may be difficult to differentiate prenatally between Ebstein anomaly and tricuspid valve dysplasia. The origin of the tricuspid regurgitant jet may help in differentiating these two lesions. In tricuspid valve dysplasia, the jet arises from the regularly inserted tricuspid valve at the level of the annulus, whereas in Ebstein anomaly, the origin of the regurgitant jet is displaced inferiorly within the right ventricle owing to the low insertion of the septal and posterior tricuspid valve leaflets (Fig. 14-5). Severe tricuspid regurgitation with cardiomegaly can be found in dilative cardiomyopathy and in other noncardiac lesions with fetal hemodynamic impairment. Premature closure of the ductus arteriosus may also be present with tricuspid regurgitation. Color and pulsed Doppler velocities across the ductus arteriosus help in differentiating this entity from Ebstein anomaly.

Prognosis and Outcome

Several prenatal series of Ebstein anomaly reported poor prognosis, with about 45% of fetuses dying in utero and an overall 80% to 90% mortality (13,14). Poor prognostic markers prenatally include massive cardiomegaly, decreased right ventricular outflow due to pulmonary stenosis, and fetal hydrops (13,15) (Fig. 14-9). Compression of the lungs may contribute to

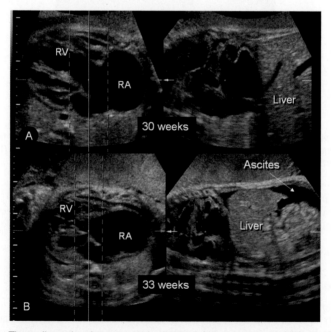

Figure 14-9. Three-dimensional tomographic display of the chest and abdomen at 30 **(A)** and 33 **(B)** weeks' gestation in a fetus with Ebstein anomaly showing the development of ascites at 33 weeks (B). This fetus died in utero at 36 weeks' gestation. RA, right atrium; RV, right ventricle.

TABLE 14-1	Echocardiographic Prognostic Score for Fetuses and Infants with Ebstein Anomaly
Score[a]	**Outcome**
Grade 1 = ratio <0.5	Very good
Grade 2 = ratio 0.5–0.99	Good—up to 92% survival
Grade 3 = ratio 1–1.49	Poor—early mortality of 10%; childhood mortality 45%
Grade 4 = ratio >1.5	Very poor—100% mortality likely

[a]Score: ratio of combined area of right atrium and atrialized right ventricle to that of the functional right ventricle and left heart in a four-chamber view at end diastole.
(From Paranon S, Acar P. Ebstein's anomaly of the tricuspid valve: from fetus to adult. *Heart* 2008;94:237–243; and Celermajer DS, Bull C, Till JA, et al. Ebstein's anomaly: presentation and outcome from fetus to adult. *J Am Coll Cardiol* 1994;23:170–176, with permission.)

pulmonary hypoplasia, a significant risk factor for the neonate. Prenatal diagnosis of Ebstein anomaly is associated with a poor outcome given an inherent selection of the most severe cases.

An echocardiographic grading score for neonates with Ebstein anomaly was proposed that involves calculating the ratio of the combined area of the right atrium and atrialized right ventricle to that of the functional right ventricle and left heart in a four-chamber view at end-diastole (16). Four grades of increasing severity were described and are shown in Table 14-1 with corresponding outcome (16). Left heart abnormalities involving the myocardium or valves were observed in 39% of primarily adult patients with Ebstein anomaly in one study, suggesting that Ebstein anomaly should not be regarded as a disease confined to the right side of the heart (17).

■ KEY POINTS: EBSTEIN ANOMALY

- The septal and posterior leaflets of the tricuspid valve are displaced inferiorly from the tricuspid valve annulus, toward the apex of the heart, and originate from the right ventricular myocardium.
- The anterior tricuspid leaflet maintains its normal attachment to the tricuspid valve annulus.
- The proximal portion of the right ventricle is continuous with the true right atrium and forms an "atrialized" portion of the right ventricle.
- Color Doppler helps in the detection of severe tricuspid regurgitation even prior to the enlargement of the right atrium.
- Tricuspid regurgitation is holosystolic with high peak velocities and typically arises from the middle of the right ventricle.
- Common associated cardiac abnormalities include an obstruction of the right ventricular outflow tract and atrial septal defects in more than 60% of cases.
- Pulmonary hypoplasia can occur with severe cardiomegaly.
- Prenatal series report poor prognosis, with about 45% of fetuses dying in utero and an overall 80% to 90% mortality.
- Poor prognostic markers prenatally include massive cardiomegaly, decreased right ventricular outflow due to pulmonary stenosis, and fetal hydrops.

TRICUSPID VALVE DYSPLASIA

Tricuspid valve dysplasia (Fig. 14-10) encompasses a heterogeneous group of malformations involving abnormalities of the tricuspid valve, where the normal anatomic insertion of the tricuspid valve leaflets is maintained at the level of the tricuspid valve annulus. The spectrum involves severe dysplastic leaflets with anomalous chordae tendineae insertion to mild lesions involving mild thickening of the valve leaflets. Similar to Ebstein anomaly, tricuspid valve dysplasia is associated with right ventricular outflow obstruction and atrial septal defects.

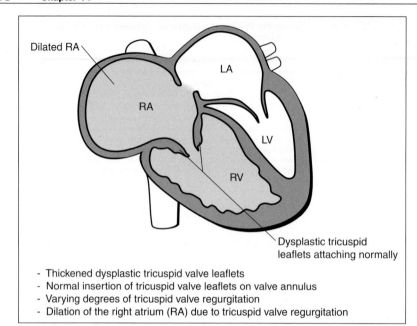

- Thickened dysplastic tricuspid valve leaflets
- Normal insertion of tricuspid valve leaflets on valve annulus
- Varying degrees of tricuspid valve regurgitation
- Dilation of the right atrium (RA) due to tricuspid valve regurgitation

Figure 14-10. Tricuspid valve dysplasia. RV, right ventricle; LA, left atrium; LV, left ventricle.

Ultrasound findings include thickened valve leaflets that do not close properly in systole and an enlarged right atrium in the four-chamber view (Fig. 14-11). Color Doppler typically shows tricuspid regurgitation with the regurgitant jet arising from the tricuspid valve annulus, a differentiating feature from Ebstein anomaly. In the presence of significant right ventricular

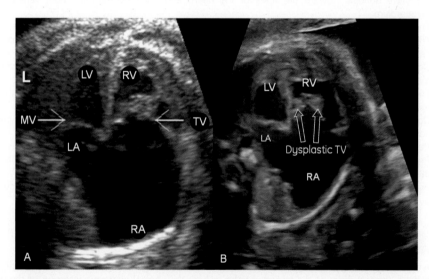

Figure 14-11. Four-chamber view in two fetuses **(A,B)** with tricuspid valve dysplasia. Tricuspid valves (TV), which are thickened, attach at their normal anatomic location on the ventricular septum near the level of the mitral valve (MV) attachment, a differentiating feature from Ebstein anomaly (see text). Dilation of the right atrium (RA) is noted. RV, right ventricle; LV, left ventricle; LA, left atrium; L, left.

outflow obstruction, color Doppler will demonstrate reverse flow in the ductus arteriosus. Three-dimensional ultrasound, in the rendered mode, may be of help in assessing tricuspid valve leaflets. Differential diagnosis of tricuspid dysplasia includes Ebstein anomaly and premature constriction of the ductus arteriosus. Associated chromosomal and nonchromosomal abnormalities are rare. The outcome of fetuses with tricuspid valve dysplasia is usually good except in its severe and rare form, which may be associated with heart failure, right ventricular outflow obstruction, severe tricuspid regurgitation, and a high rate of neonatal mortality.

■ KEY POINTS: TRICUSPID VALVE DYSPLASIA

- ■ Tricuspid valve dysplasia encompasses a heterogeneous group of malformations involving abnormalities of the tricuspid valve.
- ■ The normal anatomic insertion of the tricuspid valve leaflets is maintained at the level of the tricuspid valve annulus.
- ■ Color Doppler typically shows tricuspid regurgitation with the regurgitant jet arising from the tricuspid valve annulus, a differentiating feature from Ebstein anomaly.
- ■ Associated chromosomal and nonchromosomal abnormalities are rare.
- ■ The outcome of fetuses with tricuspid valve dysplasia is usually good.

 ## TRICUSPID REGURGITATION

The normal tricuspid valve closes during systole, preventing blood from returning to the right atrium with ventricular contraction. Tricuspid regurgitation or insufficiency is noted when blood is ejected back into the right atrium during systole (Fig. 14-12). Tricuspid regurgitation is a hemodynamic event detected by color and pulsed Doppler evaluation. Tricuspid regurgitation can be found in the fetus from 11 weeks' gestation until term (18–21). Tricuspid regurgitation varies in duration during systole and in peak velocity of the regurgitant jet. Precise description and quantification of tricuspid regurgitation is critical in understanding its pathophysiology and clinical significance.

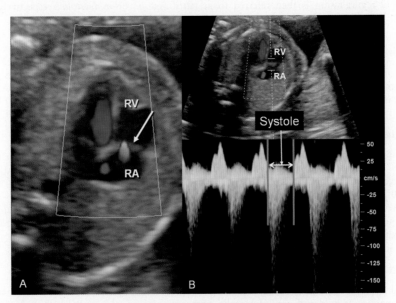

Figure 14-12. Color **(A)** and pulsed Doppler **(B)** of tricuspid regurgitation at 22 weeks' gestation demonstrating regurgitation during entire systole (holosystolic) (*double-sided arrow* in B) with peak velocities at 150 cm/sec. Color Doppler shows the regurgitation in systole in A (*arrow*). In this particular fetus, the regurgitation resolved 4 weeks later. RV, right ventricle; RA, right atrium.

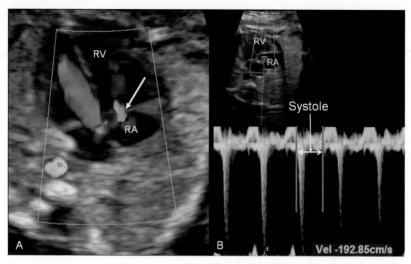

Figure 14-13. Color (*arrow* in **A**) and pulsed Doppler **(B)** of trivial tricuspid regurgitation at 22 weeks' gestation. Regurgitation occurs during the beginning of systole as "early systolic" (*double-sided arrow* in B) with peak velocities at 192 cm/sec. Spontaneous resolution occurred few weeks later. RV, right ventricle; RA, right atrium.

Duration

Tricuspid regurgitation can occur during the entire duration of systole and is thus termed *holo-systolic* (Figs. 14-6 and 14-12). When the regurgitant jet is limited to early or midsystole, tricuspid regurgitation is then referred to as *early systolic* or *midsystolic*, respectively (Fig. 14-13).

Severity

Independent from the duration of tricuspid regurgitation during systole, peak velocities of the regurgitant jet vary. Mild regurgitation has peak velocities between 30 and 70 cm/sec, whereas severe regurgitation has peak velocities between 180 and 350 cm/sec (Fig. 14-14).

Spatial Expansion

Tricuspid regurgitation can also be defined by the jet length and the right atrial area that it covers. Mild tricuspid regurgitation is defined by a jet that extends less than one third of the distance to the opposite atrial wall and covers an area less than 25% of the right atrium (19,20).

Several cardiac and noncardiac conditions in the fetus are associated with tricuspid regurgitation. Table 14-2 lists several conditions and their associated findings seen with tricuspid regurgitation in the fetus.

Trivial Tricuspid Valve Regurgitation

Trivial tricuspid regurgitation, an isolated finding in the absence of cardiac or extracardiac abnormalities, is mild and nonholosystolic, with a maximum velocity at less than 200 cm/sec (Fig. 14-13) (18). Trivial tricuspid regurgitation is a fairly common finding with a prevalence of 1% to 5% of fetuses presenting for fetal echocardiography in the second trimester of pregnancy (18). The incidence at 14 to 16 weeks' gestation was reported in 83% of fetuses in low-risk pregnancies in one study, with resolution of tricuspid regurgitation in most fetuses by

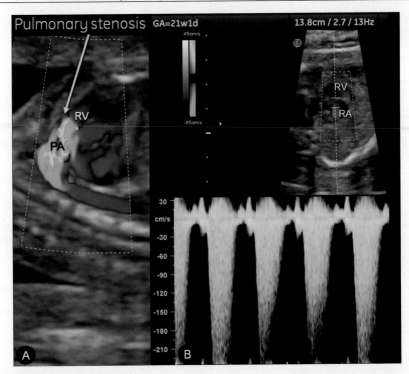

Figure 14-14. Tricuspid regurgitation at 21 weeks' gestation in a fetus with pulmonary stenosis. **A:** Color Doppler at the sagittal ductal arch view shows turbulence over the pulmonary valve. **B:** Severe holosystolic tricuspid regurgitation with peak velocities greater than 210 cm/sec. RV, right ventricle; RA, right atrium; PA, pulmonary artery.

the mid–second trimester (19). The pathogenesis of trivial tricuspid regurgitation is unknown but can be due to immature fetal myocardium (less compliant) and an increased pulmonary vascular bed pressure in early gestation. Ultrasound follow-up is recommended, and resolution of the regurgitation later in pregnancy is expected in the majority of cases.

Structural Cardiac Defects

Tricuspid regurgitation is a significant component of dysplastic tricuspid valves seen in Ebstein anomaly and tricuspid dysplasia. Fetal cardiac lesions with right ventricular outflow tract obstruction such as pulmonary atresia with intact ventricular septum, pulmonary stenosis (Fig. 14-14), and constriction of the ductus arteriosus commonly show tricuspid regurgitation. A compensatory dilation of the right ventricle with subsequent tricuspid regurgitation can also be found in aortic coarctation, hypoplastic left heart syndrome, double outlet right ventricle, and absent pulmonary valve syndrome. Rare anomalies of the right ventricle with tricuspid regurgitation include the absent tricuspid valve (called *unguarded tricuspid orifice*) (22) as well as the very rare *Uhl anomaly*, with a parchmentlike right ventricle wall.

Volume Overload

Volume overload of the right ventricle may lead to tricuspid regurgitation. Volume overload can be seen in fetal anemia (e.g., Rhesus disease, parvovirus), in peripheral arteriovenous fistula (e.g., vein of Galen aneurysm [Fig. 14-15], sacrococcygeal teratoma, chorioangioma), in the recipient twin in twin-to-twin transfusion syndrome, and in fetal arrhythmias. Some of these conditions can be associated with mitral regurgitation as well.

TABLE 14-2	Differential Diagnoses of Tricuspid Regurgitation (TR) in the Fetus	

Category	Etiology	Hints and associated findings
Trivial	Unknown	• Mild TR • Resolution with follow-up • Isolated
Heart defects with dysplastic TV	Ebstein anomaly	• Apical displacement of TV • Severe TR • Cardiomegaly, right atrial dilation
	TV dysplasia	• Thickened TV • Moderate to severe TR • Cardiomegaly, right atrial dilation
	Unguarded tricuspid orifice	• No tricuspid valve • "To and fro" flow in right heart
Heart diseases with right ventricular outflow obstruction	Pulmonary stenosis	• Thickened RV myocardium • Thickened pulmonary valve leaflets • Turbulent antegrade flow at pulmonary valve
	Pulmonary atresia with intact ventricular septum	• Hypoplastic RV • Thickened RV wall • Retrograde flow in ductus arteriosus
	Constriction of the ductus arteriosus	• Dilated RV • High velocities in ductus arteriosus with low pulsatility • History of nonsteroidal anti-inflammatory drug ingestion
Heart defects with "facultative" TV regurgitation		• Atrioventricular septal defect • Hypoplastic left heart syndrome • Coarctation of the aorta • Double outlet right ventricle • Absent pulmonary valve syndrome
Volume overload	Recipient in twin–twin transfusion syndrome	• Ultrasound markers of twin–twin transfusion syndrome
	Fetal anemia	• Increased peak velocity in middle cerebral artery
	Peripheral arteriovenous fistula	• Evidence of high-output cardiac failure
	Sustained arrhythmia	• Fetal cardiac arrhythmia
Impaired myocardial contractility	Myocarditis	• Ultrasound signs of infection • Maternal autoimmune disease (SLE)
	Cardiomyopathy	• Cardiomegaly • Poor contractility
	Fetal hypoxemia	• Severe IUGR • Abnormal Doppler studies

TV, tricuspid valve; RV, right ventricle; SLE, systemic lupus erythematosus; IUGR, in utero growth restriction.

Impairment of Myocardial Function

Impairment of myocardial function can be associated with tricuspid atresia. This is observed in cardiomyopathies, in severe intrauterine growth restriction with fetal hypoxemia, and in infectious (e.g., cytomegalovirus, parvovirus) or autoimmune (e.g., systemic lupus erythematosus) myocarditis.

Chromosomal Abnormalities

The presence of tricuspid regurgitation in the fetus at 11 to 14 weeks' gestation has been associated with chromosomal abnormalities (23) (Fig. 14-16). When the presence of tricuspid regurgitation was assessed in 1557 fetuses at 11 + 0 to 13 + 6 weeks, prior to chorionic

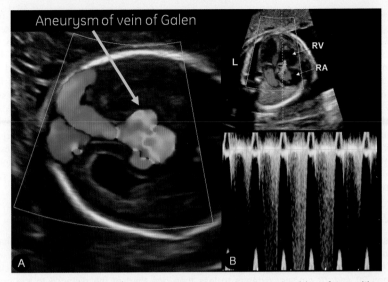

Figure 14-15. Tricuspid regurgitation resulting from volume overload in a fetus with aneurysm of vein of Galen. **A:** A large vein of Galen aneurysm (arteriovenous malformation). **B:** Dilation of right atrium (RA) and ventricle (RV) with holosystolic tricuspid regurgitation on pulsed Doppler evaluation. L, left.

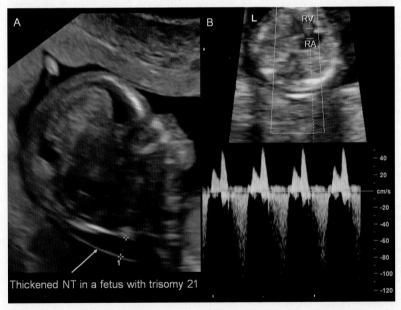

Figure 14-16. Tricuspid regurgitation at 12 weeks' gestation in a fetus with a thickened nuchal translucency (NT) **(A)** and trisomy 21. Criteria for tricuspid regurgitation include a Doppler sample volume of 2 to 3 mm, positioned across the tricuspid valve where one cross-bar is located in the right atrium (RA) and the other cross-bar located in the right ventricle (RV), in an apical four-chamber view such that the angle to the direction of flow is less than 20 degrees **(B).** Tricuspid regurgitation is diagnosed if the peak systolic velocity of the regurgitant jet is greater than 60 cm/sec and the duration of the jet involves at least half of systole as seen in B. L, left.

villous sampling, tricuspid regurgitation was found in less than 5% of chromosomally normal fetuses, in more than 65% of fetuses with trisomy 21, and in more than 30% of fetuses with trisomy 18 (23). The technical parameters of tricuspid regurgitation at 11 to 14 weeks' gestation include a Doppler sample volume of 2 to 3 mm, positioned across the tricuspid valve where one cross-bar is located in the right atrium and the other cross-bar is located in the right ventricle, in an apical four-chamber view such that the angle to the direction of flow is less than 20 degrees (Fig. 14-16) (23). Tricuspid regurgitation is diagnosed if the peak systolic velocity of the regurgitant jet is greater than 60 cm/sec and the duration of the jet involves at least half of systole (23) (Fig. 14-16). Examination of tricuspid flow in the first and early second trimesters, after screening by fetal nuchal translucency and serum biochemistry, may improve the performance of screening by reducing the false-positive rate from 5% to less than 3% while retaining the high detection rate of 90% (24,25). Tricuspid regurgitation was reported in 28% of Down syndrome fetuses in the second trimester in a high-risk referral population, albeit not in an isolated form (26).

▓ KEY POINTS: TRICUSPID REGURGITATION

- ▪ Tricuspid regurgitation varies in duration during systole, in peak velocity of the regurgitant jet, and in spatial expansion into the right atrium.
- ▪ Mild tricuspid regurgitation typically is limited to early or midsystole, has peak velocities between 30 and 70 cm/sec, extends to less than one third of the distance to the opposite atrial wall, and covers an area less than 25% of the right atrium.
- ▪ Trivial tricuspid regurgitation has a prevalence of 1% to 5% of fetuses presenting for fetal echocardiography.
- ▪ Tricuspid regurgitation occurs as a transient finding in the fetus and also with structural cardiac defects, cardiac volume overload, and impaired myocardial function.
- ▪ In first-trimester risk assessment for aneuploidy, tricuspid regurgitation is diagnosed if the peak systolic velocity of the regurgitant jet is greater than 60 cm/sec and the duration of the jet involves at least half of systole.

References

1. Fyler DC, Buckley LP, Hellenbrand WE, et al. Report of the New England Regional Infant Cardiac Program. *Pediatrics* 1980;65:375–461.
2. Bialostosky D, Horitz S, Espino-Vela J. Ebstein's malformation of the tricuspid valve: a review of 65 cases. *Am J Cardiol* 1972;29:826–830.
3. Copel JA, Pilo G, Green J, et al. Fetal echocardiographic screening for congenital heart disease: the importance of the four-chamber view. *Am J Obstet Gynecol* 1987;157:648–655.
4. Sharland GK, Chita SK, Allan LD. Tricuspid valve dysplasia or displacement in intrauterine life. *J Am Coll Cardiol* 1991;17(4):944–949.
5. Chaoui R, Bollmann R, Goldner B, et al. Fetal cardiomegaly: echocardiographic findings and outcome in 19 cases. *Fetal Diagn Ther* 1994;9(2):92–104.
6. Chaoui R, McEwing R. Three cross-sectional planes for fetal color Doppler echocardiography. *Ultrasound Obstet Gynecol* 2003;21(1):81–93.
7. Acar P, Dulac Y, Taktak A, et al. Real-time three-dimensional fetal echocardiography using matrix probe. *Prenat Diagn* 2005;25(5):370–375.
8. Goncalves LF, Romero R, Espinoza J, et al. Four-dimensional ultrasonography of the fetal heart using color Doppler spatiotemporal image correlation. *J Ultrasound Med* 2004;23(4):473–481.
9. Watson H. Natural history of Ebstein's anomaly of tricuspid valve in childhood and adolescence. An international cooperative study of 505 cases. *Br Heart J* 1974;36:417–427.
10. Cappato R, Hebe J, Weib C, et al. Radiofrequency current ablation of accessory pathways in Ebstein's anomaly. *J Am Coll Cardiol* 1993;21(Suppl A):172A.
11. Paranon S, Acar P. Ebstein's anomaly of the tricuspid valve: from fetus to adult. *Heart* 2008;94:237–243.
12. Gucer S, Ince T, Kale G, et al. Noncardiac malformations in congenital heart disease: a retrospective analysis of 305 pediatric autopsies. *Turk J Pediatr* 2005;47(2):159–166.
13. Hornberger LK, Sahn DJ, Kleinman CS, et al. Tricuspid valve disease with significant tricuspid insufficiency in the fetus: diagnosis and outcome. *J Am Coll Cardiol* 1991;17(1):167–173.
14. Roberson DA, Silverman NH. Ebstein's anomaly: echocardiographic and clinical features in the fetus and neonate. *J Am Coll Cardiol* 1989;14:1300–1307.
15. McElhinney DB, Salvin JW, Colan SD, et al. Improving outcomes in fetuses and neonates with congenital displacement (Ebstein's malformation) or dysplasia of the tricuspid valve. *Am J Cardiol* 2005;96(4):582–586.
16. Celermajer DS, Bull C, Till JA, et al. Ebstein's anomaly: presentation and outcome from fetus to adult. *J Am Coll Cardiol* 1994;23:170–176.

17. Attenhofer-Jost CH, Connolly HM, O'Leary PW, et al. Left heart lesions in patients with Ebstein anomaly. *Mayo Clin Proc* 2005;80(3):361–368.
18. Respondek ML, Kammermeier M, Ludomirsky A, et al. The prevalence and clinical significance of fetal tricuspid valve regurgitation with normal heart anatomy. *Am J Obstet Gynecol* 1994;171:1265–1270.
19. Messing B, Porat S, Imbar T, et al. Mild tricuspid regurgitation: a benign fetal finding at various stages of pregnancy. *Ultrasound Obstet Gynecol* 2005;26:606–610.
20. Gembruch U, Smrcek JM. The prevalence and clinical significance of tricuspid regurgitation in normally grown fetuses and those with intrauterine growth retardation. *Ultrasound Obstet Gynecol* 1997;9:374–382.
21. Huggon IC, DeFigueiredo DB, Allan LD. Tricuspid regurgitation in the diagnosis of chromosomal anomalies in the fetus at 11–14 weeks of gestation. *Heart* 2003;89:1071–1073.
22. Indrani S, Vijayalakshmi R, Suresh S. Color Doppler flow pattern in antenatal diagnosis of unguarded tricuspid valve. *Ultrasound Obstet Gynecol* 2005;25:514–516.
23. Falcon O, Faiola S, Huggon I, et al. Fetal tricuspid regurgitation at the 11 + 0 to 13 + 6 week scan: association with chromosomal defects and reproducibility of the method. *Ultrasound Obstet Gynecol* 2006;27:609–612.
24. Falcon O, Auer M, Gerovassili A, et al. Screening for trisomy 21 by fetal tricuspid regurgitation, nuchal translucency and maternal serum free β-hCG and PAPP-A at 11 + 0 to 13 + 6 weeks. *Ultrasound Obstet Gynecol* 2006;27:151–155.
25. Nicolaides KH, Spencer K, Avgidou K, et al. Multicenter study of first-trimester screening for trisomy 21 in 75 821 pregnancies: results and estimation of the potential impact of individual risk-orientated two-stage first-trimester screening. *Ultrasound Obstet Gynecol* 2005;25:221–226.
26. DeVore GR. Trisomy 21: 91% detection rate using second-trimester ultrasound markers. *Ultrasound Obstet Gynecol* 2001;16:133–141.

ATRIAL, VENTRICULAR, AND ATRIOVENTRICULAR SEPTAL DEFECTS

ATRIAL SEPTAL DEFECT

Definition, Spectrum of Disease, and Incidence

An atrial septal defect (ASD) is an opening of the atrial septum leading to a communication between the left and right atrium. According to its location, an ASD is classified into septum primum, septum secundum, sinus venosus, and coronary sinus defect (Fig. 15-1). Septum secundum defect (ASD II), which is due to lack of tissue in the region of the foramen ovale, is the most common, accounting for about 80% of all ASDs (1). Septum primum defect (ASD I), the second most common, represents a gap in the embryologic septum primum region, adjacent to both atrioventricular valves (Fig. 15-2) and is considered a partial atrioventricular septal defect (discussed later in this chapter). Sinus venosus atrial septal defect is found posterior and superior to the foramen ovale and inferior to the connections of the superior and inferior vena cava within the right atrium (Fig. 15-1). The rare coronary sinus atrial septal defect is located at the site of the coronary sinus ostium in the right atrium and is often associated with coronary sinus abnormalities (Fig. 15-1). The incidence of an ASD in postnatal series is high, accounting for 7% of all infants with congenital heart defects and occurring in 1 per 1500 live births with a 2:1 female-to-male ratio (2,3). ASD II and sinus venosus defects are practically inexistent in prenatal series (4). ASD I, detectable prenatally, is discussed in the section on atrioventricular septal defect.

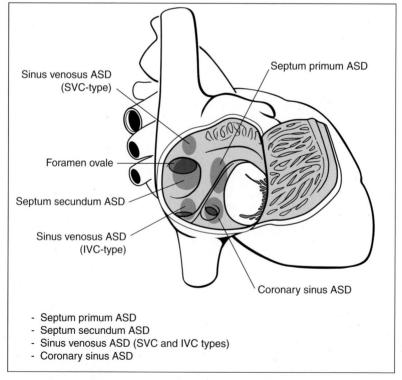

Figure 15-1. Types and anatomic locations of atrial septal defects (ASD) as seen from the right atrium. SVC, superior vena cava; IVC, inferior vena cava.

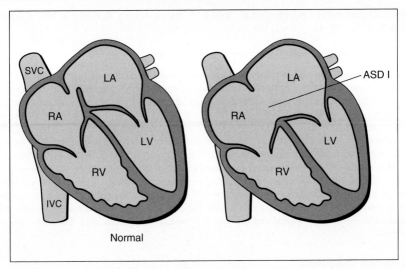

Figure 15-2. Septum primum atrial septal defect (ASD), also known as ASD type I or incomplete atrioventricular septal defect. The atrial septal defect is in the septum primum region, and the atrioventricular valves show a linear insertion. The figure on the left represents normal anatomy. LA, left atrium; RA, right atrium; LV, left ventricle; RV, right ventricle; IVC, inferior vena cava; SVC, superior vena cava.

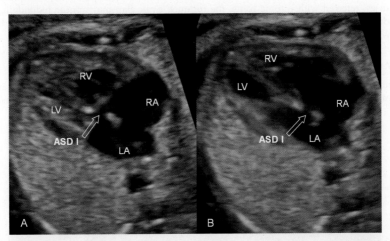

Figure 15-3. Septum primum atrial septal defect (ASD I) in systole **(A)** and diastole **(B)** in the same fetus at the four-chamber view. Note the gap in the septum primum region (*open arrows*) seen in systole (A) and diastole (B). The closed atrioventricular valves in systole (A) are shown in a linear insertion. LA, left atrium; LV, left ventricle; RA, right atrium; RV, right ventricle.

Ultrasound Findings

The diagnosis of an isolated atrial septal defect is very difficult in the fetus. ASD II is located in the foramen ovale region, and whether or not a large foramen ovale will close postnatally is difficult to predict. An attempt of a "prenatal diagnosis" of ASD II is commonly associated with a high false-positive and false-negative rate. Sinus venosus defects are difficult to image even on postnatal examination and to our knowledge have yet to be diagnosed prenatally. ASD I can be identified in the fetus by the gap in the septum primum region, which is generally accompanied with a linear insertion of both atrioventricular valves (Fig. 15-3). Color

Doppler can confirm the presence of an ASD I by demonstrating shunting of blood across the septal defect (Fig. 15-4).

Associated Cardiac and Extracardiac Findings

Associated cardiac malformations are common and include atrioventricular septal defect, isomerism, abnormal pulmonary venous connection, single ventricle, or anomalies of obstructive right ventricle and outflow tract such as Ebstein anomaly, tricuspid atresia with ventricular septal defect, and pulmonary atresia with intact ventricular septum. Abnormalities of the venous system are common, as 10% to 15% of ASD II and 80% to 90% of the sinus venosus–superior vena cava-type defects are associated with partial anomalous venous connection (5,6). Coronary sinus defects are commonly associated with persistent left superior vena cava.

ASDs are described in numerous extracardiac anomalies and syndromes, such as trisomy 21. Since their detection as an isolated finding is unlikely prenatally, the authors will not enumerate all possible associated syndromes but will mention in particular Holt-Oram syndrome, which is associated with an 85% to 95% risk for cardiac anomalies, most commonly ASD II and muscular ventricular septal defects (see Chapter 2 for details and for other associated syndromes).

Differential Diagnosis

Once an ASD is suspected, associated cardiac findings should be ruled out, mainly the presence of an associated atrioventricular septal defect or a single ventricle. In the authors' experience, the presence of a dilated coronary sinus with a persistent left superior vena cava associated with left-to-right atrial shunting on color Doppler is a common reason for referral with a false-positive diagnosis of ASD (see Chapter 23 for details) (Fig. 15-5). Furthermore, in few fetuses, referred with ectopic beats, the foramen ovale flap may appear redundant, previously described as "aneurysm of the foramen ovale" (7,8) (Fig. 15-6), and this may be confused with an atrial septal defect.

Prognosis and Outcome

Postnatally, some small ASDs may be followed up conservatively given a significant chance for spontaneous closure, especially for the ASD II type. Moderate to large ASD II and other forms

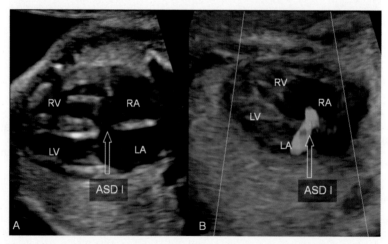

Figure 15-4. Gray scale **(A)** and color Doppler **(B)** in a fetus with septum primum atrial septal defect (ASD I). Note the gap in the septum primum region in A (*open arrow*) and shunting across the defect from the right atrium (RA) to the left atrium (LA) shown on color Doppler in B (*open arrow*) (unlike coronary sinus flow, which is from left to right). LV, left ventricle; RV, right ventricle.

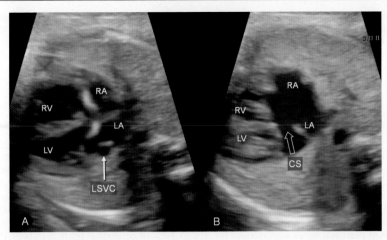

Figure 15-5. Transverse planes of the fetal chest at the level of the four-chamber view **(A)** and just inferior to the four-chamber view **(B)** in a fetus with a persistent left superior vena cava (LSVC, *arrow* in A) and dilated coronary sinus (CS, *open arrow* in B). Note the appearance of the CS in B, which can be mistaken for a septum primum defect. RV, right ventricle; LV, left ventricle; RA, right atrium; LA, left atrium.

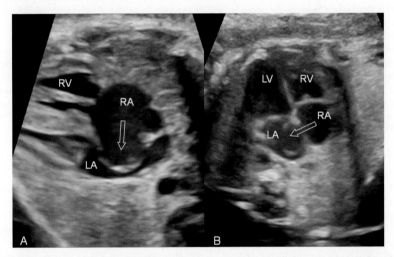

Figure 15-6. Transverse planes **(A, B)** at the level of the four-chamber view in two fetuses with redundant flaps of the foramen ovale (*open arrows*), an isolated finding that should not be mistaken for an atrial septal defect. RV, right ventricle; LV, left ventricle; RA, right atrium; LA, left atrium.

require closure in order to avoid left-to-right blood shunting with volume overload of the right atrium and subsequently the lungs. Closure is achieved either surgically or with nonsurgical techniques such as percutaneous catheter closure devices. Short- and long-term outcomes are excellent for all forms when isolated. Prognosis of ASD associated with other cardiac malformations or genetic syndromes is dependent primarily on the severity of the associated abnormality.

■ KEY POINTS: ATRIAL SEPTAL DEFECTS

- ASDs are classified into septum primum, septum secundum, sinus venosus, and coronary sinus defects based on their anatomic location.
- Septum secundum defect is the most common, accounting for about 80% of all ASDs.

- The diagnosis of an isolated atrial septal defect is very difficult or impossible in the fetus.
- Partial anomalous venous connection is associated with 10% to 15% of ASD II and 80% to 90% of the sinus venosus–superior vena cava-type ASD.
- Coronary sinus defects are commonly associated with persistent left superior vena cava.
- Holt-Oram syndrome is associated with an 85% to 95% risk for cardiac anomalies, most commonly ASD II and muscular ventricular septal defects.

 VENTRICULAR SEPTAL DEFECT

Definition, Spectrum of Disease, and Incidence

A ventricular septal defect (VSD) is an opening in the ventricular septum leading to a hemodynamic communication between the left and right ventricle. VSDs are common congenital heart defects, second only to bicuspid aortic valves. Isolated VSDs account for 30% of children born with congenital heart defects and are associated with other cardiac anomalies in about 30% of cases (9). Postnatal echocardiographic evaluation reports the prevalence of VSD to be as high as 50 per 1000 live births (10). In fetal series the incidence of isolated VSDs is much lower than postnatal series and account for 5% to 10% of congenital heart defects (4,11).

Four anatomic components of the ventricular septum exist: The *inlet septum* separates the two atrioventricular valves, the *outlet septum* includes the conal and infundibular septum and relates to the region below the arterial valves and above the crista supraventricularis, the *membranous septum* is the small thin region in the left ventricular outflow tract just beneath the aortic valve and under the crista supraventricularis, and the thick *trabecular (or muscular) septum* is the largest part of the septum, which extends from the attachments of the tricuspid valves to the apex. Many classifications of VSDs have been proposed, and typically VSDs are reported based on their anatomic locations on the septum (Figs. 15-7 and 15-8). Perimembranous VSDs are the most common, accounting for about 80% of cases (12). Muscular, inlet, and outlet VSDs account for 5% to 20%, 5% to 8%, and 5% of the remainder of cases, respectively (12,13) (Table 15-1). VSDs are frequently associated with various cardiac anomalies, as they are obligatory in some and occasionally or frequently found in others, as shown in Table 15-2. VSDs tend to have a high recurrence rate and are slightly more common in girls (14). Figure 15-9 shows two anatomic specimens of fetal hearts with VSDs.

Ultrasound Findings

Gray Scale
A VSD can be detected in the second and third trimester of pregnancy with two-dimensional (2-D) ultrasound when the size of the defect is more than 2 to 3 mm (Fig. 15-10). Smaller VSDs are often overseen on prenatal ultrasound and are occasionally detected by the routine use of color Doppler. The majority of reported VSDs in fetal series are detected when an extracardiac or cardiac anomaly is found and the heart is carefully examined.

Inlet VSDs are found in the region of the atrioventricular valves in the four-chamber plane (Fig. 15-11) and often are difficult to differentiate from a mild form of complete or partial atrioventricular septal defects. Dropout artifacts on 2-D ultrasound and overlapping of color Doppler (bleeding artifact) can lead to false-positive diagnoses. The lateral or transverse view of the heart on 2-D ultrasound can be of help in reducing false-positive and false-negative diagnoses. The presence of linear insertion of the atrioventricular valves may be very suspicious for the presence of a mild form of an atrioventricular septal defect.

Muscular VSDs are rarely detected on 2-D ultrasound unless their size is large (>2 to 3 mm) (Fig. 15-10). They can be identified in the apical or transverse four-chamber views. In such cases, the borders of the VSD commonly appear echogenic (Fig. 15-10), which can be an important hint in differentiating a true muscular VSD from artifact. The majority of muscular VSDs are detected accidentally by the routine use of color Doppler (Figs. 15-12 and 15-13). The shunt on color Doppler is typically bidirectional, and the most common location of VSDs is in the apical and midportion of the septum (Figs. 15-12 and 15-13).

The most common VSD detected on 2-D ultrasound is the *perimembranous* type, visualized in the five-chamber view. The first clue to its presence is in the interruption of the continuity between the ventricular septum and the ascending aorta (Figs. 15-14 and 15-15).

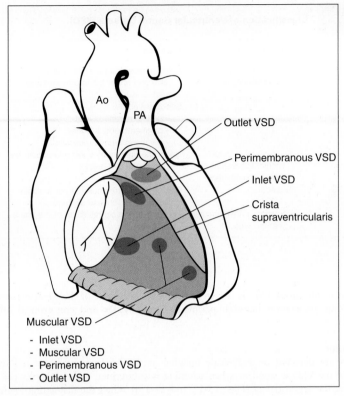

Figure 15-7. Ventricular septal defect (VSD)—types and anatomic locations as seen from the right ventricle. PA, pulmonary artery; Ao, aorta.

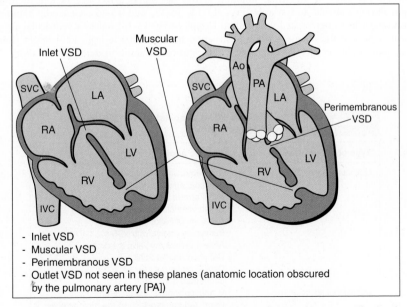

Figure 15-8. Ventricular septal defect (VSD)—anatomic locations as seen at the level of the four-chamber view and the outflow tracts. Ao, aorta; RA, right atrium; RV, right ventricle; LA, left atrium; LV, left ventricle; SVC, superior vena cava; IVC, inferior vena cava.

| TABLE 15-1 | Classification of Ventricular Septal Defects (VSD) | | |

Type	Also called	Location	Frequency
Perimembranous VSD	Infracristal, conoventricular	In the outflow tract beneath the aortic valve and under the supraventricular crest Subclassified as: – perimembranous inlet – perimembranous outlet – perimembranous muscular	70%–80%
Outlet VSD	Supracristal, subpulmonic, subarterial, doubly committed	Under the pulmonary valve and above the supraventricular crest	5%–7%
Muscular VSD	Trabecular	Can be apical, midmuscular, or multiple (called Swiss cheese septum)	5%–20%
Inlet VSD	Posterior, atrioventricular septum type	Posterior to the septal leaflet of the tricuspid valve	5%–8%

When a perimembranous VSD is detected, detailed assessment of the great arteries is critical given a strong association between perimembranous VSDs and conotruncal abnormalities (Table 15-2).

Color Doppler

Large VSDs are detected on gray-scale imaging at the level of the four- and five-chamber views. When the VSD is small or when scanning is suboptimal, color Doppler can be of help in identifying the septal defect (Figs. 15-12 and 15-13). When the insonating angle is perpendicular to the ventricular septum, motion and dropout artefacts are reduced and true shunting of blood is demonstrated at the septal defect level (Figs. 15-12 and 15-15). Despite near-equal ventricular pressures in the fetus, shunting across the septal defect occurs due to pressure changes during diastole and systole (Figs. 15-12, 15-13, and 15-15). Generally shunting is bidirectional when interrogated with pulsed Doppler (Fig. 15-16) unless a ventricular pressure gradient is present due to an outflow obstruction in one ventricle (e.g., left-to-right shunt in double outlet right ventricle or coarctation and right-to-left shunt in tetralogy of Fallot).

| TABLE 15-2 | Cardiac Anomalies Associated with Ventricular Septal Defects (VSDs) |

Type of association	Cardiac anomaly
Obligatory association	Atrioventricular septal defect Tricuspid atresia + VSD Mitral atresia +VSD Single ventricle (double inlet ventricle) Tetralogy of Fallot Pulmonary atresia with VSD Absent pulmonary valve syndrome Common arterial trunk Double outlet right ventricle Interrupted aortic arch
Occasional association	D-transposition of the great arteries Corrected transposition of the great arteries Aortic coarctation

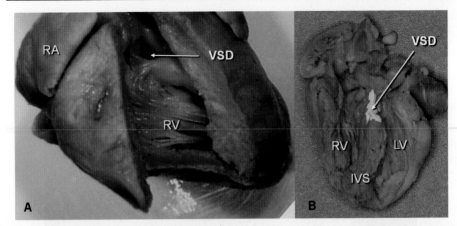

Figure 15-9. Two anatomic specimens of fetal hearts with ventricular septal defects (VSD). **A:** The heart is opened from the right ventricle (RV) and a perimembranous VSD is seen (*arrow*). **B:** The heart is opened at the four-chamber view and a large inlet VSD is noted (*arrow*—colored white for better demonstration). RA, right atrium; LV, left ventricle; IVS, interventricular septum.

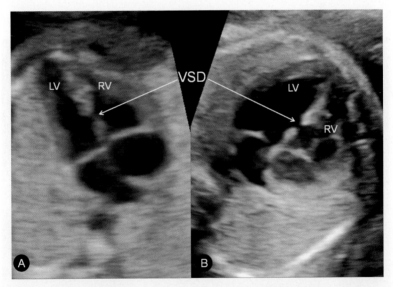

Figure 15-10. Apical four-chamber views in two fetuses **(A,B)** with large (>2 mm) muscular ventricular septal defects (VSDs) located in the middle of the septum. Note in B the echogenic borders of the VSD. LV, left ventricle; RV, right ventricle.

Early Gestation

VSDs are generally too small to be reliably detected as isolated anomalies at 11 to 14 weeks' gestation. Caution should be made in diagnosing VSDs in early gestation given a significant false-positive diagnosis from echo dropout and color overlapping. VSD, on the other hand, can be reliably demonstrated when it is associated with another cardiac anomaly or when the four-chamber view anatomy is abnormal.

Three-dimensional Ultrasound

Tomographic ultrasound imaging applied to a three-dimensional (3-D) volume acquired at the level of the four-chamber view allows for the demonstration of the VSD in different

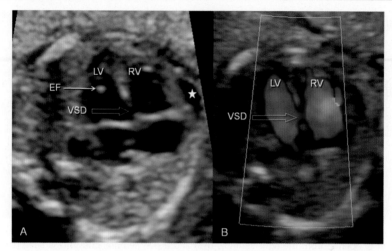

Figure 15-11. Inlet ventricular septal defect (VSD) demonstrated on gray scale (**A**, *open arrow*) and color Doppler (**B**, *open arrow*) at the four-chamber view. Echogenic intracardiac focus (EF) and pericardial effusion (*star*) is also shown in A. This fetus was found to have trisomy 21 on karyotypic analysis. LV, left ventricle; RV, right ventricle.

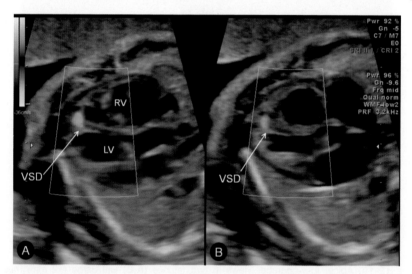

Figure 15-12. Five-chamber view with color Doppler in a fetus with a small muscular ventricular septal defect (VSD) at the cardiac apex demonstrating bidirectional flow across the VSD from the left ventricle (LV) to the right ventricle (RV) in **A** and from the RV to the LV in **B**. The small muscular VSD is not visible without color Doppler.

adjacent planes of the septum rather than a single plane on conventional 2-D sonography. The orthogonal 3-D display can be used in combination with color spatio-temporal image correlation (STIC) to demonstrate the presence of a VSD in all three planes, by placing the intersection dot on the shunting VSD (Fig. 15-17) (15). The *en face* view of the interventricular septum in a 3-D volume allows a direct view of the size of a large VSD on surface rendering (Fig. 15-18) (16) as well as blood shunting when combined with color STIC (Fig. 15-19) (17).

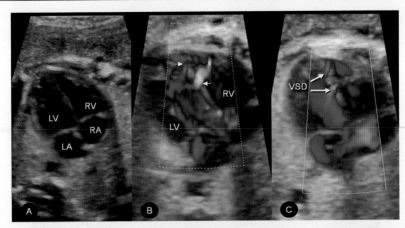

Figure 15-13. Apical four-chamber views in gray scale **(A)** and color Doppler during systole **(B)** and diastole **(C)** in a fetus with two small muscular ventricular septal defects (VSDs). The apical four-chamber view appears normal on gray scale (A). Color Doppler demonstrates two apical muscular VSDs (*arrows*) with left-to-right shunting in B and right-to-left shunting in C. LA, left atrium; LV, left ventricle; RA, right atrium; RV, right ventricle.

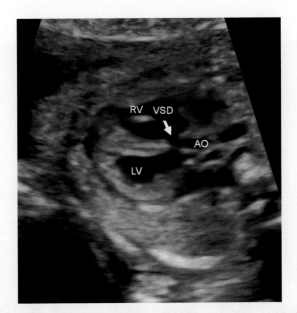

Figure 15-14. Five-chamber view in a fetus with perimembranous ventricular septal defect (VSD). The ascending aorta is seen (AO) with an interruption in the septal-aortic continuity (*arrow*) at the VSD location. LV, left ventricle; RV, right ventricle.

Differential Diagnosis

Dropout artefact, primarily in the perimembranous region of the septum, is a common false-positive diagnosis of VSD before 20 weeks' gestation. Harmonic and compound imaging designed to improve the gray-scale 2-D image may result in reducing echo reflection from the thin

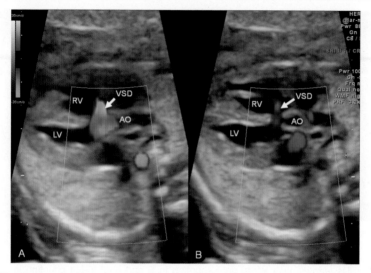

Figure 15-15. Five-chamber view with color Doppler in a fetus with perimembranous ventricular septal defect (VSD; same fetus as in Fig. 15-14). Color Doppler shows the bidirectional shunting with left-to-right shunting during systole **(A)** and right-to-left-shunting in diastole **(B)**. LV, left ventricle; RV, right ventricle; AO, aorta.

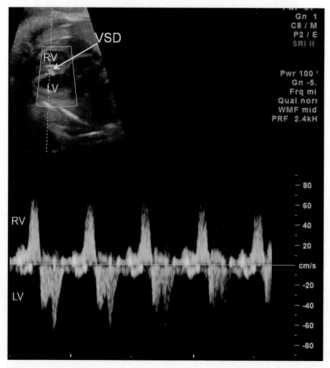

Figure 15-16. Color and pulsed Doppler in a fetus with a ventricular septal defect (VSD) demonstrating bidirectional shunting on pulsed Doppler, thus confirming the presence of a VSD. LV, left ventricle; RV, right ventricle.

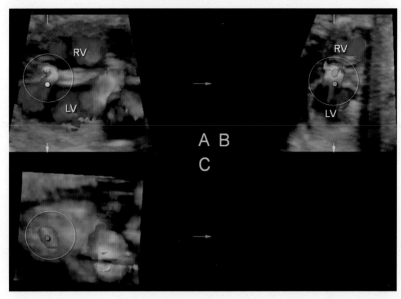

Figure 15-17. Muscular ventricular septal defect (VSD) demonstrated in three-dimensional ultrasound in orthogonal planes display. The dot (shown in the *circle*) represents the intersection of the three planes. The dot is placed on the VSD in **plane A** (transverse view at level of the four-chamber view) and is seen in **plane B** (short-axis view of the ventricles) and **plane C** (*en face* view of the interventricular septum). LV, left ventricle; RV, right ventricle.

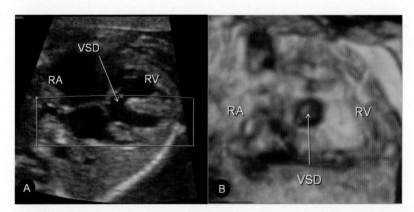

Figure 15-18. Large perimembranous ventricular septal defect (VSD) shown in three-dimensional (3-D) ultrasound in the *en face* surface-rendering mode. The 3-D box is placed over the interventricular septum on two-dimensional ultrasound as shown in **plane A.** Surface-rendering mode shown in **plane B** demonstrates the VSD in an *en face* view from the right ventricle (RV). RA, right atrium.

perimembranous region and thus misdiagnose a VSD. The false-positive diagnosis of a VSD is more common in the apical approach to the ventricular septum. The transverse approach to the septum and the use of sensitive color Doppler may be of help in confirming the diagnosis.

Associated Cardiac and Extracardiac Findings

Associated cardiac anomalies are common and are typically diagnosed prior to the diagnosis of the VSD. When an apparently isolated large (>2 to 3 mm) VSD is detected in midgestation,

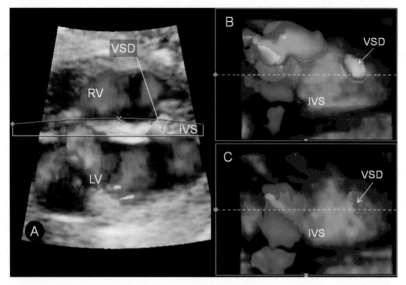

Figure 15-19. Three-dimensional (3-D) spatio-temporal image correlation (STIC) volume with color Doppler in surface-rendering mode showing a muscular ventricular septal defect (VSD). In **plane A,** the 3-D box is placed over the interventricular septum (IVS) with the VSD seen on color Doppler. In **planes B** and **C,** the VSD is imaged in surface view from the right ventricle (RV), showing left-to-right shunting (*red color*) in plane B and right-to-left shunting (*blue color*) in plane C. LV, left ventricle.

careful attention should be given to the outflow tracts given a high association of VSD with conotruncal anomalies. Table 15-2 summarizes the most common cardiac anomalies associated with VSD.

Extracardiac anomalies are associated with VSD and are not specific. The association of an extracardiac abnormality with a VSD increases the risk for the presence of a syndrome or chromosomal aberration. Chromosomal abnormalities, such as trisomy 21, have been reported in more than 20% of fetuses with VSD (4,18). Conversely, VSDs are the most common lesion in many chromosomal abnormalities such as trisomies 21, 18, and 13 (see Chapter 2). The association of an isolated muscular VSD with chromosomal abnormalities is still controversial.

Prognosis and Outcome

The long-term outcome of fetuses with VSD is dependent on the size and location of the defect and the associated cardiac and extracardiac malformations. Small muscular VSDs detected by color Doppler have an excellent outcome and up to 80% close spontaneously before birth or by the first 2 years of life (19,20). When a muscular VSD is diagnosed in the second trimester, the authors recommend follow-up in the third trimester to confirm its presence and to rule out additional small VSDs or other cardiac anomalies.

When the VSD is moderate or large, hemodynamic changes may necessitate surgical closure in order to reduce long-term morbidities. Hemodynamic changes include left-to-right shunting in the infant, which may lead to heart failure. Medical management of mild to moderate-size VSDs has been associated with good long-term outcome (19). Early repair of large VSDs in the first year of life has been shown to result in higher rates of enhanced left ventricular function and regression of hypertrophy than those repaired in childhood (21,22).

■ KEY POINTS: VENTRICULAR SEPTAL DEFECTS

- VSDs are common congenital heart defects, second only to bicuspid aortic valves.
- Four anatomic types of VSDs exist: inlet, outlet, (peri)membranous, and trabecular (or muscular).

- Perimembranous VSDs are the most common, accounting for about 80% of cases.
- Dropout artifacts on 2-D ultrasound and overlapping of color Doppler (bleeding artifact) can lead to false-positive diagnoses of VSD.
- The lateral or transverse view of the heart on 2-D ultrasound can be of help in reducing false-positive and false-negative diagnoses of VSD.
- When the borders of the VSD appear echogenic, it helps in differentiating a true muscular VSD from artifact.
- When a perimembranous VSD is detected, detailed assessment of the great arteries is critical given a strong association with conotruncal abnormalities.
- Chromosomal abnormalities have been reported in more than 20% of fetuses with VSD.
- VSDs are the most common lesion in many chromosomal abnormalities such as trisomies 21, 18, and 13.
- About 80% of small muscular VSDs spontaneously close before birth or by the first 2 years of life.

ATRIOVENTRICULAR SEPTAL DEFECT

Definition, Spectrum of Disease, and Incidence

Complete atrioventricular septal defect (AVSD) is a cardiac malformation that combines an atrial septum primum defect and a ventricular septal defect with an abnormal common atrioventricular valve, which connects to the right and left ventricles (Fig. 15-20). The common atrioventricular valve usually has five leaflets. Synonyms for AVSD include endocardial cushion defect and atrioventricular canal defect. Partial AVSD includes an atrial septum primum defect and a cleft in the mitral valve. In partial AVSD, two distinct mitral and tricuspid valve annuli exist. AVSD can also be classified as balanced or unbalanced. In unbalanced AVSD the atrioventricular connection predominantly drains to one of the two ventricles, resulting in ventricular size disproportion. Unbalanced AVSD is typically found in association with heterotaxy syndrome (see Chapter 22).

AVSD results from failure of fusion of the endocardial cushions during embryogenesis of the heart. It is a common cardiac malformation found in 4% to 5% of all infants with congenital heart disease and occurs in 0.19 per 1000 live births (23,24). AVSD is also commonly diagnosed in the fetus, accounting for 18% of cardiac abnormalities in one large series (4). AVSD is slightly more common in girls (23) and has a high association with chromosomal abnormalities, primarily Down syndrome. Figure 15-21 represents an anatomic specimen of a fetal heart with AVSD.

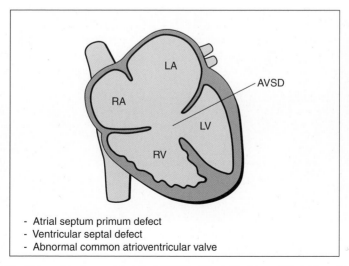

- Atrial septum primum defect
- Ventricular septal defect
- Abnormal common atrioventricular valve

Figure 15-20. Atrioventricular septal defect (AVSD). RA, right atrium; RV, right ventricle; LV, left ventricle; LA, left atrium.

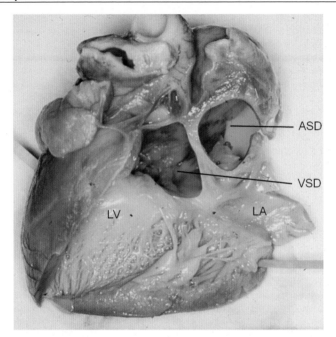

Figure 15-21. Anatomic specimen of a fetal heart with atrioventricular septal defect. The heart is opened from the left atrium (LA) and left ventricle (LV). Large interatrial septum primum defect (ASD) as well as an interventricular septal defect (VSD) are seen.

Ultrasound Findings

Gray Scale
AVSD is best detected in the apical four-chamber view. In diastole, when the common valve is open, a defect in the center of the heart (also referred to as *crux*) can be identified due to lack of tissue (Fig. 15-22). This defect in the center of the heart results from the large atrial and

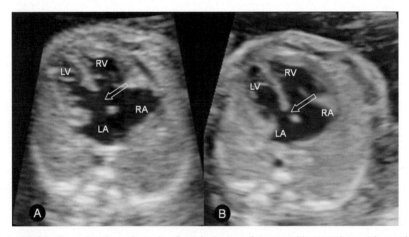

Figure 15-22. Four-chamber views in diastole in two fetuses with complete atrioventricular septal defects (AVSDs). **A:** The AVSD is large and clearly visible (*open arrow*). **B:** The AVSD is small (*open arrow*) and difficult to detect. The diagnosis was confirmed in systole owing to the linear insertion of the valves as seen in Figure 15-23. LA, left atrium; LV, left ventricle; RA, right atrium; RV, right ventricle.

ventricular septal defects at the atrioventricular region. In systole, when the common AV valve is closed, the normal apical offset of the tricuspid valve insertion on the septum is lost and the common valve appears as a linear line across (Fig. 15-23). The four-chamber view allows for the evaluation of ventricular size for an unbalanced AVSD (Fig. 15-24). In partial AVSD, the linear AV valve insertion is seen, combined with an atrial septum primum defect but without a large ventricular septal defect. Mild forms of AVSD can be overlooked, especially in the lateral four-chamber view, where the AV valve insertion cannot be adequately assessed. Interestingly, the authors have recently noted that the atrioventricular length ratio (AVL) is increased in fetuses with AVSD (normal 0.5), and this finding can be used to facilitate AVSD detection (25) (Fig. 15-25). A cutoff value for the AVL ratio over 0.6 detects AVSD in 83% of cases,

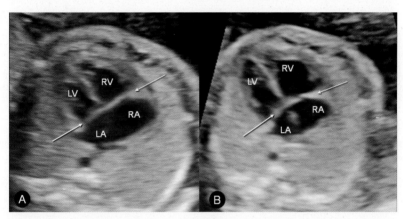

Figure 15-23. Four-chamber views in systole in two fetuses with complete atrioventricular septal defects (same fetuses as in Fig. 15-22). Note the linear insertion of the common atrioventricular valves when closed (*arrows*). Compare with findings during diastole in Figure 15-22. LA, left atrium; LV, left ventricle; RA, right atrium; RV, right ventricle.

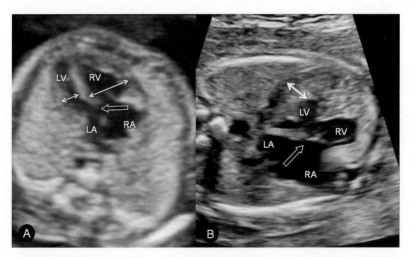

Figure 15-24. Two fetuses with unbalanced atrioventricular septal defects (AVSDs) (*open arrows*) and diminutive left ventricles. **A:** The AVSD is associated with a diminutive left ventricle (*double-sided arrows*) but normal-appearing cardiac walls in a fetus with trisomy 21. **B:** The AVSD is associated with left isomerism and heart block with thickened myocardium (*double-sided arrow*). LA, left atrium; LV, left ventricle; RA, right atrium; RV, right ventricle.

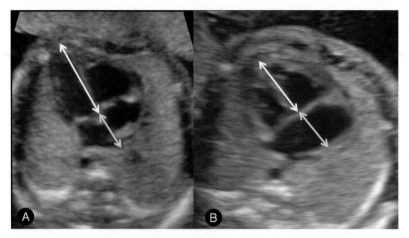

Figure 15-25. Atrioventricular length ratio (AVL ratio) in a normal fetus **(A)** and a fetus with atrioventricular septal defect (AVSD) **(B).** Note an increase in atrial length (*yellow arrows*) in the fetus with AVSD (B) as compared to the normal fetus (A). See text for details.

with a false-positive rate of 5.7% (25) (Fig. 15-26). Evaluation of the ventriculoarterial connection is needed in order to assess for the presence of conotruncal abnormalities, a common association with AVSD.

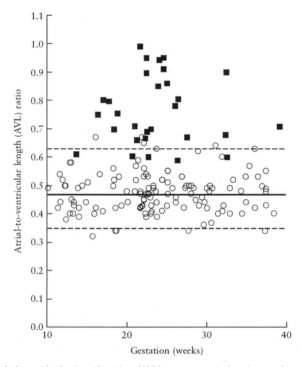

Figure 15-26. Atrioventricular length ratios (AVL) versus gestational ages in normal fetuses (*o*) and fetuses with atrioventricular septal defects (AVSDs) (*solid squares*). The solid line represents the mean AVL ratio in normal fetuses. The dashed lines mark the 95% reference range. See text for details. (From Machlitt A, Heling KS, Chaoui R. Increased cardiac atrial-to-ventricular length ratio in the fetal four-chamber view: a new marker for atrioventricular septal defects. *Ultrasound Obstet Gynecol* 2004;24(6):618–622, with permission.)

Color Doppler

Color Doppler is helpful in confirming the diagnosis of AVSD. In AVSD, color Doppler at the four-chamber view during diastole will demonstrate a single channel of blood flow to the ventricles that divides over the remnant of the ventricular septum (Fig. 15-27). The degree of ventricular hypoplasia in unbalanced AVSD can also be assessed by color Doppler (Fig. 15-28). During systole, color Doppler will demonstrate common valve regurgitation in the majority of

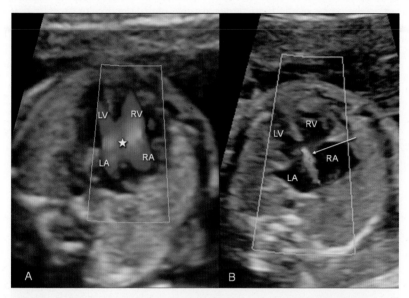

Figure 15-27. Color Doppler at the level of the four-chamber views in two fetuses with complete atrioventricular septal defects during diastole **(A)** and systole **(B).** In diastole (A), a single channel of blood entering the ventricles is noted over a common atrioventricular valve (*star*). In systole (B), a regurgitant jet (*arrow*) from the dysplastic common atrioventricular valve is noted. LA, left atrium; LV, left ventricle; RA, right atrium; RV, right ventricle.

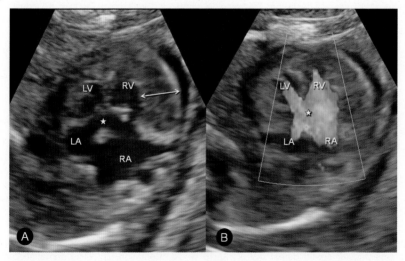

Figure 15-28. Gray scale **(A)** and color Doppler **(B)** at the four-chamber view in a fetus with an unbalanced atrioventricular septal defect (*star*); a thickened, primitive myocardium (*double-sided arrow*); and a diminutive left ventricle (LV). Color Doppler (B) highlights the diminutive size of the LV, best demonstrated in diastole. LA, left atrium; RA, right atrium; RV, right ventricle.

complete AVSD cases (Fig. 15-27). The regurgitant jet generally originates from the center of the valve and is rarely severe enough to cause atrial dilation. A regurgitant jet, which appears to arise from the left ventricle, should alert for the presence of a complete or partial AVSD, given the rarity of mitral regurgitation in the fetus.

Early Gestation

AVSD may be recognized in early gestation at the 11- to 14-week scan by demonstrating the defect in the center of the heart during diastole on 2-D and color Doppler evaluation (Fig. 15-29). This is best achieved by transvaginal ultrasound if possible, and a common indication for the targeted cardiac evaluation is a thickened nuchal translucency (Fig. 15-29).

Care should be given to the proper use of color Doppler settings in order to avoid artifacts. The presence of common valve regurgitation on color Doppler should help in confirming the diagnosis (Fig. 15-30).

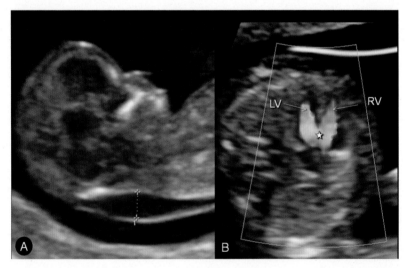

Figure 15-29. Thickened nuchal translucency **(A)** and atrioventricular septal defect (AVSD) **(B)** in a fetus at 12 weeks' gestation. Transvaginal ultrasound with color Doppler (B) confirms the presence of complete AVSD (*star*). Trisomy 18 was noted on chorionic villous sampling. LV, left ventricle; RV, right ventricle.

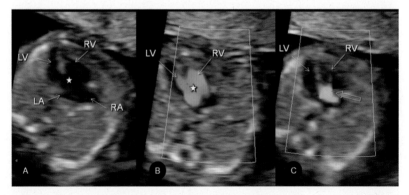

Figure 15-30. Gray scale **(A)** and color Doppler during diastole **(B)** and systole **(C)** in a fetus with atrioventricular septal defect (AVSD) at 16 weeks' gestation. AVSD is demonstrated in A and B (*star*), central channel of ventricular filling is demonstrated in diastole in B, and common atrioventricular valve regurgitation is seen in systole in C (*open arrow*). LA, left atrium; LV, left ventricle; RA, right atrium; RV, right ventricle.

Three-dimensional Ultrasound

The tomographic ultrasound imaging mode applied to a 3-D volume acquired at the level of the four-chamber view allows for the demonstration of the anatomic characteristics of AVSD in multiple planes (26,27). Surface rendering at the four-chamber-view level may emphasize the size of the gap in the crux of the heart (Fig. 15-31). The *en face* view of the common AV valve can be visualized from either the atrial (Fig. 15-32) or the ventricular region, the latter having the advantage of providing valuable information on the anatomy of the valve apparatus (28).

Associated Cardiac and Extracardiac Findings

Associated cardiac abnormalities in AVSD include tetralogy of Fallot, double outlet ventricle, right aortic arch, and other conotruncal anomalies. Pulmonary atresia and anomalies of the pulmonary and systemic veins can also be found, mainly in association in both left and right

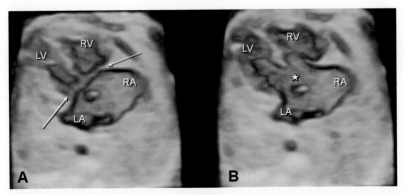

Figure 15-31. Three-dimensional ultrasound in surface-rendering mode at the four-chamber view in systole **(A)** and diastole **(B)** in a fetus with a complete atrioventricular septal defect. The typical linear arrangement of the common valve in noted in systole (A) (*arrows*) and the gap in the crux of the heart is demonstrated in diastole (B) (*star*). LA, left atrium; LV, left ventricle; RA, right atrium; RV, right ventricle.

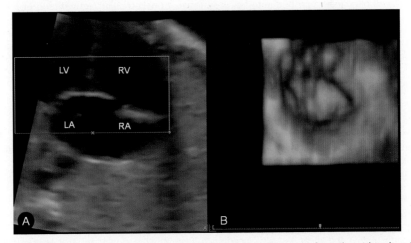

Figure 15-32. *En face* view of a common atrioventricular valve, seen from the atrium in a fetus with atrioventricular septal defect in a four-dimensional volume. The rendering box is placed over the common valve with the rendering line (*green*) in the atria **(A)**. Surface rendering of the common valve is shown in **B.** In real time, opening and closing of the common valve can be demonstrated. LA, left atrium; LV, left ventricle; RA, right atrium; RV, right ventricle.

isomerism. Unbalanced AVSD results in ventricular disproportion with hypoplasia of one ventricle. Aortic coarctation may also be associated with AVSD, resulting in a small left ventricle and on occasion a severely hypoplastic aortic arch, which is hemodynamically similar to hypoplastic left heart syndrome.

Extracardiac anomalies in AVSD primarily include chromosomal abnormalities, mainly trisomy 21 and much less commonly trisomies 18 and 13. About 40% to 45% of children with Down syndrome have congenital heart disease and of these, 40% are AVSD, commonly of the complete type (23,29). Antenatal diagnosis of AVSD, when isolated, is associated with trisomy 21 in 58% of cases (30). The additional presence of an intracardiac echogenic focus increases the risk of aneuploidy. AVSD diagnosed prenatally is part of heterotaxy syndrome in about a third of cases (31). When AVSD is associated with heterotaxy, the risk of chromosomal abnormality is virtually absent, but the outcome is worsened due to the severity of the cardiac and extracardiac malformations (see Chapter 22).

Differential Diagnosis

Isolated inlet VSD can be misdiagnosed as AVSD if attention is not paid to the normal atrial septum and the normal attachment of the tricuspid valve. AVSD can be mimicked by the presence of a dilated coronary sinus in a left persistent superior vena cava (32). The linear insertion of both atrioventricular valves can also be present without a septal defect as described in common association with trisomy 21 (33). Differentiating a large AVSD or an unbalanced AVSD from a single-ventricle heart can be difficult. Furthermore, an unbalanced AVSD can be difficult to differentiate from a hypoplastic left heart syndrome or tricuspid atresia based on a hypoplastic left or right ventricle, respectively. Clues for the diagnosis of AVSD are presented in Table 15-3.

Prognosis and Outcome

Prenatal diagnosis of complete AVSD has been associated with an overall survival rate of 32%, excluding pregnancy terminations and those lost to follow-up, at a regional fetal medicine center (34). This poor prognosis is primarily due to a high incidence of cardiac and extracardiac abnormalities in prenatally diagnosed AVSD (34).

Long-term outcome of isolated cases has been excellent, with a cumulative 20-year survival of 95% and a very low operative mortality (<2%) (35,36). Reoperation occurs in about a quarter of patients primarily due to left progressive atrioventricular regurgitation or left ventricular outflow obstruction (37). The operation consists of closing the interventricular and interatrial septal defects and reconstructing the atrioventricular valve apparatus. In unbalanced AVSD, a biventricular repair may be impossible due to the severe hypoplasia of one ventricle. Palliative surgery, such as in cases involving a univentricular heart, is typically performed.

■ KEY POINTS: ATRIOVENTRICULAR SEPTAL DEFECT

- AVSD combines an atrial septum primum defect and a ventricular septal defect with an abnormal common atrioventricular valve.
- The common atrioventricular valve in AVSD usually has five leaflets.
- Partial AVSD includes an atrial septum primum defect and a cleft in the mitral valve with two distinct mitral and tricuspid valve annuli.
- In unbalanced AVSD the atrioventricular connection predominantly drains to one of the two ventricles, resulting in ventricular size disproportion.
- Unbalanced AVSD is typically found in association with heterotaxy syndrome.
- AVSD is best detected in the apical four-chamber view (Table 15-3).
- In systole, in AVSD, the common valve appears as a linear line across.
- In partial AVSD, the linear AV valve insertion is seen, combined with an atrial septum primum defect but without a large ventricular septal defect.
- During systole, color Doppler will demonstrate common valve regurgitation in the majority of complete AVSD cases.
- AVSD is present in 40% of congenital heart disease in Down syndrome.

TABLE 15-3	Clues for the Diagnosis of Atrioventricular (AV) Septal Defect in the Four-chamber View
Diastole (AV valve opened)	Two-dimensional: Gap in the center of the heart
	Color: Single inflow channel with mixture of blood in both atria and ventricles
Systole (AV valve closed)	Two-dimensional: Common AV valve with both leaflets at one level, showing a linear line
	Two-dimensional: AV length ratio >0.6 (long atrium)
	Color: AV valve regurgitation

■ When AVSD is associated with heterotaxy, the risk of chromosomal abnormality is virtually absent.

■ Prenatal diagnosis of complete AVSD has been associated with an overall low survival rate due to associated cardiac and extracardiac abnormalities.

■ Long-term outcome of isolated AVSD cases is excellent.

References

1. Feldt RH, Avasthey P, Yoshim ASVF, et al. Incidence of congenital heart disease in children born to residents of Olmsted County, Minnesota 1950–1969. *Mayo Clin Proc* 1971;46:794–799.
2. Hoffman JIE, Christianson MA. Congenital heart disease in a cohort of 19,502 births with long term follow-up. *Am J Cardiol* 1978;42:641–647.
3. Samanek M. Children with congenital heart disease: probability of natural survival. *Pediatr Cardiol* 1992;13:152–158.
4. Allan LD, Sharland GK, Milburn A, et al. Prospective diagnosis of 1006 consecutive cases of congenital heart disease in the fetus. *J Am Coll Cardiol* 1994;23:1452–1458.
5. Gotsman MS, Astley R, Parsons CG. Partial anomalous pulmonary venous drainage in association with atrial septal defect. *Br Heart J* 1965;27:566.
6. Ettedgui JA, Sievers RD, Anderson RH, et al. Diagnostic echocardiographic features of the sinus venosus defect. *Br Heart J* 1990;64:329.
7. Stewart PA, Wladimiroff JW. Fetal atrial arrhythmias associated with redundancy/aneurysm of the foramen ovale. *J Clin Ultrasound* 1988;16(9):643–650.
8. Rice MJ, McDonald RW, Reller MD. Fetal atrial septal aneurysm: a cause of fetal atrial arrhythmias. *J Am Coll Cardiol* 1988;12(5):1292–1297.
9. Ferencz C, Rubin JD, Loffredo CA, et al. *Epidemiology of congenital heart disease: the Baltimore-Washington infant study 1981–1989.* Austin, TX: Futura Publishing, 1993;38
10. Roguin N, Du Z-D, Barak M, et al. High prevalence of muscular ventricular septal defect in neonates. *J Am Coll Cardiol* 1995;26:1545–1548.
11. Mavroudis C, Backer CL, Idriss FS. Ventricular septal defect. In: C Mavroudis, CL Backer CL, eds. *Pediatric cardiac surgery*, 2nd ed. St. Louis: Mosby-Year Book, 1994;201–221.
12. Lincoln C, Jamieson S, Shinebourne E, et al. Transatrial repair of ventricular septal defects with reference to their anatomic classification. *J Thorac Cardiovasc Surg* 1977;74:183–190.
13. Soto B, Becker AE, Moulaert AJ, et al. Classification of ventricular septal defects. *Br Heart J* 1980;43:332–343.
14. Hoffman JLE, Rudolph AM. The natural history of ventricular septal defects in infancy. *Am J Cardiol* 1965;16:634–653.
15. Chaoui R, Hoffmann J, Heling KS. Three-dimensional (3D) and 4D color Doppler fetal echocardiography using spatio-temporal image correlation (STIC). *Ultrasound Obstet Gynecol* 2004;23(6):535–545.
16. Paladini D, Russo MG, Vassallo M, et al. The 'in-plane' view of the inter-ventricular septum. A new approach to the characterization of ventricular septal defects in the fetus. *Prenat Diagn* 2003;23(13):1052–1055.
17. Yagel S, Valsky DV, Messing B. Detailed assessment of fetal ventricular septal defect with 4D color Doppler ultrasound using spatio-temporal image correlation technology. *Ultrasound Obstet Gynecol* 2005;25(1):97–98.
18. Axt-Fliedner R, Schwarze A, Smrcek J, et al. Isolated ventricular septal defects detected by color Doppler imaging: evolution during fetal and first year of postnatal life. *Ultrasound Obstet Gynecol* 2006;27(3):266–273.
19. Kidd I, Driscoll DJ, Gersony WM, et al. Second natural history study of congenital heart defects: results of treatment of patients with ventricular septal defects. *Circulation* 1993;87(suppl I): I38–I51.
20. Paladini D, Palmieri S, Lamberti A, et al. Characterization and natural history of ventricular septal defects in the fetus. *Ultrasound Obstet Gynecol* 2000;16(2):118–122.
21. Cordell D, Graham TP Jr, Arwood GF, et al. Left heart volume characteristics following ventricular septal defect closure in infancy. *Circulation* 1976;54:294–298.
22. Graham TP Jr, Cordell GD, Bender HA Jr. Ventricular function following surgery. In: RD Rowe, BSL Kidd, eds. *The child with congenital heart disease after surgery*. Mt. Kisco, NY: Futura Publishing, 1976;277–293.
23. Fyler DC, Buckley LP, Hellenbrand WE, et al. Endocardial cushion defect. Report of the New England Regional infant cardiac program. *J Pediatr* 1980;65:441–444.
24. Samanek M. Prevalence at birth, "natural" risk and survival with atrioventricular septal defect. *Cardiol Young* 1991;1:285–289.
25. Machlitt A, Heling KS, Chaoui R. Increased cardiac atrial-to-ventricular length ratio in the fetal four-chamber view: a new marker for atrioventricular septal defects. *Ultrasound Obstet Gynecol* 2004;24(6):618–622.

26. Paladini D, Vassallo M, Sglavo G, et al. The role of spatio-temporal image correlation (STIC) with tomographic ultrasound imaging (TUI) in the sequential analysis of fetal congenital heart disease. *Ultrasound Obstet Gynecol* 2006;27(5):555–561.
27. Chaoui R, Heling KS. New developments in fetal heart scanning: three- and four-dimensional fetal echocardiography. *Semin Fetal Neonatal Med* 2005;10(6):567–577.
28. Vinals F, Pacheco V, Giuliano A. Fetal atrioventricular valve junction in normal fetuses and in fetuses with complete atrioventricular septal defect assessed by 4D volume rendering. *Ultrasound Obstet Gynecol* 2006;28(1):26–31.
29. DeBiase L, Di Ciommo V, Ballerini L, et al. Prevalence of left-sided obstructive lesions in patients with atrioventricular canal without Down syndrome. *J Thorac Cardiovasc Surg* 1986;91:467–472.
30. Delisle MF, Sandor GG, Tessier F, et al. Outcome of fetuses diagnosed with atrioventricular septal defect. *Obstet Gynecol* 1999;94:763–767.
31. Huggan IC, Cook AC, Smeetan NC, et al. Atrioventricular septal defects diagnosed in fetal life: associated cardiac and extra-cardiac abnormalities and outcome. *J Am Coll Cardiol* 2000;36:593–601.
32. Park JK, Taylor DK, Skeels M, et al. Dilated coronary sinus in the fetus: misinterpretation as an atrioventricular canal defect. *Ultrasound Obstet Gynecol* 1997;10:126–129.
33. Fredouille C, Piercecchi-Marti MD, Liprandi A, et al. Linear insertion of atrioventricular valves without septal defect: a new anatomical landmark for Down's syndrome? *Fetal Diagn Ther* 2002;17(3):188–192.
34. Rasiah SV, Ewer AK, Miller P, et al. Outcome following prenatal diagnosis of complete atrioventricular septal defect. *Prenat Diagn* 2008;28:95–101.
35. Aubert S, Henaine R, Raisky O, et al. Atypical forms of isolated partial atrioventricular septal defect increase the risk of initial valve replacement and reoperation. *Eur J Cardiothorac Surg* 2005;28:223–228.
36. Studer M, Blackstone EH, Kirklin JW, et al. Determinants of early and late results of repair of atrioventricular septal (canal) defects. *J Thorac Cardiovasc Surg* 1982;84:523–542.
37. McGrath LB, Gonzalez-lavin L. Actuarial survival, freedom from reoperation, and other events after repair of atrioventricular septal defects. *J Thorac Cardiovasc Surg* 1987;94:582.

UNIVENTRICULAR ATRIOVENTRICULAR CONNECTION, DOUBLE INLET VENTRICLE, AND TRICUSPID ATRESIA WITH VENTRICULAR SEPTAL DEFECT

16

UNIVENTRICULAR ATRIOVENTRICULAR CONNECTION

Univentricular atrioventricular connection describes a group of cardiac malformations where the atrioventricular connection is completely or predominantly to a single ventricular chamber. Embryologically, this malformation is thought to result from failure of the development of the bulboventricular loop stage. Much debate still exists today on the various subclassifications of cardiac anomalies within this group and what should be included or excluded. From a clinical point of view, a congenital heart defect with a univentricular atrioventricular connection, *single ventricular physiology*, describes a heart with one functioning ventricle with inflow from one or both atria. Numerous terms were used to describe this malformation, including univentricular heart, primitive ventricle, common ventricle, single ventricle, cor triloculare biatriatum, cor biloculare, dominant ventricle, and double inlet ventricle (1). The classic Van Praagh's classification (2), which was later modified by Hallermann et al. (3), described one or two atrioventricular valves that empty into a single ventricle and excluded mitral or tricuspid atresia. Anderson's simpler classification described a single ventricular mass with or without a rudimentary chamber and allowed for the inclusion of mitral or tricuspid atresia (4,5). In Anderson's classification, the rudimentary chamber, if present, should not have an inlet but may have an outlet (4,5). Within univentricular atrioventricular connection, three subgroups can be identified: *double inlet*, where two atria connect to a single ventricle through two patent atrioventricular valves; *single inlet*, where one atrium connects to a single ventricle through a single atrioventricular valve; and *common inlet*, where both atria connect to a single ventricle through a single atrioventricular valve (6). The morphology of the ventricle is generally a left ventricular morphology with a rudimentary right chamber. On rare occasions, a right ventricular morphology with a rudimentary left chamber, or a ventricle of indeterminate morphology without a rudimentary chamber, can be seen. A *single ventricle heart*, which results from a surgical repair of a congenital heart anomaly, should not be classified as univentricular atrioventricular connection. Table 16-1 lists several cardiac anomalies that may show a *single ventricle* on fetal echocardiography. Of those, double inlet ventricle and tricuspid atresia with ventricular septal defect have been commonly classified in the univentricular atrioventricular connection and will be discussed in this chapter. Figure 16-1 represents four-chamber views in two fetuses with single ventricle anatomy.

DOUBLE INLET VENTRICLE

Definition, Spectrum of Disease, and Incidence

Double inlet ventricle (DIV) is considered a classic and most common form of univentricular atrioventricular connection (6). It is characterized by two normally developed right and left

TABLE 16-1	Cardiac Anomalies That May Show a *Single Ventricle* on Fetal Echocardiography

Hypoplastic left heart syndrome
Pulmonary atresia with intact septum
Atrioventricular septal defect (unbalanced)
Single ventricle in right and left isomerism
Corrected transposition with tricuspid atresia
Mitral atresia with ventricular septal defect
Double inlet ventricle
Tricuspid atresia with ventricular septal defect

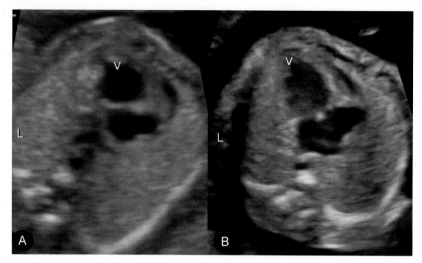

Figure 16-1. Four-chamber view showing a "single ventricle anatomy" in two fetuses. **A:** The fetus has a hypoplastic left heart syndrome with absent left ventricle and mitral and aortic atresia. **B:** The fetus has a hypoplastic right ventricle in pulmonary atresia with intact septum. The detection of one ventricle on fetal echocardiography is not synonymous with a single ventricle. See text and Table 16-1 for details. L, left; V, ventricle.

atria that connect via separate right and left atrioventricular valves to a common ventricle (Fig. 16-2). The most common form of DIV is a double inlet to a morphologic left ventricle, representing about 80%, and the anomaly is also called double inlet left ventricle (DILV) (2). In DILV, a small underdeveloped right ventricle (not shown in Fig. 16-2) is commonly present and connects to the single ventricle with a ventricular septal defect. This "remnant" ventricle is a small outlet chamber and the septal defect is usually called bulboventricular foramen. The aorta and pulmonary arteries usually arise in D- or L-malposition, and depending on the looping, one or both vessels (double outlet) may commonly arise from the small outlet chamber. In

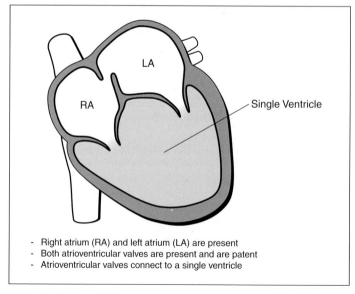

- Right atrium (RA) and left atrium (LA) are present
- Both atrioventricular valves are present and are patent
- Atrioventricular valves connect to a single ventricle

Figure 16-2. Double inlet ventricle.

cases where the bulboventricular foramen (septal defect) is restrictive, the corresponding arising vessel(s) from the remnant chamber may be diminutive (pulmonary stenosis or aortic coarctation). Other forms of DIV include a double inlet right ventricle, a double inlet ventricle of mixed morphology, and a double inlet ventricle of undetermined or undifferentiated morphology (2). DIV is rare and is found in 0.1 per 1000 live births (7). The prevalence is more common in fetal series due to the easy detection of DIV on the four-chamber view of the heart.

Ultrasound Findings

Gray Scale

The four-chamber view is abnormal in DIV as it shows a single ventricle with a missing ventricular septum (Fig. 16-3). Identifying the morphology of the single ventricle on ultrasound is based on the anatomic characteristic of the morphologic right and left ventricles as discussed in Chapter 5. The left ventricular myocardium appears smooth with fine trabeculations, whereas the right ventricular myocardium is coarse with an irregular surface. Assessment of atrioventricular valve anatomy and/or insertion of papillary muscles cannot be used to determine ventricular morphology in univentricular atrioventricular connection. The rudimentary right ventricle and the septal defect (bulboventricular foramen) in DILV are not visualized in the four-chamber plane but in a more cranial plane, when an attempt to visualize the great vessels is made (Fig. 16-4). The rudimentary outlet chamber in DILV is more commonly located on the left side of the main ventricle (L-looping) but can be located on the right side (D-looping) (8). The great arteries are generally in L-malposition if the small outlet chamber is on the left side of the ventricle. When the small outlet chamber is localized on the right side, the great arteries arise either in D-malposition or are normally related with the pulmonary artery arising from the small outlet chamber (8). Outflow tract obstructions are recognized due to size discrepancy rather than flow disturbances, which may be absent (Fig. 16-4). A narrow pulmonary artery suggests the presence of pulmonary stenosis, whereas a narrow ascending aorta may be associated with coarctation of the aorta or tubular aortic arch hypoplasia.

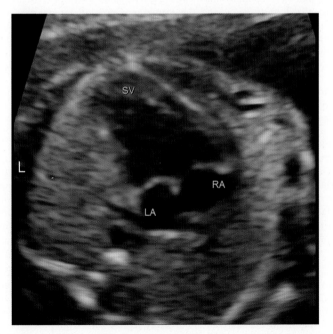

Figure 16-3. Four-chamber view in a fetus with double inlet ventricle. Note the presence of the right (RA) and left atrium (LA) draining through two atrioventricular valves into a single ventricle (SV). L, left.

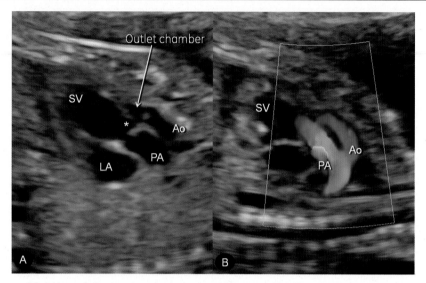

Figure 16-4. Long-axis view in two-dimensional **(A)** and color Doppler **(B)** imaging in a fetus with double inlet ventricle (same fetus as in Fig. 16-3) showing a remnant ventricle as small outlet chamber connected to the single ventricle (SV) by a ventricular septal defect (*asterisk*). The aorta (Ao) and pulmonary artery (PA) arise in a parallel course; the aorta appears narrow due to the small ventricular septal defect. LA, left atrium.

Color Doppler

Color Doppler may be misleading since two atrioventricular valves are patent and two color stripes are visualized, thus mimicking the virtual presence of a separation or septum (9) (Fig. 16-5). Diagnosis is typically made on two-dimensional (2-D) ultrasound, and color Doppler provides additional information on the patency of the left and right atrioventricular valves, flow across the ventricular septal defect, and great vessels (Fig. 16-4). Restrictive ventricular septal defect, which may occur in this condition, is better evaluated using color Doppler.

Early Gestation

DIV can be detected in early gestation by noting the absence of a ventricular septum on the four-chamber view as well as abnormally arising great vessels.

Three-dimensional Ultrasound

The combination of three-dimensional ultrasound with tomographic imaging permits the simultaneous visualization of the abnormality in the four-chamber plane and the demonstration of the rudimentary ventricle with the course of the great vessels. Navigating through the volume in an offline setting may facilitate the evaluation of the spatial orientation of the great arteries. Surface rendering shows the large ventricle with inflow from two atrioventricular valves and a rudimentary outlet chamber (Fig. 16-6) and may help in identifying the spatial relationship of the great vessels.

Associated Cardiac and Extracardiac Findings

Associated malformations in DIV are atresia, hypoplasia or straddling of the atrioventricular valves, pulmonary (or subpulmonic) outflow obstruction, (sub)aortic outflow obstruction, and conduction abnormalities, primarily due to the anatomic disruption of the conduction system (10).

The most important extracardiac abnormality to rule out is the presence of right or left isomerism (see Chapter 22), especially in the presence of a common inlet ventricle (11). The sequential approach to the ultrasound examination of the heart may permit detection of corresponding abnormalities. Chromosome anomalies and other extracardiac anomalies are possible but unusual.

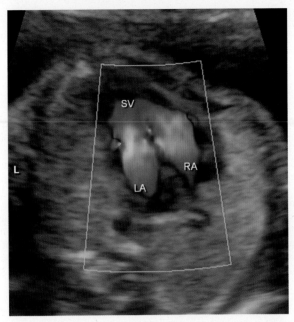

Figure 16-5. Four-chamber view with color Doppler in a fetus with double inlet ventricle demonstrating blood flow during diastole from the right (RA) and left atrium (LA) into a single ventricle (SV). L, left.

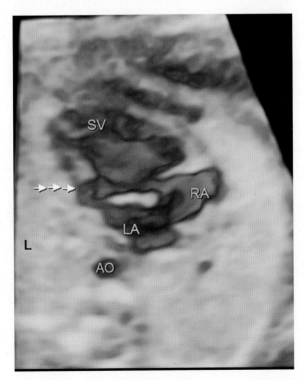

Figure 16-6. Surface rendering mode of the four-chamber view in a fetus with double inlet ventricle showing the right (RA) and left atrium (LA) as well as the single ventricle (SV). The small rudimentary ventricle can also be identified (*arrows*). L, left; AO, descending aorta.

Differential Diagnosis

Table 16-1 lists several cardiac malformations in the differential diagnosis of DIV. DIV may be missed on prenatal ultrasound in a lateral view of the heart in diastole because the papillary muscles may mimic a ventricular septum in a single ventricle.

Prognosis and Outcome

DIV with patent atrioventricular valves is well tolerated in the fetus. Follow-up ultrasound is important prenatally as outflow tract obstruction may develop or worsen due to reduced flow and lack of vessel growth. The neonatal course of DIV is dependent on the presence of associated malformations such as obstruction of the great vessels or atrioventricular valve abnormalities. Surgical treatment corresponds to a single ventricular repair. The type of surgical repair (pulmonary artery banding, Fontan procedure, or other) mainly depends on detailed evaluation of the great vessel arrangement and perfusion.

An overall mortality rate of 29% with follow-up up to 25 years of age was noted in an outcome study on 105 patients with DILV and transposed arteries (12). Multivariate analysis showed the presence of arrhythmia and pacemaker requirement as independent risk factors for mortality, whereas pulmonary atresia or stenosis and pulmonary artery banding were associated with decreased mortality (12). Gender, era of birth, aortic arch anomaly, and systemic outflow obstruction were not risk factors for long-term outcome (12).

■ KEY POINTS: DOUBLE INLET VENTRICLE

- Double inlet ventricle is the most common form of univentricular atrioventricular connection.
- It is characterized by two normally developed right and left atria that connect via separate right and left atrioventricular valves to a common ventricle.
- The most common form is a double inlet to a morphologic left ventricle, representing about 80% of cases.
- The four-chamber view is abnormal.
- Outflow tract obstruction is often present and affects the vessel arising from the rudimentary ventricle.
- Associated malformations are atresia, hypoplasia or straddling of the atrioventricular valves, pulmonary (or subpulmonic) outflow obstruction, (sub)aortic outflow obstruction, and conduction abnormalities.

■ TRICUSPID ATRESIA WITH VENTRICULAR SEPTAL DEFECT

Definition, Spectrum of Disease, and Incidence

Tricuspid atresia (TA) is characterized by the absence of the right atrioventricular connection, resulting in lack of communication between the right atrium and ventricle (Fig. 16-7). The right ventricle is therefore diminutive in size. In most cases, the tricuspid valve apparatus does not develop and the right atrioventricular junction appears as echogenic thickened tissue on ultrasound examination. An inlet-type ventricular septal defect (VSD), typically perimembranous, is always present, and the size of the right ventricle is related to the size of the VSD (Fig. 16-7). A large interatrial communication, in the form of a widely patent foramen ovale or atrial septal defect, is necessary given an obstructed tricuspid valve. TA is classified into three types based on the spatial orientation of the great vessels (13,14). TA type 1 occurs in 70% to 80% of cases and is associated with normally oriented great arteries (aorta from left ventricle and pulmonary artery from right ventricle) (Fig. 16-7). TA type 2 occurs in 12% to 25% of cases and is associated with D-transposition of the great vessels. TA type 3, an uncommon malformation, is seen in the remainder of TA cases and usually denotes complex great vessel abnormalities such as truncus arteriosus or L-transposition. TA is rare, with an incidence of 0.08 per 1000 live births (7). TA is reported in about 4% of congenital heart disease prenatally and is more common in prenatal series primarily as it belongs to the group of cardiac anomalies associated with an abnormal four-chamber view (15–18). Figure 16-8 is an anatomic specimen of a fetal heart with TA.

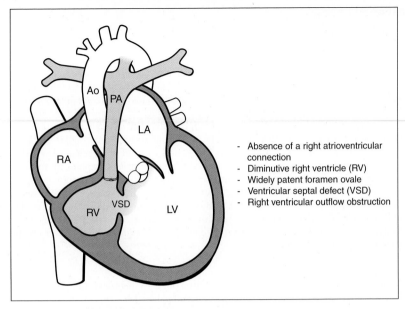

- Absence of a right atrioventricular connection
- Diminutive right ventricle (RV)
- Widely patent foramen ovale
- Ventricular septal defect (VSD)
- Right ventricular outflow obstruction

Figure 16-7. Tricuspid atresia with ventricular septal defect. RA, right atrium; LV, left ventricle; LA, left atrium; PA, pulmonary artery; Ao, aorta.

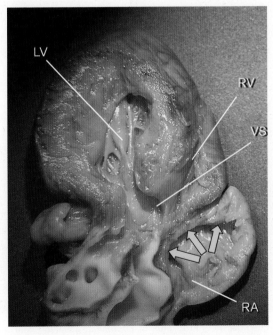

Figure 16-8. Anatomic specimen of a fetal heart with tricuspid atresia and ventricular septal defect opened at the four-chamber-view plane. The right ventricle (RV) is small and is connected to the left ventricle (LV) by a ventricular septal defect (VS) with absent right atrioventricular junction. The atretic tricuspid valve (*yellow arrows*) appears as thickened tissue. RA, right atrium.

Ultrasound Findings

Gray Scale

The four-chamber view in TA is diagnostic and reveals a diminutive right ventricle, a ventricular septal defect, and the absence of a right-sided atrioventricular junction (Fig. 16-9). The right ventricle is small and its size is primarily related to the size of the VSD: the smaller the VSD, the smaller the right ventricle (Figs. 16-9 and 16-10). Right ventricular contractility is normal with no myocardial thickening. The atretic right atrioventricular junction appears as an echogenic thickened tissue and the right atrium is slightly dilated (Fig. 16-9). The interatrial communication is large, and there is often a redundant flap of the septum secundum that bulges into the left atrium (Fig. 16-9). The interatrial and interventricular septa are malaligned (Fig. 16-9). In the five-chamber-, short-axis, and three-vessel-trachea views, the ventriculoarterial connections can be evaluated for discordance (see Chapter 20 for details on ultrasound diagnosis of transposition of the great arteries). The size of the great vessel arising from the right ventricle should be carefully evaluated for the presence of stenosis, a fairly common association. The severity of right outflow obstruction is directly related to the size of the right ventricle and the VSD. Pulmonary or aortic atresia can be found on occasion. A right aortic arch can be present and noted to course to the right of the trachea on the three-vessel-trachea view.

Color Doppler

Color Doppler confirms the diagnosis on 2-D ultrasound by demonstrating the lack of blood flow across the tricuspid valve and a patent mitral valve (Fig. 16-11). Aliasing is typically noted across the mitral valve on color Doppler due to increased blood flow (Fig. 16-11). The presence of mitral valve regurgitation on color Doppler prenatally has been associated with poor outcome. The right ventricular cavity is filled in late diastole from the left ventricle as left-to-right shunting through the VSD and flow across the VSD can be visualized on color

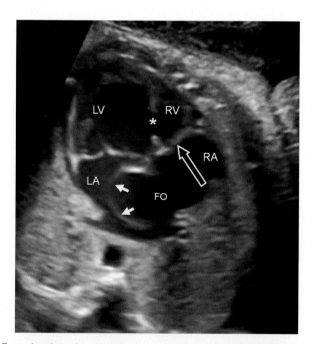

Figure 16-9. Four-chamber view in a fetus at 29 weeks' gestation with tricuspid atresia and ventricular septal defect. The right ventricle (RV) is small and is connected to the left ventricle (LV) with a ventricular septal defect (*asterisk*). Open arrow points to the atretic, thickened tricuspid valve. Note the wide foramen ovale (FO) with a redundant flap of the interatrial septum (*small arrows*). Interatrial and interventricular septae are malaligned. LA, left atrium; RA, right atrium.

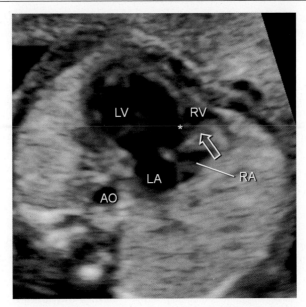

Figure 16-10. Four-chamber view in a fetus at 22 weeks' gestation with tricuspid atresia and a restrictive ventricular septal defect (*asterisk*) with an underdeveloped right ventricle (RV). Open arrow points to the atretic, thickened tricuspid valve. RA, right atrium; LA, left atrium; LV, left ventricle; AO, descending aorta.

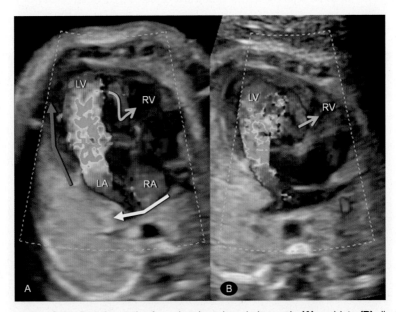

Figure 16-11. Color Doppler at the four-chamber view during early **(A)** and late **(B)** diastole in a fetus with tricuspid atresia and ventricular septal defect (same fetus as in Fig. 16-9). In early diastole (A), blood entering the right atrium (RA) passes across the wide foramen ovale to the left atrium (LA) (*white arrow*) and through the mitral valve to the left ventricle (LV) (*red arrow*). Color aliasing is seen across the mitral valve due to increased blood flow (A and B). The right ventricle (RV) receives blood from the left ventricle (LV) across the VSD (*blue arrow*) primarily in late diastole (B) and systole.

Doppler (Fig. 16-11). Color Doppler is also helpful in the evaluation of flow across the great arteries. Flow across the pulmonary artery is generally antegrade and nonturbulent. The suspicion of pulmonary stenosis is generally achieved by a diminutive size of the vessel rather than the demonstration of turbulent flow on color Doppler, which is typically absent in these cases. Flow across the ductus arteriosus in the three-vessel-trachea view is usually antegrade, but the demonstration of retrograde flow in the arterial duct is a sign of ductal-dependent pulmonary circulation with possible cyanosis in the newborn (Fig. 16-12B). Ductal-dependent circulation in TA is usually seen in severe pulmonary stenosis or atresia in association with a small right ventricle.

Early Gestation

Due to the abnormal four-chamber view, TA can be detected in early gestation either on 2-D imaging or when combined with color Doppler (Fig. 16-13). TA has been associated with an enlarged nuchal translucency in early gestation (19). Since reverse flow in the ductus venosus has been reported in the second and third trimesters in association with TA, this finding may be present at 11 to 14 weeks' gestation and may represent an early sign of right ventricular disease (20).

Three-dimensional Ultrasound

Tomographic and orthogonal display may demonstrate the main features of TA such as the abnormal four-chamber view, the size of the small right ventricle, the VSD, and the relationship and size of the great arteries (21,22). Volume rendering in surface mode or other displays (inversion mode, glass body mode) may help in the evaluation of ventricular size (Fig. 16-14) and great vessel spatial relationship.

Associated Cardiac and Extracardiac Findings

Associated cardiac findings include a large interatrial communication such as a patent foramen ovale or an atrial septal defect, a ventricular septal defect, transposition of the great

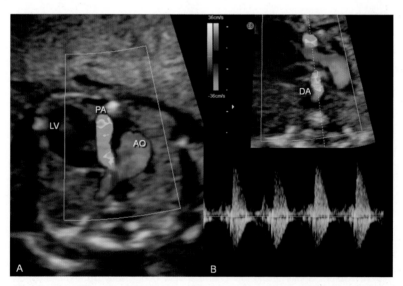

Figure 16-12. Color **(A)** and pulsed Doppler **(B)** of the three-vessel-trachea view in a fetus with tricuspid atresia, restrictive ventricular septal defect, and pulmonary stenosis (same fetus as in Fig. 16-10). Plane A shows a small pulmonary artery (PA) in comparison to the dilated aorta (AO). Pulsed Doppler interrogation of the ductus arteriosus (DA) **(B)** reveals retrograde flow, a sign of severe outflow obstruction and postnatal ductal-dependent pulmonary circulation. LV, left ventricle.

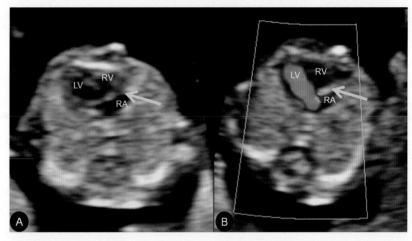

Figure 16-13. Gray scale **(A)** and color Doppler **(B)** at the four-chamber view in a fetus with tricuspid atresia at 13 weeks' gestation. Plane A shows an abnormal four-chamber view with a diminutive right ventricle (RV) with a ventricular septal defect. Plane B shows absence of flow across the tricuspid valve (*arrow*) on color Doppler during diastole. RA, right atrium; LV, left ventricle.

vessels, and various degrees of right ventricular outflow obstruction. Right ventricular outflow obstruction varies, from a patent pulmonary artery to stenosis and atresia and from patent aortic arch to aortic stenosis, coarctation, or interruption of the aortic arch. In a multicenter study on the cardiac anatomy in 60 fetuses with TA, 9 fetuses had patent great vessels, 16 had pulmonary stenosis, 11 had pulmonary atresia, 6 had aortic stenosis, 4 had coarctation of the aorta, 9 had aortic hypoplasia, 2 had interrupted aorta, and 3 had a common arterial trunk, or undefined ventriculoarterial connection (23). Interestingly, all fetuses with pulmonary outflow obstruction had ventriculoarterial concordance and almost all fetuses with aortic outflow obstruction had a ventriculoarterial discordance (23). Other associated cardiac lesions include persistent left superior vena cava, right aortic arch, pulmonary venous abnormalities, and juxtaposition of the atrial appendages (23). On very rare occasions, the great vessels are in a corrected transposition orientation, which was found in 6 of 60 cases in the series described previously (23). Due to the atrioventricular discordance, the right ventricle is on the left side and the atretic valve is found on the left side, which may erroneously suggest mitral atresia with VSD.

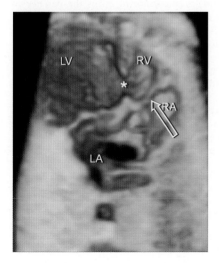

Figure 16-14. Surface-rendering mode of a three-dimensional volume in a fetus with tricuspid atresia and ventricular septal defect at the four-chamber-view plane showing a dilated left (LV) and a hypoplastic right ventricle (RV) with a ventricular septal defect (*asterisk*). Open arrow points to the atretic tricuspid valve. LA, left atrium; RA, right atrium.

TABLE 16-2	Differentiating Features of Tricuspid Atresia with Ventricular Septal Defect (TA-VSD) and Pulmonary Atresia with Intact Ventricular Septum (PA-IVS)	
	TA-VSD	**PA-IVS**
Right ventricle	Always hypoplastic	Generally hypoplastic, but may be of normal size or dilated
Right ventricular wall	Normal	Hypertrophic
Interventricular septum	Ventricular septal defect	Intact septum bulging to the left ventricle
Interatrial septum	Large interatrial communication with redundant foramen ovale	Normal foramen ovale
Tricuspid valve	Thickened echogenic tissue and no valve apparatus	Generally dysplastic tricuspid valve with limited valve excursion occasionally with tricuspid regurgitation
Right atrium	Normal size with a large interatrial communication	May be dilated due to severe tricuspid regurgitation
Pulmonary artery and valve	Patent valve (rarely atretic), narrow pulmonary artery	Atretic valve, narrow pulmonary artery
Ductus arteriosus	Generally antegrade flow	Always retrograde flow
Great vessels	In 80% of cases concordant, in 20% transposed	Concordant
Other features	No ventriculocoronary arterial communications	Ventriculocoronary arterial communications may be present
Postnatally	May be stable without cyanosis	Always cyanotic

Extracardiac anomalies can be found in TA, and fetal karyotyping should be offered despite a rare association with chromosomal aberration including 22q11 microdeletion (23).

Differential Diagnosis

Two cardiac malformations are commonly involved in the differential diagnosis of TA: pulmonary atresia with intact septum and double inlet ventricle. Double inlet ventricle was previously discussed in this chapter. Table 16-2 differentiates TA with VSD from pulmonary atresia with intact septum, both presenting with hypoplastic right ventricle in the four-chamber view.

Prognosis and Outcome

Prenatal follow-up with serial ultrasound examination is important to assess the patency of the foramen ovale and the presence of right ventricular outflow obstruction. Ductus venosus flow will show reverse flow during diastole in almost all cases, but this is a reflection of right ventricular dysfunction rather than a poor prognostic sign (20). Pregnancy termination is reported in about 28% in a multicenter series of TA diagnosed prenatally (23).

Postnatal outcome is dependent on associated cardiac and extracardiac findings. An outcome study of prenatally diagnosed TA estimated an 83% survival at 1 year of age following active management (23).

Surgical correction of TA revolves around bypassing the right ventricle and creating a conduit between the systemic venous blood and the pulmonary circulation. Most TA patients are treated with the Fontan procedure, which primarily consists of a cavopulmonary shunt. If the pulmonary artery is of normal size, preventing pulmonary overcirculation and pulmonary hypertension is achieved by banding the pulmonary artery. The overall mortality rate in patients who were treated with the Fontan procedure was between 7% and 10% in pediatric series (24,25).

■ KEY POINTS: TRICUSPID ATRESIA WITH VENTRICULAR SEPTAL DEFECT

■ Tricuspid atresia is characterized by the absence of the right atrioventricular connection, resulting in lack of communication between the right atrium and ventricle.

- An inlet-type VSD, typically perimembranous, is always present.
- Interatrial communication is large with a redundant septum secundum valve.
- Ventriculoarterial connections are concordant in 70% to 80% and discordant in 12% to 25% of cases.
- Associated cardiac findings include a large interatrial communication such as a patent foramen ovale or an atrial septal defect, a ventricular septal defect, transposition of the great vessels, and various degrees of right ventricular outflow obstruction.
- Prenatal follow-up with serial ultrasound examination is important to assess the patency of the foramen ovale and the presence of right ventricular outflow obstruction.
- An outcome study of prenatally diagnosed TA estimated an 83% survival at 1 year of age following active management.

References

1. Freedom RM, Smallhorn JF. Hearts with a univentricular atrioventricular connection. In: RM Freedom, LN Benson, JF Smallhorn, eds. *Neonatal heart disease.* New York: Springer-Verlag, 1992;497–521.
2. Van Praagh R, Van Praagh S, Vlad P, et al. Diagnosis of the anatomic types of single or common ventricle. *Am J Cardiol* 1965;15:345–366.
3. Hallermann FJ, Davis GD, Ritter DG, et al. Roentgenographic features of common ventricle. *Radiology* 1966;87:409–423.
4. Anderson RH, Tynan M, Freedom RM, et al. Ventricular morphology in the univentricular heart. *Herz* 1979;4(2):184–197.
5. Anderson RH, Becker AE, Tynan M, et al. The univentricular atrioventricular connection: getting to the root of a thorny problem. *Am J Cardiol* 1984;54(7):822–828.
6. Hagler DJ, Edwards WD. Univentricular atrioventricular connection. In: GC Emmanouilides, HD Allen, TA Riemenschneider, et al., eds. *Moss & Adams heart disease in infants, children and adolescents.* Baltimore: Williams & Wilkins, 1995;1278–1306.
7. Hoffman JI, Kaplan S. The incidence of congenital heart disease. *Circ Res* 2004;94:1890–1900.
8. Hornberger LK. Double-inlet ventricle in the fetus. In: L Allan, L Hornberger, G Sharland, eds. *Textbook of fetal cardiology.* London: Greenwich Medical Media Limited, 2000;174–182.
9. Chaoui R, McEwing R. Three cross-sectional planes for fetal color Doppler echocardiography. *Ultrasound Obstet Gynecol* 2003;21(1):81–93.
10. Allen HD, Driscoll DJ, Shaddy RE, et al., eds. *Moss and Adam's heart disease in infants, children and adolescents: including the fetus and young adult,* 7th ed. Baltimore: Williams & Wilkins, 1995;1131.
11. Van Praagh R, Ongley PA, Swan HJC. Anatomic types of single or common ventricle in man: morphologic and anatomic aspects of sixty necropsied cases. *Am J Cardiol* 1964;13:367–386.
12. Lan YT, Chang RK, Laks H. Outcome of patients with double-inlet left ventricle or tricuspid atresia with transposed great arteries. *J Am Coll Cardiol* 2004;43:113–119.
13. Kuhne M, Uber zwei falle kongenitaler atresie des ostium venosum dextrum. *Jahrb F Kinderh* 1906;63:235–249.
14. Tandon R, Edwards JE. Tricuspid atresia: a re-evaluation and classification. *J Thorac Cardiovasc Surg* 1974;67:530–542.
15. Sharland GK. Tricuspid valve abnormalities. In: L Allan, LK Hornberger, GK Sharland, eds. *Textbook of fetal cardiology.* London: Greenwich Medical Media Limited, 2000;133–147.
16. De Vore GR, Siassi B, Platt LD. Fetal echocardiography: the prenatal diagnosis of tricuspid atresia (type Ic) during the second trimester of pregnancy. *J Clin Ultrasound* 1987;15(5):317–324.
17. Garne E. Prenatal diagnosis of six major cardiac malformations in Europe—a population based study. *Acta Obstet Gynecol Scand* 2001;80(3):224–228.
18. Tongsong T, Sittiwangkul R, Wanapirak C, et al. Prenatal diagnosis of isolated tricuspid valve atresia: report of 4 cases and review of the literature. *J Ultrasound Med* 2004;23(7):945–950.
19. Galindo A, Comas C, Martinez JM, et al. Cardiac defects in chromosomally normal fetuses with increased nuchal translucency at 10–14 weeks of gestation. *J Matern Fetal Neonatal Med* 2003;13(3):163–170.
20. Berg C, Kremer C, Geipel A, et al. Ductus venosus blood flow alterations in fetuses with obstructive lesions of the right heart. *Ultrasound Obstet Gynecol* 2006;28(2):137–142.
21. Chaoui R, Hoffmann J, Heling KS. Three-dimensional (3D) and 4D color Doppler fetal echocardiography using spatio-temporal image correlation (STIC). *Ultrasound Obstet Gynecol* 2004;23(6):535–545.
22. Goncalves LF, Lee W, Chaiworapongsa T, et al. Four-dimensional ultrasonography of the fetal heart with spatiotemporal image correlation. *Am J Obstet Gynecol* 2003;189(6):1792–1802.
23. Wald RM, Tham EB, McCrindle BW, et al. Outcome after prenatal diagnosis of tricuspid atresia: a multicenter experience. *Am Heart J* 2007;153(5):772–778.
24. Sharma R, Iyer KS, Airan B, et al. Univentricular repair: early and midterm results. *J Thorac Cardiovasc Surg* 1995;110:1692–1701.
25. Gentles TL, Mayer JE Jr, Gauvreau K, et al. Fontan operation in five hundred consecutive patients: factors influencing early and late outcomes. *J Thorac Cardiovasc Surg* 1997;114:376–391.

TETRALOGY OF FALLOT, PULMONARY ATRESIA WITH VENTRICULAR SEPTAL DEFECT, AND ABSENT PULMONARY VALVE SYNDROME

TETRALOGY OF FALLOT

Definition, Spectrum of Disease, and Incidence

Tetralogy of Fallot (TOF) is characterized by a subaortic (malaligned) ventricular septal defect (VSD), an aortic root that overrides the VSD, and infundibular pulmonary stenosis (Fig. 17-1). Right ventricular hypertrophy, which represents the fourth anatomic feature of the "tetralogy," is typically not present prenatally. The spectrum of TOF includes severe forms, such as pulmonary atresia with VSD and absent pulmonary valve, both of which will be discussed in more detail later in this chapter. TOF is one of the most common forms of cyanotic congenital heart disease (CHD) and is found in about 1 in 3600 live births and accounts for 3% to 7% of infants with CHD (1). The classic form of TOF with pulmonary stenosis accounts for about 80% of all newborns with TOF (2).

Ultrasound Findings

Gray Scale

In TOF the four-chamber view appears normal unless the VSD is large and visible in this plane. TOF is typically detected in the five-chamber view, which demonstrates a perimembranous subaortic VSD with an aortic root override (Fig. 17-2). This aortic override is due to a discontinuity between the interventricular septum and the medial aortic wall, with a partial connection of the aorta to the right ventricle. The aorta is thus slightly shifted to the right, a condition termed *aortic dextroposition*. Generally the aortic root, which receives blood from both the right and left ventricles, appears dilated, especially in the third trimester, which may provide the first hint to the presence of TOF. Furthermore, in TOF, the overriding aorta

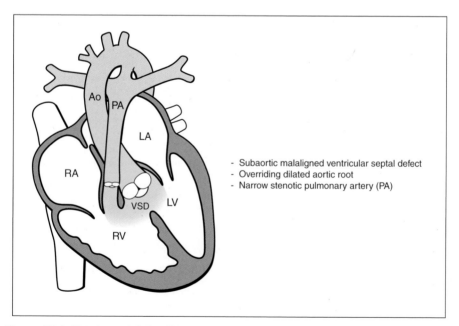

- Subaortic malaligned ventricular septal defect
- Overriding dilated aortic root
- Narrow stenotic pulmonary artery (PA)

Figure 17-1. Tetralogy of Fallot. RA, right atrium; RV, right ventricle; LA, left atrium; LV, left ventricle; Ao, aorta.

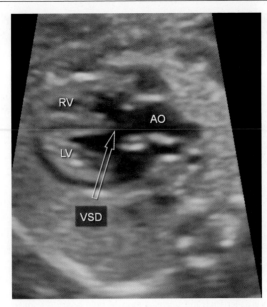

Figure 17-2. Transverse plane of the fetal chest at the level of the five-chamber view showing the ventricular septal defect (VSD) (*arrow*) and the dilated overriding aorta (AO). LV, left ventricle; RV, right ventricle.

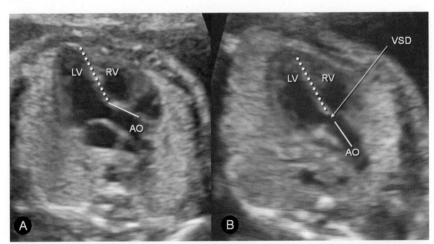

Figure 17-3. Comparison of the apical five-chamber view in a normal fetus **(A)** and a fetus with tetralogy of Fallot with aortic override **(B).** In the normal fetus (A), the ascending aorta (AO) points to the right fetal shoulder with a wide angle between the direction of the ventricular septum (*dashed line*) and the anterior wall of the ascending aorta (*solid line*) (see also Fig. 6-4). In the fetus with aortic override (B), the course of the ascending aorta (*solid line*) is parallel to the ventricular septum (*dashed line*). This finding is also noted in other anomalies involving aortic override. RV, right ventricle; LV, left ventricle; VSD, ventricular septal defect.

assumes a parallel course to the ventricular septum in contrast to the ascending aorta in a normal heart (Fig. 17-3). The diagnosis of TOF also requires the demonstration of a narrow but patent main pulmonary artery "pulmonary stenosis," which is best demonstrated in the short-axis or the three-vessel view (Fig. 17-4). In some milder forms of TOF, especially in midgestation, the size discrepancy between the pulmonary trunk and the aorta may be subtle. The discrepancy in size, however, becomes more obvious with advancing gestation.

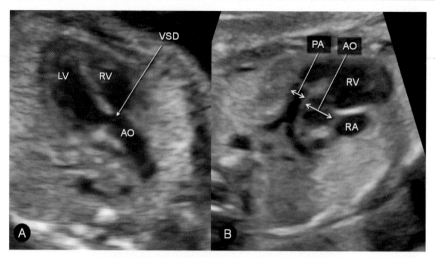

Figure 17-4. Two diagnostic planes for tetralogy of Fallot: the five-chamber-view plane **(A)** and the three-vessel-view plane **(B).** In the five-chamber view (A), the ventricular septal defect (VSD) is demonstrated with an overriding aorta (AO). In the three-vessel-view plane (B), the main pulmonary artery (PA) is smaller than the aorta, a sign of pulmonary stenosis. LV, left ventricle; RV, right ventricle; RA, right atrium.

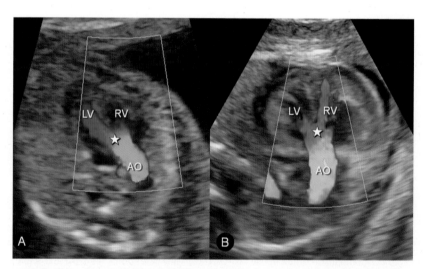

Figure 17-5. Color Doppler in the apical five-chamber-view plane in fetus **A** with simple tetralogy of Fallot (TOF) and in fetus **B** with atrioventricular septal defect, thickened myocardium, and TOF. Color Doppler demonstrates blood filling the slightly dilated AO from both right (RV) and left (LV) ventricles; *star* denotes the site of aortic override.

Color Doppler

Color Doppler facilitates the demonstration of VSD (shunting of blood across the VSD) and confirms the presence of an overriding aorta with blood draining from both ventricles into the aortic root (Fig. 17-5). Color Doppler at the three-vessel-trachea view can also demonstrate a small pulmonary artery (Fig. 17-6). Often, the inflow into the aorta appears aliased on color Doppler due to the high perfusion (Fig. 17-5). Color and pulsed Doppler velocities in the pulmonary artery are generally normal or only mildly increased in the fetus, in contrast to

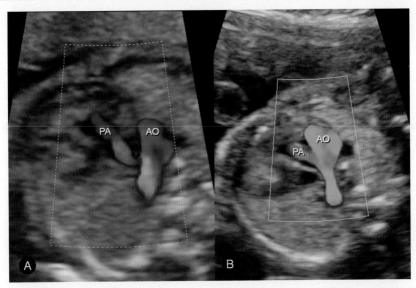

Figure 17-6. Color Doppler at the three-vessel-trachea-view plane in the same two fetuses presented in Figure 17-5. Color Doppler demonstrates in **A** and **B** a small pulmonary artery (PA) when compared to the size of the aorta (AO). Pulmonary stenosis is diagnosed based on size discrepancy rather than Doppler velocities across the pulmonary valves (see Fig. 17-7).

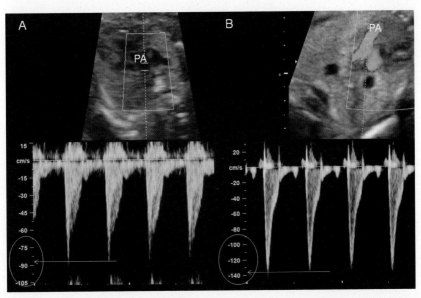

Figure 17-7. Color and pulsed Doppler across the pulmonary valve in two fetuses with tetralogy of Fallot. In fetus **A,** Doppler velocities are 85 cm/sec, within the normal range, and in fetus **B,** Doppler velocities are 130 cm/sec, slightly increased. PA, pulmonary artery.

postnatal findings (3) (Fig. 17-7). Flow across the ductus arteriosus is antegrade in mild TOF, but can also be reversed in more severe cases (Fig. 17-8). In such cases, postnatal ductus dependency of the pulmonary circulation can be associated with cyanosis of the newborn.

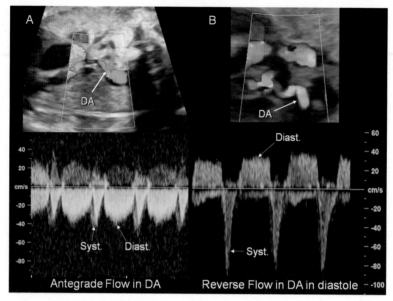

Figure 17-8. Color and pulsed Doppler across the ductus arteriosus (DA) in two fetuses showing a small DA in fetus **A** with antegrade flow throughout the cardiac cycle and reverse flow in the DA during diastole in fetus **B.** Fetus B is at risk for ductal-dependent circulation postnatally. Syst, systolic; Diast, diastolic.

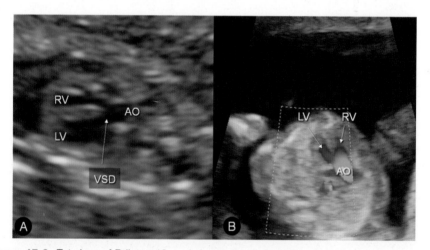

Figure 17-9. Tetralogy of Fallot at 13 weeks' gestation in fetus **A** and at 14 weeks' gestation in fetus **B.** The ventricular septal defect (VSD) and aortic override are demonstrated in fetus A on gray scale. Color Doppler shows aortic filling from both left (LV) and right ventricles (RV) in fetus B. AO, aorta.

Early Gestation

In the late first and early second trimesters, the diagnosis of TOF is possible but in many cases difficult (4). Clues to the diagnosis include a large aortic root in the five-chamber view on gray scale and color (Fig. 17-9) and/or a small pulmonary artery. The aortic override may not be easily detected. The discrepant size between the aorta and pulmonary artery with antegrade flow in both vessels on color Doppler is an important sign at this early gestation. There is a strong association between an increased nuchal translucency measurement and the diagnosis of tetralogy of Fallot, even in the absence of chromosomal abnormalities, with almost half of the cases in one study showing this association (5).

Three-dimensional Ultrasound

The tomographic mode applied to a three-dimensional (3-D) volume acquired at the level of the four-chamber view allows the demonstration of the VSD, aortic overriding, and the stenotic pulmonary artery in a single view of multiple planes (Fig. 17-10). Spatio-temporal image correlation (STIC) with color Doppler displayed in glass body mode provides a clear demonstration of the lesion in the three-vessel-trachea view (Fig. 17-11).

Associated Cardiac and Extracardiac Findings

Associated cardiac abnormalities are common with TOF. Variations in coronary artery anatomy are occasionally seen, which may have an impact on the surgical approach to repair (6). A patent foramen ovale or an atrial septal defect has been reported in 83% and a persistent left superior vena cava in 11% of newborns with TOF (7). The presence of a right-sided aortic arch, with a course to the right of the trachea, is seen in 25% of cases with TOF (8). Occasionally an atrioventricular septal defect coexists with TOF, and this increases the risk of chromosomal abnormalities (9).

In general, a higher incidence of extracardiac malformations, chromosomal anomalies, and genetic syndromes is seen in the fetus with TOF when compared to the neonate. Associated extracardiac congenital anomalies are fairly common with no specific organ involvement. The rate of chromosomal abnormalities is around 30%, with trisomies 21, 13, and 18 accounting for the majority of cases (5). The rate of deletion 22q11 is found in 10% to 15% of fetuses and neonates with TOF (5,10). The risk of deletion 22q11 in cases of TOF increases when the thymus is hypoplastic, the aortic arch is right sided, extracardiac anomalies are noted, or polyhydramnios is found. Table 17-1 lists common cardiac and extracardiac abnormalities associated with TOF.

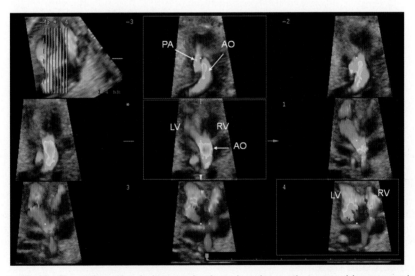

Figure 17-10. Three-dimensional ultrasound volume in color spatio-temporal image correlation (STIC) shown in tomographic display in a fetus with tetralogy of Fallot demonstrating in one view ventricular filling in diastole (*box in lower row*), aortic override with filling from both ventricles (*box in middle row*), and a small pulmonary artery (PA) as compared to the aorta (AO) (*box in upper row*). RV, right ventricle; LV, left ventricle.

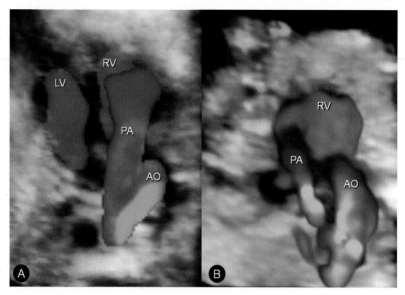

Figure 17-11. Three-dimensional ultrasound volume in color spatio-temporal image correlation (STIC) in glass body mode display at the three-vessel-trachea view in a normal fetus **(A)** and in a fetus with tetralogy of Fallot **(B)**. Note the small pulmonary artery (PA) in fetus B when compared to the dilated aorta (AO). RV, right ventricle; LV, left ventricle.

TABLE 17-1	Common Cardiac and Extracardiac Abnormalities Associated with Tetralogy of Fallot

Associated cardiac abnormalities	
- Patent foramen ovale/atrial septal defect	83%
- Right-sided aortic arch	25%
- Persistent left superior vena cava	11%
- Atrioventricular septal defect	<5%
- Abnormal coronary circulation	<5%
- Anomaly of pulmonary venous connection	<1%
Associated extracardiac abnormalities	
- Chromosomal abnormalities	30%
- Deletion 22q11	10%–15%
- Congenital anomaly of anatomic organs	Common

Differential Diagnosis

Differential diagnosis of TOF includes pulmonary atresia with VSD, absent pulmonary valve, common arterial trunk, and double outlet right ventricle. The differential diagnosis can be typically achieved by the correct evaluation of the size and origin of the pulmonary trunk. Table 17-2 lists various diagnostic tools in the differential diagnosis of these cardiac lesions.

Prognosis and Outcome

Serial prenatal ultrasound examinations to document fetal pulmonary artery growth and flow across the ductus arteriosus are critical for counseling and appropriate care of the newborn, as pulmonary artery growth has been shown to be variable and unpredictable (3,11). In general, prenatally diagnosed cases of TOF have a worse prognosis than postnatal cases due to

TABLE 17-2	**Differential Diagnosis of a Great Vessel Override Over a Ventricular Septal Defect (VSD)**	
	Diagnostic clue	**Additional signs**
Tetralogy of Fallot	• Patent, narrow PA • Antegrade flow in PA	• Antegrade or retrograde flow in DA
Pulmonary atresia with VSD	• Very narrow PA • No antegrade flow in PA	• DA tortuous with retrograde flow
Absent pulmonary valve	• Very large PA • To-and-fro blood flow in PA	• No DA generally • Aortic root is more narrow than the PA
Common arterial trunk	• PA arises from the overriding vessel	• Valve of the overriding vessel may show regurgitation
Double outlet right ventricle	• PA is overriding and aorta courses in parallel	• Mimics a TGA with VSD • Aorta or PA may be of normal size or narrow

PA, pulmonary artery; DA, ductus arteriosus; TGA, transposition of great arteries.

an increased association with chromosomal aberrations, associated syndromes, or complex extracardiac anomalies (5). Case series and analysis of cardiac surgery databases suggest a short- and long-term survival of infants with TOF upward of 90% (12,13). Poor prognostic signs include decelerated growth of the pulmonary artery, accelerated growth of the ascending aorta, cessation of forward flow through the pulmonary valve, and reversed flow through the ductus arteriosus (3). TOF with an atresia of the pulmonary valve (pulmonary atresia with VSD) or cases of absent pulmonary valve are acknowledged to have a worse prognosis. Table 17-3 lists poor prognostic signs associated with TOF.

■ KEY POINTS: TETRALOGY OF FALLOT

■ TOF is characterized by subaortic ventricular septal defect, aortic root override, and infundibular pulmonary stenosis.

■ TOF is one of the most common forms of cyanotic congenital heart disease.

■ The classic form with pulmonary stenosis accounts for about 80% of all cases.

■ The four-chamber view appears normal unless the ventricular septal defect is large and visible in this plane.

■ TOF is typically detected in the five-chamber view, demonstrating a perimembranous sub-aortic VSD with an aortic root override.

■ The aortic root appears dilated, especially in the third trimester.

■ There is a strong association between an increased nuchal translucency measurement and the diagnosis of tetralogy of Fallot.

■ Associated cardiac and extracardiac abnormalities are common.

■ A patent foramen ovale or an atrial septal defect is found in 83% of cases.

TABLE 17-3	**Poor Prognostic Signs of Tetralogy of Fallot (TOF)**

- Decelerated growth of the pulmonary artery
- Accelerated growth of the ascending aorta
- Cessation of forward flow through the pulmonary valve
- Reversed flow through the ductus arteriosus
- TOF with atresia of the pulmonary valve (pulmonary atresia with ventricular septal defect)
- Absent pulmonary valve
- Associated chromosomal aberrations
- Associated extracardiac congenital malformations
- Small left ventricle
- Associated abnormal venous connection

- A right-sided aortic arch and a persistent left superior vena cava have been found in 25% and 11% of cases, respectively.
- The rate of chromosomal abnormalities is around 30%.
- Microdeletion of 22q11 is found in 10% to 15% of fetuses.
- Poor prognostic signs include decelerated growth of the pulmonary artery, accelerated growth of the ascending aorta, cessation of forward flow through the pulmonary valve, and reversed flow through the ductus arteriosus.

PULMONARY ATRESIA WITH VENTRICULAR SEPTAL DEFECT

Definition, Spectrum of Disease, and Incidence

Pulmonary atresia with ventricular septal defect (PAVSD) is characterized by atresia of the pulmonary valve, hypoplasia of the pulmonary tract, membranous or infundibular ventricular septal defect, and an overriding aorta (Fig. 17-12). PAVSD was previously referred to as "severe tetralogy of Fallot." Distinct features of PAVSD that differentiate it from TOF include no right ventricular outflow and severe abnormalities of the pulmonary circulation, where the blood supply to the lungs is entirely from the systemic arterial circulation. Sources of pulmonary blood flow include the ductus arteriosus and systemic-pulmonary collateral circulation, or a combination of both. Systemic-pulmonary collateral circulation typically includes collateral arteries from the descending aorta to the lungs, called *major aortopulmonary collateral arteries* (MAPCAs) (Figs. 17-12 and 17-13). PAVSD accounts for about 20% of all TOF cases, represents about 2% of congenital heart disease, and has a prevalence of 0.07 per 1000 live births (2,14). A 10-fold increased risk for PAVSD is seen in infants of diabetic mothers (14). Figure 17-14 demonstrates an anatomic specimen of a fetal heart with pulmonary atresia and ventricular septal defect.

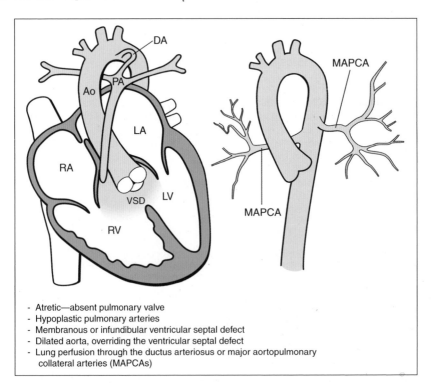

- Atretic—absent pulmonary valve
- Hypoplastic pulmonary arteries
- Membranous or infundibular ventricular septal defect
- Dilated aorta, overriding the ventricular septal defect
- Lung perfusion through the ductus arteriosus or major aortopulmonary collateral arteries (MAPCAs)

Figure 17-12. Pulmonary atresia with ventricular septal defect. RA, right atrium; RV, right ventricle; LA, left atrium; LV, left ventricle; Ao, aorta; PA, pulmonary artery; DA, ductus arteriosus; VSD, ventricular septal defect.

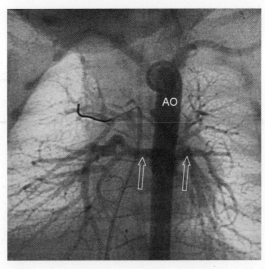

Figure 17-13. Angiogram of the descending aorta in a newborn with pulmonary atresia with ventricular septal defect, demonstrating major aortopulmonary collateral arteries (*arrows*). Compare with Figure 17-12.

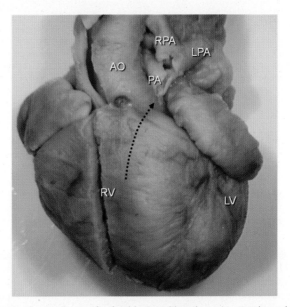

Figure 17-14. Anatomic specimen of a fetal heart with pulmonary atresia and ventricular septal defect. The ascending aorta (AO) is large and the pulmonary artery (PA) is diminutive with small right (RPA) and left pulmonary arteries (LPA). Note that the main pulmonary artery is underdeveloped with no connection (*arrow*) to the right ventricle (RV). LV, left ventricle.

Ultrasound Findings

Gray Scale

The four-chamber view is typically normal. PAVSD is suspected on the five-chamber view where the VSD and the aortic override are detected (Fig. 17-15A). The aortic root in PAVSD

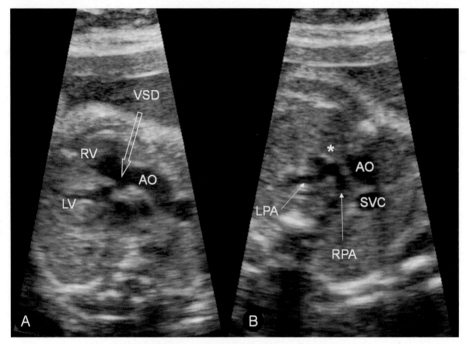

Figure 17-15. Pulmonary atresia with ventricular septal defect (VSD) shown in the five-chamber view **(A)** and the three-vessel view **(B).** In the five-chamber view (A), the VSD is seen with a large overriding aorta (AO). The three-vessel view (B) demonstrates the absence of the main pulmonary artery (*asterisk*) and right (RPA) and left pulmonary arteries (LPA) drained retrograde by a tortuous ductus arteriosus (DA). The DA is demonstrated in Figure 17-16. RV, right ventricle; LV, left ventricle; SVC, superior vena cava.

has a larger diameter than in TOF, since the entire right ventricular stroke volume drains into the aorta across the VSD (Fig. 17-15A). In the three-vessel view the hypoplastic pulmonary artery can occasionally be visualized, but this could be difficult on two-dimensional ultrasound in severe cases (Fig. 17-15B). In some cases a closed pulmonary valve can be seen, and on occasion the proximal pulmonary trunk may be absent. The ductus arteriosus may be small and is often tortuous, but when it is the source of pulmonary circulation, it can be dilated, which facilitates its detection on gray-scale imaging in the three-vessel-trachea view.

Color Doppler

Aortic override with blood draining from both ventricles can be easily demonstrated by color Doppler (Fig. 17-16A). Color Doppler can help differentiate PAVSD from TOF. In PAVSD, color Doppler confirms the absence of blood draining from the right ventricle into the pulmonary trunk, and demonstrates retrograde filling of the right and left pulmonary arteries (Fig. 17-16B). Color Doppler can also show reverse flow in the tortuous, occasionally dilated, ductus arteriosus in PAVSD (Fig. 17-16B). Once PAVSD is suspected, the examiner should seek, using low Doppler velocity settings, the presence of MAPCAs, which typically arise from the descending aorta (Fig. 17-17). A longitudinal view of the aorta from an anterior or lateral approach may enhance visualization (Fig. 17-18). Generally more than one MAPCA is found. Even if not detected at first attempt, MAPCAs should be sought on follow-up ultrasound examinations.

Early Gestation

PAVSD may be detected in early gestation by demonstrating an enlarged, overriding aortic root and the absence of a normal-size pulmonary artery (Fig. 17-19). Color Doppler can facilitate recognition of PASVD by confirming the absence of right ventricular–pulmonary flow.

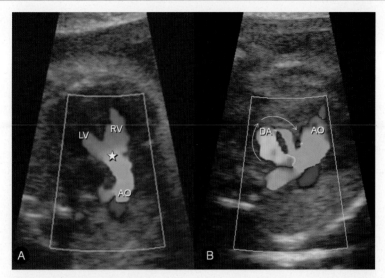

Figure 17-16. Pulmonary atresia with ventricular septal defect (VSD) shown in the five-chamber view **(A)** and the three-vessel view **(B)** in color Doppler (same fetus as shown in Fig. 17-15). In the five-chamber view (A), the large overriding aorta (AO) is shown with aortic filling from both the right (RV) and left ventricles (LV). The star marks the location of the VSD. In the three-vessel view (B), the tortuous ductus arteriosus (DA) (*curved arrow*) is shown with retrograde drainage into the pulmonary arteries (not seen in this plane).

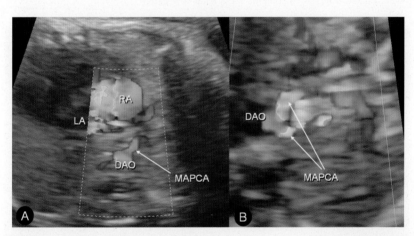

Figure 17-17. Transverse planes of the fetal chest with color Doppler in two fetuses with pulmonary atresia with ventricular septal defect, demonstrating major aortopulmonary collateral arteries (MAPCAs) arising from the descending aorta (DAO). In fetus **A,** one MAPCA is seen arising to the right side, and in fetus **B,** two MAPCAs are detected coursing into the lungs. MAPCAs are best detected with low-color Doppler velocity settings. RA, right atrium; LA, left atrium.

MAPCAs may also be detected in early gestation, particularly when vessel size is large enough to demonstrate blood flow on color Doppler.

Three-dimensional Ultrasound

The application of tomographic imaging on a three-dimensional volume was discussed in the TOF section. The benefit of three-dimensional ultrasound with rendering modes (B-flow or color/power Doppler) is primarily in the spatial demonstration of the MAPCAs (Fig. 17-20).

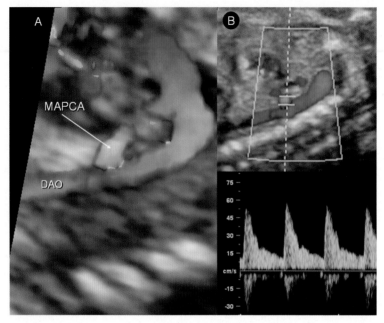

Figure 17-18. Color **(A)** and pulsed **(B)** Doppler of major aortopulmonary collateral artery (MAPCA) arising from the descending aorta (DAO) and visualized in a longitudinal view of the aortic arch. Pulsed Doppler (B) confirms the arterial flow pattern.

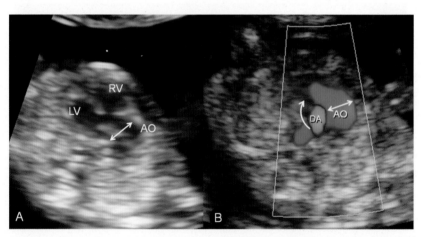

Figure 17-19. Transvaginal ultrasound at the level of the five-chamber view **(A)** and the transverse ductal arch view **(B)** in a fetus at 12 weeks' gestation with pulmonary atresia and ventricular septal defect. The five-chamber view (A) shows a large overriding aorta (AO) (*double-sided arrow*). Reverse flow in the ductus arteriosus (DA) is demonstrated on color Doppler (*curved arrow*) at the transverse ductal view (B). RV, right ventricle; LV, left ventricle.

Associated Cardiac and Extracardiac Findings

A right-sided aortic arch can be present in 20% to 50% of all cases (15). Secundum-type atrial septal defect or a patent foramen ovale is seen in about half the cases postnatally (15). Absence of the ductus arteriosus is also reported in about half the cases. MAPCAs, when present, are associated with stenosis in about 60% of cases (16).

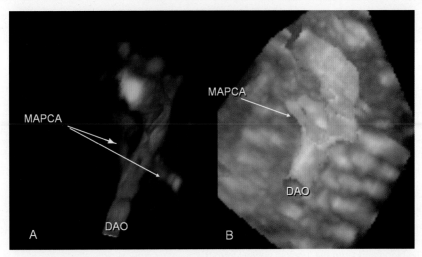

Figure 17-20. Three-dimensional ultrasound in power Doppler **(A)** and color Doppler **(B)** modes of a fetus with major aortopulmonary collateral arteries (MAPCAs). DAO, descending aorta.

Associated extracardiac findings include a high incidence of chromosomal aberrations. In the Baltimore-Washington Infant Study, 8.3% of children with PAVSD had chromosomal anomalies (14). The incidence of 22q11 microdeletion is high and is found in 20% of fetuses with PAVSD, with an increased association in the presence of MAPCAs and/or a right aortic arch (17,18). The 22q11 microdeletion was more commonly detected in PAVSD than in TOF in some series (19,20). Other nonchromosomal extracardiac anomalies are infrequent in PAVSD.

Differential Diagnosis

The primary differential diagnosis of PAVSD is TOF, as the two anomalies are often discussed together. Table 17-4 lists differentiating features of both entities. Differentiating PAVSD from common arterial trunk (CAT) may be difficult and based on the authors' experience is a common referral diagnosis for PAVSD. The presence of a normal aortic valve, retrograde blood flow in the ductus arteriosus, and branch pulmonary arteries and demonstration of MAPCAs help differentiate PAVSD from CAT (21). Previous type IV CAT, with both pulmonary arteries arising directly from the descending aorta, is currently classified as PAVSD. Other

TABLE 17-4	Differentiating Features of Tetralogy of Fallot (TOF) and Pulmonary Atresia with Ventricular Septal Defect (PAVSD)	
	TOF	**PAVSD**
VSD + aortic override	Present	Present
Aortic root size	Normal to dilated	More dilated than in TOF
Pulmonary trunk	Narrow, patent pulmonary valve, antegrade flow on color Doppler	Hypoplastic or absent, no recognized pulmonary valve, no antegrade flow
Ductus arteriosus	Narrow, antegrade flow or even reverse flow if pulmonary trunk very narrow. Difficult to visualize with right aortic arch	Tortuous and occasionally dilated due to reverse flow
Major aortopulmonary collateral arteries	Typically absent	Present
Chromosomal aberrations	22q11 deletion in 10%–15% Trisomies in 30%	22q11 deletion in 20% Trisomies in 8%–9%
Prognosis	Good if no associated malformations	Guarded

differential diagnoses include double outlet right ventricle with pulmonary stenosis or atresia, single ventricle with pulmonary stenosis or atresia, and total anomalous venous connection with pulmonary venous obstruction.

Prognosis and Outcome

Prognosis of PAVSD is primarily dependent on the adequacy of the pulmonary circulation and associated abnormalities. The natural history of PAVSD can vary greatly based on the anatomic components of this malformation. In general, if the ductus arteriosus is the primary source of pulmonary flow, long-term outcome is enhanced. In a reported series of 495 surgical patients, long-term survival of 61% and 75% was noted for palliative and complete repair, respectively (22). The presence of MAPCAs was a significant risk factor for late mortality (22). The identification of PAVSD in the fetus carries a worse prognosis.

▓ KEY POINTS: PULMONARY ATRESIA WITH VENTRICULAR SEPTAL DEFECT

- PAVSD is characterized by atresia of the pulmonary valve, hypoplasia of the pulmonary tract, membranous or infundibular ventricular septal defect, and an overriding aorta.
- The blood supply to the lungs is entirely from the systemic arterial circulation.
- A 10-fold increased risk is seen in infants of diabetic mothers.
- The four-chamber view is typically normal.
- The overriding aorta, which appears dilated, is a leading diagnostic sign.
- A right-sided aortic arch can be present in 20% to 50% of cases.
- Secundum-type atrial septal defect or a patent foramen ovale is seen in about half the cases postnatally.
- Absence of the ductus arteriosus is reported in about half the cases.
- MAPCAs, when present, are associated with stenosis in about 60% of cases.
- There is a high incidence of numerical chromosomal aberrations, in the range of 8.3%.
- The incidence of 22q11 microdeletion is found in 20% of fetuses.
- Prognosis is primarily dependent on the adequacy of the pulmonary circulation and associated abnormalities.
- The presence of MAPCAs is a significant risk factor for late mortality.

▓ ABSENT PULMONARY VALVE SYNDROME

Definition, Spectrum of Disease, and Incidence

Absent pulmonary valve syndrome (APVS) is a rare cardiac malformation characterized by absent, dysplastic, or rudimentary pulmonary valve leaflets, in association with an outlet VSD and an overriding aorta (Fig. 17-21). Most cases of APVS are also associated with an absent patent ductus arteriosus, which has been postulated as a cause of pathogenesis of APVS (23). The main, right, and left pulmonary arteries become severely dilated, and the main pulmonary valve annulus shows signs of stenosis with severe insufficiency. Other clinical features include a common association of airway abnormalities, which may lead to severe respiratory compromise. A rare variant of APVS has been reported with an intact ventricular septum, a less dilated pulmonary trunk, and a patent ductus arteriosus.

APVS is typically classified as a subgroup of tetralogy of Fallot. The incidence of APVS is rare as it accounts for 3% to 6% of all patients with TOF and for 0.2% to 0.4% of liveborn infants with congenital heart disease (24,25). The incidence of APVS is higher in fetal life, with figures close to 15% to 20% of all prenatal TOF cases and 1% of fetal congenital heart disease (26). Figure 17-22 demonstrates an anatomic specimen of a fetal heart with APVS.

Ultrasound Findings

Gray Scale

In APVS the four-chamber view typically shows a dilated right ventricle due to volume overload from the insufficient pulmonary valve. The five-chamber view reveals the VSD with the

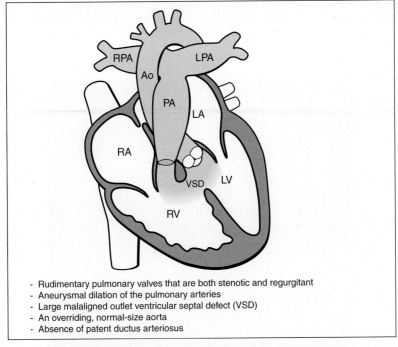

- Rudimentary pulmonary valves that are both stenotic and regurgitant
- Aneurysmal dilation of the pulmonary arteries
- Large malaligned outlet ventricular septal defect (VSD)
- An overriding, normal-size aorta
- Absence of patent ductus arteriosus

Figure 17-21. Absent pulmonary valve syndrome. RPA, right pulmonary artery; LPA, left pulmonary artery; RA, right atrium; RV, right ventricle; LA, left atrium; LV, left ventricle; Ao, aorta; PA, pulmonary artery; LPA, left pulmonary artery; RPA, right pulmonary artery.

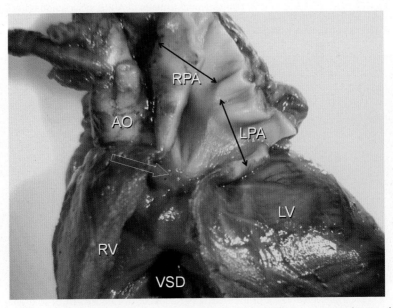

Figure 17-22. Anatomic specimen of a heart with absent pulmonary valve syndrome, showing an opened right ventricular outflow tract with a large ventricular septal defect (VSD). The region of the pulmonary valvular ring shows absence of valve leaflets (*open arrow*) and dilated right (RPA) and left pulmonary arteries (LPA). AO, aorta; LV, left ventricle; RV, right ventricle.

overriding aorta, but in APVS, conversely to the classic TOF, the aortic root is not dilated (Fig. 17-23). The short-axis view or the three-vessel-trachea view reveals the impressive, massively dilated main, right, and left pulmonary arteries (Fig. 17-24). Instead of diameters between 2 and 6 mm for the pulmonary arteries and trunk, measurements in the range of

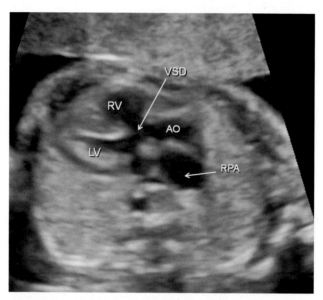

Figure 17-23. Transverse five-chamber view of a fetus with absent pulmonary valve syndrome (APVS) showing the ventricular septal defect (VSD) with the overriding aorta (AO), similar to tetralogy of Fallot and pulmonary atresia with ventricular septal defect discussed in this chapter (compare with Figs. 17-2 and 17-15). Differentiating features of APVS include a massively dilated right pulmonary artery (RPA) seen in this plane. The overriding aorta is not as dilated as in tetralogy of Fallot or in pulmonary atresia with VSD. LV, left ventricle; RV, right ventricle.

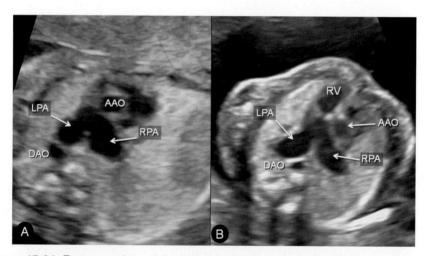

Figure 17-24. Transverse views of the fetal upper chest in two fetuses **(A,B)** with absent pulmonary valve syndrome (APVS) in a plane between the right ventricular short axis and the three-vessel view demonstrating dilated left (LPA) and right pulmonary arteries (RPA), a characteristic finding in APVS. Ductus arteriosus is not seen as it is absent in almost all cases (compare with findings in Fig. 17-25). AAO, ascending aorta; DAO, descending aorta; RV, right ventricle.

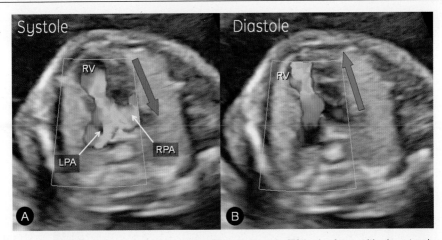

Figure 17-25. Color Doppler during systole **(A)** and diastole **(B)** in the fetus with absent pulmonary valve syndrome shown in Figure 17-24B with the characteristic dilated left (LPA) and right pulmonary arteries (RPA). In systole (A), turbulent blood flow streams from the right ventricle (RV) across the pulmonary ring with absent or remnant pulmonary valves into the LPA and RPA (*blue arrow*). In diastole (B), blood flows back (*red arrow*) from the pulmonary arteries into the RV. Note the aliased color in A and B, a sign of high velocities. See pulsed Doppler in Figure 17-26.

10 to 18 mm can be obtained. In most cases no ductus arteriosus is found (Fig. 17-24). In the presence of a right aortic arch, the descending aorta can be found to be on the right side and ventral to the spine.

Color Doppler
Main findings on color and pulsed Doppler include high velocities across the pulmonary valve annulus, with a typical to-and-fro flow, as a sign of stenosis and severe insufficiency (Fig. 17-25). Velocities around 200 to 250 cm/sec are generally obtained across the main pulmonary valves on pulsed Doppler evaluation (Fig. 17-26). Color Doppler may also show tricuspid valve regurgitation.

Early Gestation
The main feature of APVS, a markedly dilated pulmonary artery, may not be evident before 22 weeks of gestation (27). It is not uncommon, therefore, to see a normal-size pulmonary artery in fetuses with APVS in early gestation. Anatomic and hemodynamic abnormalities show significant progression prenatally, and the full spectrum of APVS may not be manifested until late in gestation (28).

Diagnosis of APVS is very difficult in the first trimester, but this entity has been reported in early gestation (28) with pulmonary valve insufficiency as the only sonographic feature. An increased nuchal translucency has been noted in up to 40% of fetuses with APVS in some series, and this may facilitate the recognition of this syndrome in early gestation (27). Reverse end-diastolic flow of the umbilical artery was noted in 5 of 614 fetuses in a prospective study between 10 and 14 weeks; three of these five fetuses had TOF with APVS and a patent ductus arteriosus (29).

Three-dimensional Ultrasound
The application of three-dimensional tomographic imaging enables the demonstration of slightly discrepant ventricles in the four-chamber view as well as severely dilated pulmonary arteries. The combination of color Doppler and three-dimensional tomographic imaging reveals the impressive turbulent flow across the right ventricular outflow tract (Fig. 17-27).

Associated Cardiac and Extracardiac Findings

Associated cardiac findings include a right-sided aortic arch and the presence of major aorto-pulmonary collateral arteries. Coronary artery variation may also exist with APVS.

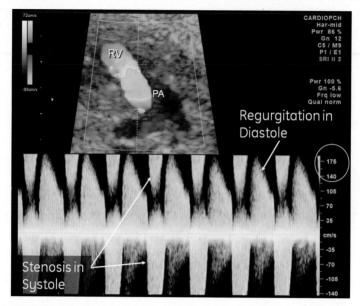

Figure 17-26. Pulsed Doppler across the dysplastic or absent pulmonary valve in the fetus with absent pulmonary valve syndrome, also shown in Figures 17-25 and 17-24B. The spectral Doppler across the pulmonary artery (PA) demonstrates to-and-fro flow as shown on color Doppler in Figure 17-25. Note the stenosis in systole with peak velocities greater than 200 cm/sec and regurgitation in diastole with regurgitant velocities reaching 175 cm/sec. RV, right ventricle.

Extracardiac findings include a high association with chromosomal anomalies, primarily the 22q11 microdeletion. This association is in the order of 20% to 25% of fetuses with APVS, and this rate has been fairly consistent between various series (27,30,31). Other chromosomal anomalies can be found but are often related to the presence of associated extracardiac malformations. The APVS variant with a patent ductus arteriosus is rarely associated with chromosomal or extracardiac anomalies (27,30,31). A common and serious association with APVS is bronchomalacia primarily due to bronchial compression by the dilated pulmonary trunk (31,32).

Differential Diagnosis

APVS is easily diagnosed when the pathognomic sign of aneurysmal dilatation of the pulmonary artery is seen on ultrasound. Nevertheless, differential diagnosis of an overriding aorta is presented in Table 17-2.

Prognosis and Outcome

Prenatally diagnosed APVS typically represents the severe end of the spectrum and is commonly associated with a poor outcome. Survival in the order of 15% to 20% has been reported in such series (27,30,31). The high mortality has been related to both cardiac failure and associated bronchomalacia (31). The occurrence of bronchomalacia is common in the presence of cardiomegaly and marked pulmonary dilatation, which represents a poor prognostic sign. Prenatal counseling should take into account the progression of this lesion in utero. Fetuses with a patent ductus arteriosus and less dilated pulmonary arteries may have a better outcome.

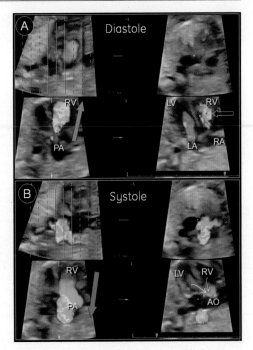

Figure 17-27. Three-dimensional ultrasound volume in color spatio-temporal image correlation (STIC) in tomographic display in a fetus with absent pulmonary valve syndrome. **A** shows the diastolic part of the cardiac cycle with the filling of both ventricles from the atria in the four-chamber view (*lower right*) and the severe regurgitation across the absent pulmonary valve (*red arrow*) in the right ventricular outflow tract (*lower left*). Note the turbulent flow in the right ventricle (RV) (*open arrow*) owing to the combined filling on one hand from the right atrium and on the other from the regurgitant flow from the right outflow tract. **B** shows the systolic part with the overriding aorta (AO) (*two curved arrows*) and blood flow from both right and left ventricles (LV) (*lower right*) and the turbulent flow across the absent pulmonary valve (*lower left, blue arrow*). Compare with findings in Figure 17-25. PA, pulmonary artery.

■ KEY POINTS: ABSENT PULMONARY VALVE SYNDROME

- APVS is characterized by absent, dysplastic, or rudimentary pulmonary valve leaflets, in association with an outlet ventricular septal defect.
- The four-chamber view typically shows a dilated right ventricle due to volume overload.
- The aortic root is not dilated, unlike in the classic form of tetralogy of Fallot.
- In most cases no ductus arteriosus is found.
- An increased nuchal translucency has been noted in up to 40% of fetuses.
- Associated cardiac findings include a right-sided aortic arch and the presence of major aorto-pulmonary collateral arteries.
- Microdeletion of 22q11 is found in about 20% to 25% of fetuses.
- Bronchomalacia, due to bronchial compression by the dilated pulmonary trunk, is a common and serious association.
- Prenatal diagnosis carries a poor outcome.

References

1. Fyler DC. Tetralogy of Fallot. In: AS Nadas, DC Fyler, eds. *Nadas' pediatric cardiology*, 4th ed. Philadelphia: Hanley & Belfus, 1992;471–491.
2. Perry LW, Neil CA, Ferencz C, et al. Infants with congenital heart disease: the cases. In: C Ferencz, JD Rubin, CA Loffredo, et al., eds. *Perspectives in pediatric cardiology. Epidemiology of congenital heart disease: the Baltimore-Washington Infant Study 1981–1989.* Armonk, NY: Futura Publishing, 1993;33–62.
3. Hornberger LK, Sanders SP, Sahn DJ, et al. In utero pulmonary artery and aortic growth and potential for progression of pulmonary outflow tract obstruction in tetralogy of Fallot. *J Am Coll Cardiol* 1995;25:739–745.
4. Achiron R, Rotstein Z, Lipitz S, et al. First-trimester diagnosis of fetal congenital heart disease by transvaginal ultrasonography. *Obstet Gynecol* 1994;84(1):69–72.
5. Poon LCY, Huggon IC, Zidere V, et al. Tetralogy of Fallot in the fetus in the current era. *Ultrasound Obstet Gynecol* 2007;29:625–627.
6. Need LR, Powell AJ, del Nido P, et al. Coronary echocardiography in tetralogy of Fallot: diagnostic accuracy, resource utilization and surgical implications over 13 years. *J Am Coll Cardiol* 2000;36:1371–1377.

7. Rao BN, Anderson RC, Edwards JE. Anatomic variations in the tetralogy of Fallot. *Am Heart J* 1971;81:361–371.

8. Silverman N, Sinder A. Conditions with override of the ventricular septum by the systemic artery. In: G Hachtel, ed. *Two-dimensional echocardiography in congenital heart disease*. Norwalk, CT: Appleton-Century-Crofts, 1982;149–155.

9. Uretzky G, Puga FJ, Danielson GK, et al. Complete atrioventricular canal associated with tetralogy of Fallot. *J Thorac Cardiovasc Surg* 1984;87:756–780.

10. Shinebourne EA, Babu-Narayan SV, Carvalho JS. Tetralogy of Fallot: from fetus to adult. *Heart* 2006;92;1353–1359.

11. Pepas LP, Savis A, Jones A, et al. An echocardiographic study of tetralogy of Fallot in the fetus and infant. *Cardiol Young* 2003;13:240–247.

12. Gibbs JL, Monro JL, Cunningham D, et al. Survival after surgery or therapeutic catheterisation for congenital heart disease in children in the United Kingdom: analysis of the central cardiac audit database for 2000–1. *BMJ* 2004;328:611.

13. Murphy JG, Gersh BJ, Mair DD, et al. Long-term outcome in patients undergoing surgical repair of tetralogy of Fallot. *N Engl J Med* 1993;329:593–599.

14. Ferencz C, Loffredo CA, Correa-Villasenor A, et al., eds. *Malformations of the cardiac outflow tract in genetic and environmental risk factors of major cardiovascular malformations. The Baltimore-Washington Infant Study 1981–1989*. Armonk, NY: Futura Publishing, 1997;59–102.

15. Bharati S, Paul MH, Idriss FS, et al. The surgical anatomy of pulmonary atresia with ventricular septal defect: pseudotruncus. *J Thorac Cardiovasc Surg* 1975;69:713–721.

16. Liao PK, Edwards WD, Julsrud PR, et al. Pulmonary blood supply in patients with pulmonary atresia and ventricular septal defect. *J Am Coll Cardiol* 1985;6:1343–1350.

17. Goldmuntz E, Clark BJ, Mitchell LE, et al. Frequency of 22q11 deletions in patients with conotruncal defects. *J Am Coll Cardiol* 1998;32:492–498.

18. Momma K, Kondo C, Matsuoka R. Tetralogy of Fallot with pulmonary atresia associated with chromosome 22q11 deletion. *J Am Coll Cardiol* 1996;27:198–202.

19. Digilio MC, Marino B, Grazioli S, et al. Comparison of occurrence of genetic syndromes in ventricular septal defect with pulmonic stenosis (classic tetralogy of Fallot) versus ventricular septal defect with pulmonic atresia. *Am J Cardiol* 1996;77:1375–1376.

20. Chessa M, Butera G, Bonhoeffer P, et al. Relation of genotype 22q11 deletion to phenotype of pulmonary vessels in tetralogy of Fallot and pulmonary atresia-ventricular septal defect. *Heart* 1998;79:186–190.

21. Volpe P, Paladini D, Marasini M, et al. Common arterial trunk in the fetus: characteristics, associations, and outcome in a multicentre series of 23 cases. *Heart* 2003;89:1437–1441.

22. Cho JM, Puga FJ, Danielson GK, et al. Early and long-term results of the surgical treatment of tetralogy of Fallot with pulmonary atresia, with or without major aortopulmonary collateral arteries. *J Thorac Cardiovasc Surg* 2002;124:70–81.

23. Yeager SB, Van Der Velde ME, Waters BL, et al. Prenatal role of the ductus arteriosus in absent pulmonary valve syndrome. *Echocardiography* 2002;19:489–493.

24. Ferencz C. A case-control study of cardiovascular malformations in liveborn infants: the morphogenetic relevance of epidemiologic findings. In: EB Clark, A Takao, eds. *Developmental cardiology: morphogenesis and function*. Mount Kisco, NY: Futura Publishing, 1990;523–539.

25. Allan LD, Sharland GK, Milburn A, et al. Prospective diagnosis of 1006 consecutive cases of congenital heart disease in the fetus. *J Am Coll Cardiol* 1994;23:1452–1458.

26. Wisniewsky KB. Tetralogy of Fallot. In: JA Drose, ed. *Fetal echocardiography*. Philadelphia: WB Saunders, 1998;185–194.

27. Galindo A, Gutierrez-Larraya F, Martintz JM, et al. Prenatal diagnosis and outcome for fetuses with congenital absence of the pulmonary valve. *Ultrasound Obstet Gynecol* 2006;28:32–39.

28. Becker R, Schmitz L, Guschmann M, et al. Prenatal diagnosis of familial absent pulmonary valve syndrome: case report and review of the literature. *Ultrasound Obstet Gynecol* 2001;17:263–267.

29. Berg C, Thomsen Y, Geipel A, et al. Reversed end-diastolic flow in the umbilical artery at 10-14 weeks of gestation is associated with absent pulmonary valve syndrome. *Ultrasound Obstet Gynecol* 2007;30:254–258.

30. Volpe P, Paladini D, Marasini M, et al. Characteristics, associations and outcome of absent pulmonary valve syndrome in the fetus. *Ultrasound Obstet Gynecol* 2004;24:623–628.

31. Razavi RS, Sharland GK, Simpson JM. Prenatal diagnosis by echocardiogram and outcome of absent pulmonary valve syndrome. *Am J Cardiol* 2003;91:429–432.

32. Moon-Grady AJ, Tacy TA, Brook MM, et al. Value of clinical and echocardiographic features in predicting outcome in the fetus, infant, and child with tetralogy of Fallot with absent pulmonary valve complex. *Am J Cardiol* 2002;89:1280–1285.

COMMON ARTERIAL TRUNK

Definition, Spectrum of Disease, and Incidence

Common arterial trunk (CAT), also referred to as persistent truncus arteriosus, truncus arteriosus communis, and aorticopulmonary trunk, is characterized by a single arterial trunk that arises from the base of the heart and gives origin to the systemic, coronary, and pulmonary circulations (Fig. 18-1). A large ventricular septal defect (VSD) is almost always present in this anomaly. CAT results from failure of the truncus swellings, which normally divide the truncus arteriosus into the aorta and pulmonary arteries during embryogenesis, to fuse, resulting in a persistent common trunk (1). The spectrum of the disease is wide and is mainly related to the anatomic origin of the right and left pulmonary arteries, which may arise from a pulmonary trunk (Fig. 18-1A,B) or as direct branches from the CAT or the descending aorta. CAT is classified into four types by Collett and Edwards, based on the anatomic origin of the pulmonary arteries (2). In type 1, a short pulmonary trunk arises from the CAT and divides into right and left pulmonary arteries (Fig. 18-1A). In types 2 and 3, both pulmonary arteries arise separately, as individual branches, from the CAT and they are either close anatomically (type 2) or at some distance from one another (type 3). In type 4, which is now reclassified as pulmonary atresia with VSD (see Chapter 17) rather than CAT, the pulmonary arteries arise from the aortic arch or the descending aorta. Another classification, type A1 through A4, is proposed by Van Praagh and Van Praagh (3). In this classification, type A1 is similar to type 1 of Collett and Edwards's

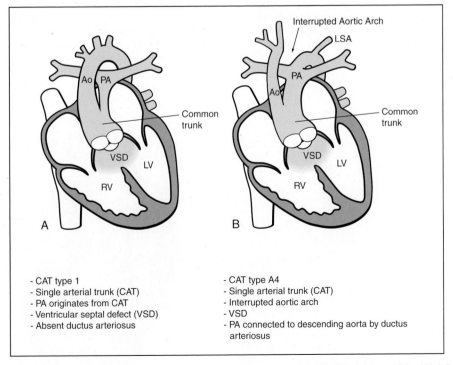

Figure 18-1. Common arterial trunk (CAT) type 1 **(A)** and type A4 **(B)**. RV, right ventricle; LV, left ventricle; PA, pulmonary artery; Ao, aorta; LSA, left subclavian artery; VSD, ventricular septal defect.

classification, type A2 combines types 2 and 3, type A3 describes a single pulmonary artery origin from the CAT with either a ductus or collateral circulation supplying the contralateral lung, and type A4 refers to abnormalities of the aortic arch including complete interruption (Fig. 18-1B). The root of the CAT is large and has a biventricular origin in most cases. In up to a third of CAT cases, however, the root appears to arise entirely from the right ventricle, and in rare cases entirely from the left ventricle. The CAT valve has three leaflets (tricuspid) in about 69% of cases, four leaflets (quadricuspid) in 22% of cases, two leaflets (bicuspid) in 9% of cases, and, on very rare occasions, one, five, or more leaflets (4). The two most commonly diagnosed types of CAT in the fetus are type 1/type A1 and type A4. Figure 18-2 shows an anatomic specimen of CAT type 1.

CAT is found in 1.6% of all newborns with congenital heart disease (5), is reported to occur in about 1.07 of 10,000 births (6), and is found more commonly in offsprings of diabetic mothers (7). CAT occurs equally in boys and girls and is more commonly prevalent in fetal series (8). Associated chromosomal anomalies, mainly deletion 22q11, are common.

Ultrasound Findings

Gray Scale

The four-chamber view appears normal in CAT (Fig. 18-3A) unless the VSD is large and visible in this plane or levorotation of the heart is present. The diagnosis is best achieved by detecting a malaligned VSD with an overriding large vessel on the five-chamber view (Fig. 18-3B) and an absence of a separate pulmonary artery and valve arising from the right ventricle. Confirming the diagnosis is usually made by identifying the pulmonary trunk (or arteries) directly arising from the overriding large vessel (Fig. 18-3B). In the five-chamber view, the root of the CAT is large and the valve leaflets are thickened (dysplastic) with lack of proper excursion (Fig. 18-4). Short-axis view may demonstrate an abnormal number of valve leaflets (Fig. 18-5). Identifying a short main pulmonary artery in the five-chamber view that arises from the large common trunk and courses to the left confirms the CAT diagnosis (type 1) and differentiates this abnormality from tetralogy of Fallot. In CAT type 1, the aorta is large and the pulmonary artery is narrow. In the CAT types 2 and 3, there is no pulmonary trunk, and the pulmonary arteries arise either posteriorly (type 2) or laterally (type 3) from the common trunk. Differentiating various CAT types is difficult and unreliable prenatally, especially in the second trimester (9). The three-vessel-trachea view is also helpful in

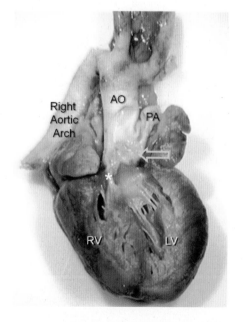

Figure 18-2. Anatomic specimen of common arterial trunk type 1 (compare to Fig. 18-1A). The common trunk (*arrow*) is open to demonstrate the dysplastic truncal valve and the bifurcation into the pulmonary artery (PA) and the aorta (AO). The ductus arteriosus is absent and a right aortic arch is noted. The asterisk shows a ventricular septal defect. RV, right ventricle; LV, left ventricle.

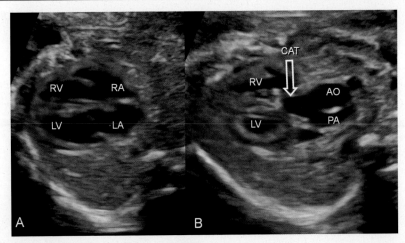

Figure 18-3. These figures represent transverse views of a fetus with common arterial trunk (CAT). **A:** A normal four-chamber view. **B:** The transverse view at the level of the five-chamber view demonstrating a large common trunk (CAT, *arrow*) giving origin to the aorta (AO) and pulmonary artery (PA). RA, right atrium; LA, left atrium; RV, right ventricle; LV, left ventricle.

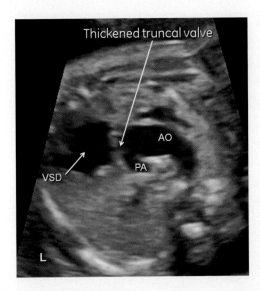

Figure 18-4. Transverse view at the level of the five-chamber view demonstrating the large overriding common arterial trunk bifurcating into the pulmonary artery (PA) and aorta (AO). Note the thickened and dysplastic truncal valve. VSD, ventricular septal defect; L, left.

the diagnosis as it will show a single large vessel, representing the aortic arch, because the ductus arteriosus is not developed in more than 50% of cases (Fig. 18-6) (8). In 70% of the cases, the aortic arch on the three-vessel-trachea view will be to the left of the trachea and in 30% to the right as the right aortic arch. The thymus gland, which is also seen in the three-vessel-trachea view between the transverse aortic arch and the anterior thorax wall, is small or absent in about one third of cases, a sign of a possible association with a 22q11 microdeletion (Fig. 18-6) (10,11).

Color Doppler

Color Doppler may be helpful but is not necessary for the diagnosis of CAT. Color Doppler helps in demonstrating shunting across the VSD and high-velocity flow across the overriding

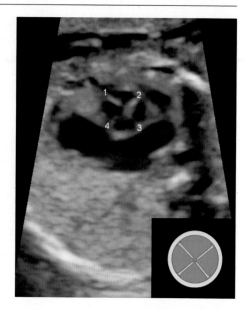

Figure 18-5. Short-axis view of the common truncal valve showing the presence of a quadricuspid (four leaflets) valve (numbered *1* to *4*).

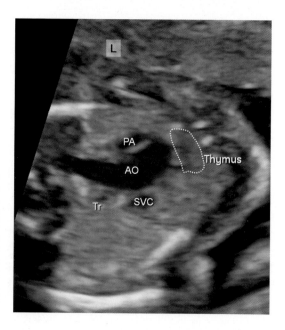

Figure 18-6. The three-vessel-tra-chea view in a fetus with common arterial trunk. Note the small pulmo-nary artery (PA) and the large aortic arch (AO) with no continuity toward the aortic isthmic region (compare to the normal anatomy of the three-ves-sel-trachea view in Chapter 6). A hypoplastic thymus is shown as part of 22q11 microdeletion in this fetus. SVC, superior vena cava; Tr, trachea; L, left.

common arterial trunk with color aliasing (Fig. 18-7). A common and characteristic finding is the demonstration of diastolic valve regurgitation on color Doppler of the dysplastic, and on few occasions stenotic, CAT valves (Fig. 18-8). In CAT types 2 and 3, color Doppler helps to identify the origin and course of the right and left pulmonary arteries.

Early Gestation

The diagnosis of CAT is possible in the late first and early second trimesters of pregnancy (12). Hints for the diagnosis in early gestation, which can be made easier by color Doppler,

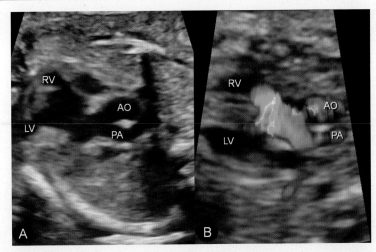

Figure 18-7. Two-dimensional **(A)** and color Doppler **(B)** of a common arterial trunk at the level of the five-chamber view. A shows a large overriding common arterial trunk bifurcating into the pulmonary artery (PA) and aorta (AO). B shows color aliasing at the valve level. RV, right ventricle; LV, left ventricle.

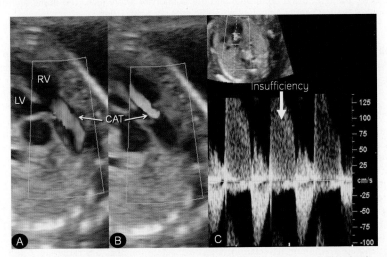

Figure 18-8. Color and spectral Doppler of a common arterial trunk with dysplastic valve. **A:** Flow on color Doppler into the common trunk during systole (*blue*). **B:** Severe regurgitation on color Doppler during diastole (*red*). **C:** Holodiastolic severe insufficiency (regurgitation) on spectral Doppler (*arrow*) with valve stenosis (peak velocity >100 cm/sec). LV, left ventricle; RV, right ventricle; CAT, common arterial trunk.

include a dilated overriding vessel in the five-chamber view and one large vessel in the three-vessel-trachea view (Fig. 18-9). Truncal valve regurgitation (when present) helps in differentiating CAT from other cardiac malformations. The demonstration of the origin of a small main pulmonary trunk is difficult in early gestation (8).

Three-dimensional Ultrasound
Tomographic ultrasound imaging allows for the demonstration of the anatomic characteristics of CAT in different planes concurrently (13). Three-dimensional rendering and reconstruction,

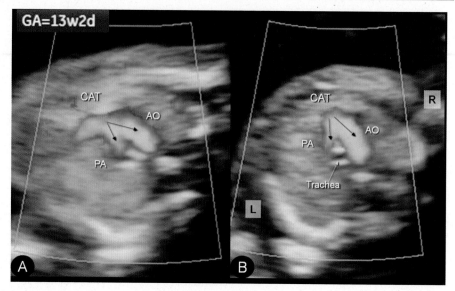

Figure 18-9. A, B: A common arterial trunk (CAT) in a fetus at 13.2 weeks' gestation. The CAT bifurcates to give rise to the aorta (AO) and the pulmonary artery (PA). The aortic arch courses to the right of the trachea as a right-sided aortic arch. R, right; L, left.

especially with power Doppler, inversion mode, or B-flow, has been shown to help in the identification of the CAT with its bifurcations (Figs. 18-10 to 18-12) and the small pulmonary branches in CAT types 2 and 3.

Associated Cardiac and Extracardiac Findings

Associated cardiac malformations are common with CAT. VSD is almost always seen and is part of this cardiac malformation. The ductus arteriosus is absent in 50% of the cases, and when present it remains patent postnatally in about two thirds of patients (14). Aortic arch abnormalities are common with CAT, with right-sided arch noted in 21% to 36% of cases, interrupted arch in about 15% of cases, and rarely hypoplasia of the arch or persistence of double aortic arch (8,14–16). Absence of one of the pulmonary arteries is described in up to 16% in one series, with the pulmonary artery absent on the side of the aortic arch (17). Variations in origins of the coronary arteries are abnormal in more than a third of CAT cases, and this information is relevant for surgical planning (18). Truncal valve dysplasia with incompetence is a common association. Other cardiac anomalies are rather rare and include atrioventricular septal defect, single ventricle, and tricuspid atresia with VSD, among others.

Extracardiac structural malformations are seen in up to 40% of CAT cases and are typically nonspecific (19,20). Chromosomal anomalies are also common and fetal karyotype should be offered when CAT is diagnosed. Numerical chromosomal anomalies are found in about 4.5% of the cases and include trisomies 21, 18, and 13 (21), and 22q11 microdeletion is reported in 30% to 40% of cases (10,11,19,22) (see Table 2-5 in Chapter 2). CAT has been reported in 21% of infants with DiGeorge syndrome (23). CAT and double outlet right ventricle are the two common cardiac abnormalities reported in fetuses of diabetic mothers (7).

Differential Diagnosis

Two cardiac anomalies should be considered in the differential diagnosis of CAT—tetralogy of Fallot and pulmonary atresia with VSD—since both have an associated VSD and an overriding aorta. Color Doppler is helpful for accurate differentiation between these entities in the fetus. The demonstration of a common origin of both the aorta and pulmonary artery from a

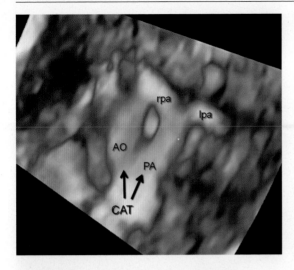

Figure 18-10. Reconstruction plane in power Doppler obtained from a three-dimensional volume in a fetus with common arterial trunk (CAT) type 1 demonstrating the bifurcation of the trunk into the aorta (AO) and the main pulmonary artery (PA). The PA is seen to divide into the right (rpa) and left pulmonary artery (lpa).

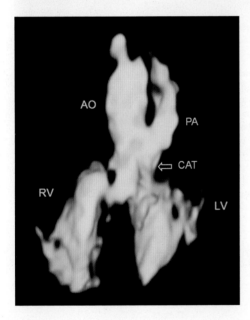

Figure 18-11. Common arterial trunk (CAT, *arrow*) type 1 with its bifurcation into the aorta (AO) and pulmonary artery (PA) is shown in a three-dimensional volume with inversion mode. Compare with Figures 18-1A and 18-2. LV, left ventricle; RV, right ventricle.

large overriding trunk is crucial for the correct diagnosis of CAT. One of the easy signs is the demonstration of a dysplastic valve with insufficiency, typical for CAT but not for tetralogy of Fallot or other conditions (see Table 17-2). Table 18-1 summarizes the main differentiating features between CAT and tetralogy of Fallot, and Tables 17-2 and 17-4 outline other differentiating features. An incorrect diagnosis of CAT for tetralogy of Fallot or pulmonary atresia with VSD is not uncommon (19,24–26).

Prognosis and Outcome

Prenatal follow-up of fetuses with CAT is important, especially when the lesion is complicated by truncal valve stenosis and insufficiency or other intracardiac anomalies given an increased risk for cardiac failure, hydrops, and fetal demise. Data from three series, summarized in

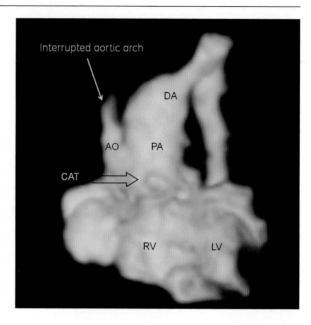

Figure 18-12. Common arterial trunk (CAT, *open arrow*) type A4 with an interrupted aortic arch is shown in three-dimensional volume with inversion mode. Note the bifurcation of the CAT into the pulmonary artery (PA) and aorta (AO). The ductus arteriosus (DA) is present but the ascending aorta is small and interrupted. (The course of the small brachiocephalic vessels is not demonstrated in this image.) Compare with Figure 18-1B. LV, left ventricle; RV, right ventricle.

Table 18-2, involving a total of 86 fetuses with CAT show pregnancy termination in 37% of cases, corrected survival after excluding pregnancy termination and in utero deaths in 58%, and an overall survival rate of 32%, much lower than reported in pediatric studies (8,19,24).

Survival beyond infancy is uncommon in the absence of corrective surgery (2), and neonatal prognosis is related to the presence of associated abnormalities. Complete surgical repair in the first 8 weeks of life is the preferred treatment option. Surgery consists of three parts: closure of the ventricular septal defect, detachment of the pulmonary arteries from the truncal root, and reattachment of the pulmonary arteries to the right ventricle with a conduit. Generally, further surgeries are required to replace the pulmonary artery conduit primarily owing to lack of growth with age. In a recent outcome study involving 50 CAT infants operated on

TABLE 18-1	Differentiating Features of Common Arterial Trunk (CAT) Type 1 and Tetralogy of Fallot (TOF)	
	CAT type 1	**TOF**
Malaligned ventricular septal defect and aortic override	Present	Present
Aortic root size	Markedly dilated	Normal to dilated
Pulmonary trunk	Arising from the common arterial trunk No pulmonary trunk arising from ventricle	Narrow, separately arising from ventricle with patent pulmonary valve
Ductus arteriosus	Absent in 50%	Narrow, antegrade flow
Aortic valve/truncal valve	Valve with one to six leaflets Often dysplastic and insufficient	Normal aortic valve No regurgitation
Chromosomal aberrations	22q11 deletion in 30%–40%, other trisomies in 4%–5%	22q11 deletion in 10%–15%, other trisomies in 30%
Prognosis in postnatal isolated cases	Good Reoperations of pulmonary conduit required	Good to excellent

TABLE 18-2	Outcome in Fetal Series of Common Arterial Trunk

	Compiled data[a]
Number of cases	87
Pregnancy termination (%)	34 (39%)
In utero deaths	4 (4.5%)
Live births	48 (55%)
Neonatal and infant deaths (%)	20 (23%)
Survival in all cases (%)	28 (32%)
Survival in continuing cases (%)	28/52 (53%)
Survival in all liveborns (%)	28/48 (58%)

[a]Data compiled from Sharland GK. Common arterial trunk. In: L Allan, ed. *Textbook of fetal cardiology*. London: Greenwich Medical Media Limited, 2000;288–303; Volpe P, Paladini D, Marasini M, et al. Common arterial trunk in the fetus: characteristics, associations, and outcome in a multicentre series of 23 cases. *Heart* 2003;89(12):1437–1441; and Swanson TM, Selamet Tierney ES, Tworetzky W, et al. Truncus arteriosus: diagnostic accuracy, outcomes, and impact of prenatal diagnosis. *Pediatr Cardiol* 2009;30:256–261.

from 2 days to 6 months of age, an actuarial survival of 96% at 3 years was reported (27). There were no deaths in patients with associated interrupted aortic arch and two deaths in patients with truncal valve regurgitation, neither of whom underwent repair (27). Conduit replacement was done in 17 patients (34%) after a mean duration of 2 years (27). In this study, interrupted aortic arch and truncal valve regurgitation, traditional risk factors for surgical repair (28), had no effect on the overall outcome (27).

KEY POINTS: COMMON ARTERIAL TRUNK

- CAT is characterized by a single arterial trunk that arises from the base of the heart and gives origin to the systemic, coronary, and pulmonary circulations.
- A large ventricular septal defect is almost always present.
- CAT is classified into four types based on the anatomic origin of the pulmonary arteries.
- The CAT root is large and has a biventricular origin in most cases.
- In up to a third of CAT cases, however, the root appears to arise entirely from the right ventricle and in rare cases entirely from the left ventricle.
- The CAT valve has three leaflets (tricuspid) in about 69% of cases, four leaflets (quadricuspid) in 22% of cases, two leaflets (bicuspid) in 9% of cases, and, on very rare occasions, one, five, or more leaflets.
- The two most commonly diagnosed types in the fetus are type 1/type A1 and type A4.
- The four-chamber view appears normal.
- Confirmation of the diagnosis is usually made by identifying the pulmonary trunk (or arteries) directly arising from the overriding large vessel.
- The three-vessel-trachea view shows a single large vessel, representing the aortic arch.
- The ductus arteriosus is absent in 50% of the cases, and when present it remains patent postnatally in about two thirds of patients.
- Aortic arch abnormalities are common, with right-sided arch noted in 21% to 36% of cases, interrupted arch in about 15% of cases, and rarely hypoplasia of the arch or persistence of double aortic arch.
- Extracardiac structural malformations are seen in up to 40% of cases.
- Numerical chromosomal anomalies are found in about 4.5% of cases.
- The 22q11 microdeletion is reported in 30% to 40% of cases.
- Prenatal series show a worse outcome than postnatal reports.

References

1. Van Mierop L, Patterson D, Schnaar W. Pathogenesis of persistent truncus arteriosus in light of observations made in a dog embryo with the anomaly. *Am J Cardiol* 1978;41:755–762.

2. Collett R, Edwards J. Persistent truncus arteriosus: a classification according to anatomic types. *Surg Clin North Am* 1949;1245–1270.
3. Van Praagh R, Van Praagh S. The anatomy of common aorticopulmonary trunk (truncus arteriosus communis) and its embryologic implications: a study of 57 necropsy cases. *Am J Cardiol* 1965;16:406–425.
4. Fuglestad S, Puga F, Danielson G. Surgical pathology of the truncal valve: a study of 12 cases. *Am J Cardiovasc Pathol* 1988;2:39–47.
5. Ferencz C. A case-control study of cardiovascular malformations in liveborn infants: the morphogenetic relevance of epidemiologic findings. In EB Clark, A Takao, eds. *Developmental cardiology: Morphogenesis and function.* Mount Kisco, NY: Futura Publishing, 1990;526.
6. Hoffman JI, Kaplan S. The incidence of congenital heart disease. *Circ Res* 2004;94:1890–1900.
7. Ferencz C, Rubin JD, McCarter RJ, et al. Maternal diabetes and cardiovascular malformations: predominance of double outlet right ventricle and truncus arteriosus. *Teratology* 1990;41:319–326.
8. Sharland GK. Common arterial trunk. In: L Allan, ed. *Textbook of fetal cardiology.* London: Greenwich Medical Media Limited, 2000;288–303.
9. Muhler MR, Rake A, Schwabe M, et al. Truncus arteriosus communis in a midtrimester fetus: comparison of prenatal ultrasound and MRI with postmortem MRI and autopsy. *Eur Radiol* 2004;14(11):2120–2124.
10. Machlitt A, Tennstedt C, Korner H, et al. Prenatal diagnosis of 22q11 microdeletion in an early second-trimester fetus with conotruncal anomaly presenting with increased nuchal translucency and bilateral intracardiac echogenic foci. *Ultrasound Obstet Gynecol* 2002;19(5):510–513.
11. Chaoui R, Kalache KD, Heling KS, et al. Absent or hypoplastic thymus on ultrasound: a marker for deletion 22q11.2 in fetal cardiac defects. *Ultrasound Obstet Gynecol* 2002;20(6):546–552.
12. Achiron R, Weissman A, Rotstein Z, et al. Transvaginal echocardiographic examination of the fetal heart between 13 and 15 weeks' gestation in a low-risk population. *J Ultrasound Med* 1994;13(10):783–789.
13. Paladini D, Vassallo M, Sglavo G, et al. The role of spatio-temporal image· correlation (STIC) with tomographic ultrasound imaging (TUI) in the sequential analysis of fetal congenital heart disease. *Ultrasound Obstet Gynecol* 2006;27(5):555–561.
14. Butto F, Lucas R, Edwards J. Persistent truncus arteriosus: pathologic anatomy in 54 cases. *Pediatr Cardiol* 1986;7:95–101.
15. Marcelleti C, McGoon D, Danielson G. Early and late results of surgical repair of truncus arteriosus. *Circulation* 1977;55:636–641.
16. Nath P, Zollikofer C, Castendeda-Zuniga W. Persistent truncus arteriosus associated with interruption of the aortic arch. *Br J Radiol* 1980;53:853–859.
17. Mair D, Ritter D, Davis G. Selection of patients with truncus arteriosus for surgical correction: anatomic and hemodynamic considerations. *Circulation* 1974;49:144–151.
18. Shrivastava S, Edwards J. Coronary arterial origin in persistent truncus arteriosus. *Circulation* 1977;55:551–554.
19. Volpe P, Paladini D, Marasini M, et al. Common arterial trunk in the fetus: characteristics, associations, and outcome in a multicentre series of 23 cases. *Heart* 2003;89(12):1437–1441.
20. Fyler DC, Buckley LP, Hellenbrand WE, et al. Report of the New England Regional Infant Cardiac Program. *Pediatrics* 1980;65:374–461.
21. Harris JA, Francannet C, Pradat P. The epidemiology of cardiovascular defects, part 2: a study based on data from three large registries of congenital malformations. *Pediatr Cardiol* 2003;24:222–235.
22. Boudjemline Y, Fermont L, Le Bidois J, et al. Prevalence of 22q11 deletion in fetuses with conotruncal cardiac defects: a 6-year prospective study. *J Pediatr* 2001;138:520–524.
23. Van Mierop LH, Kutsche LM. Cardiovascular anomalies in DiGeorge syndrome and importance of neural crest as a possible pathogenetic factor. *Am J Cardiol* 1986;58:133–137.
24. Swanson TM, Selamet Tierney ES, Tworetzky W, et al. Truncus arteriosus: diagnostic accuracy, outcomes, and impact of prenatal diagnosis. *Pediatr Cardiol* 2009;30:256–261.
25. Tometzki AJ, Suda K, Kohl T, et al. Accuracy of prenatal echocardiographic diagnosis and prognosis of fetuses with conotruncal anomalies. *J Am Coll Cardiol* 1999;33(6):1696–1701.
26. Sivanandam S, Glickstein JS, Printz BF, et al. Prenatal diagnosis of conotruncal malformations: diagnostic accuracy, outcome, chromosomal abnormalities, and extracardiac anomalies. *Am J Perinatol* 2006;23(4):241–245.
27. Jahangiri M, Zurakowski D, Mayer JE, et al. Repair of the truncal valve and associated interrupted arch in neonates with truncus arteriosus. *J Thorac Cardiovasc Surg* 2000;119:508–514.
28. Williams JM, de Leeuw M, Black MD, et al. Factors associated with outcomes of persistent truncus arteriosus. *J Am Coll Cardiol* 1999;34:545–553.

DOUBLE OUTLET RIGHT VENTRICLE

Definition, Spectrum of Disease, and Incidence

Double outlet right ventricle (DORV) refers to a heterogeneous group of cardiac anomalies where the aorta and pulmonary artery arise primarily from the morphologic right ventricle (Fig. 19-1). The consensus definition of DORV was made deliberately broad by the Congenital Heart Surgery Nomenclature and Database Project, which stated that "DORV is a type of ventriculoarterial connection in which both great vessels arise either entirely or predominantly from the right ventricle" (1). DORV therefore encompasses a family of complex cardiac malformations where both great arteries arise primarily from the morphologic right ventricle but differ with regard to the variable spatial relationship of the great arteries, the location of the ventricular septal defect that is commonly seen with DORV, and the presence or absence of pulmonary and less commonly aortic outflow obstruction. In DORV, four types of anatomic relationships of the aorta to the pulmonary artery at the level of the semilunar valves have been described (2) and include a right posterior aorta, a right anterior aorta, a left anterior aorta, and a right lateral aorta (Table 19-1). The ventricular septal defect (VSD) that is commonly associated with DORV has been described in four anatomic locations: subaortic type; subpulmonary type; subaortic and subpulmonary type (also called doubly committed); and remote type, nonrelated to both arteries (Table 19-2). The exact subtype of DORV may be hard to characterize prenatally as the position of the VSD is difficult to establish with accuracy in fetal echocardiography.

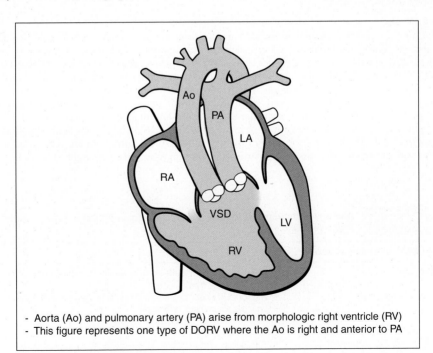

- Aorta (Ao) and pulmonary artery (PA) arise from morphologic right ventricle (RV)
- This figure represents one type of DORV where the Ao is right and anterior to PA

Figure 19-1. Double outlet right ventricle (DORV). LV, left ventricle; LA, left atrium; RA, right atrium; VSD, ventricular septal defect.

TABLE 19-1	Anatomic Relationships of the Great Arteries at the Semilunar Valves in Double Outlet Right Ventricle (DORV)

Relationships of great arteries in DORV	Description
Right posterior aorta to the pulmonary artery (tetralogy of Fallot-type DORV) Right anterior aorta to the pulmonary artery (D-transposition-type DORV)	• Rare form of DORV • Normal relationship of great arteries • Second most common type of DORV • VSD either subaortic or subpulmonary • Subgroup called Taussig-Bing form of DORV
Left anterior aorta to the pulmonary artery (L-transposition-type DORV)	• Rare form of DORV • Left course of the aorta in the thorax • VSD either subaortic or subpulmonary
Right lateral aorta to the pulmonary artery (side by side)	• Most common form of DORV • Aorta to the right of pulmonary artery • Subaortic-type VSD is most common
VSD, ventricular septal defect.	

DORV occurs in about 1% to 1.5% of children born with congenital heart disease and has an incidence of approximately 0.09 per 1000 live births (3). It is found equally in boys and girls. DORV is more common in fetal series and has been reported in up to 6% of congenital heart disease (4). In fetal series, DORV is reported either as a separate entity or within the group of conotruncal anomalies (4–11). The prevalence of DORV is increased in diabetic pregnancies (12). Figures 19-2 and 19-3 represent anatomic specimens of two types of DORV in fetal hearts.

Ultrasound Findings

Gray Scale
The aims of two-dimensional ultrasound in the diagnosis of DORV include detecting the abnormal ventriculoarterial connections, defining the anatomic relationship of the great vessels, and, if possible, describing the location of the VSD when present. The four-chamber view in DORV is usually normal in the first and second trimesters. The left ventricle may become diminutive with advancing gestation, which may result in an abnormal four-chamber view later in pregnancy. DORV is occasionally associated with abnormalities of the atrioventricular valves (e.g., mitral atresia, atrioventricular septal defect, and double inlet ventricle), and when present may lead to an abnormal four-chamber view. The five-chamber view is abnormal as it shows the VSD, the lack of continuity of the medial wall of the aorta with the ventricular septum, and the origin of both great arteries from the anterior chamber (right ventricle). The

TABLE 19-2	Anatomic Positions of Ventricular Septal Defects (VSDs) in Double Outlet Right Ventricle

Anatomic positions of VSD	Description
Subaortic type	• VSD located closer to the aortic valve than the pulmonary valve • Most common type
Subpulmonary type	• VSD located closer to the pulmonary valve than the aortic valve • Typically supracristal in location • Second most common type
Subaortic and subpulmonary type (doubly committed)	• Large VSD • VSD closely related to both semilunar valves • Rare type
Remote type (nonrelated)	• VSD is distant from and nonrelated to both semilunar valves

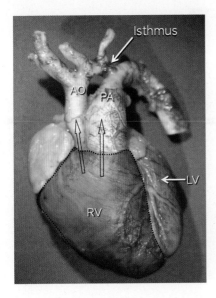

Figure 19-2. Anatomic specimen of a fetus with double outlet right ventricle. Both great arteries arise from the right ventricle (RV) (*arrows*). The aorta (AO) is on the right side to the main pulmonary artery (PA), in side-by-side position. The AO is narrow, with a small isthmus representing aortic coarctation. The left ventricle (LV) is smaller than the RV (*dashed area*).

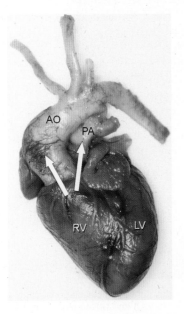

Figure 19-3. Anatomic specimen of a fetus with double outlet right ventricle with pulmonary atresia. Both great arteries arise from the right ventricle (RV) (*arrows*). The aorta (AO) is anterior and to the right of the pulmonary artery (PA) in D-malposition. The dilated aorta and the very small pulmonary artery are compatible with the diagnosis of pulmonary atresia. LV, left ventricle.

location and position of the VSD in relation to the great arteries should be described if possible. By angling the transducer between the five-chamber view and the three-vessel-trachea view, the parallel arrangement of the great vessels is demonstrated (Fig. 19-4). Even when the aorta is in a right posterior position to the pulmonary artery (see Table 19-1), the great vessels still assume a parallel course to each other (11,13). The presence of outflow tract obstruction in DORV is best assessed by size discrepancy of the great vessels rather than Doppler flow measurements (Fig. 19-5). Pulmonary artery atresia or stenosis is more common than aortic atresia or aortic coarctation in DORV (Fig. 19-5). Right-sided aortic arch may be present and can be detected on the three-vessel-trachea view. In some DORV types, the malposition of the

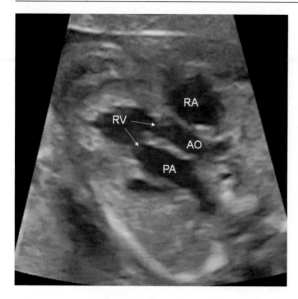

Figure 19-4. Double outlet right ventricle demonstrated in an oblique plane between the five-chamber view and three-vessel view. The aorta (AO) and pulmonary artery (PA) are shown to arise from the right ventricle (RV) (*arrows*) in a side-by-side position with the AO to the right of the PA. Note that the AO and PA are of normal size. RA, right atrium.

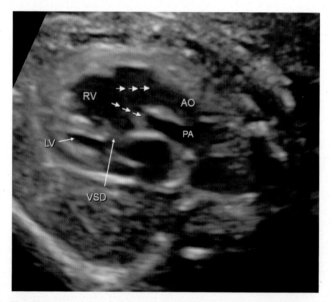

Figure 19-5. Five-chamber view of a fetus with double outlet right ventricle demonstrating a small left ventricle (LV), a dilated right ventricle (RV), both aorta (AO) and pulmonary artery (PA) arising from the RV (*arrows*), and a ventricular septal defect (VSD) in a subpulmonic location. Note that the PA is narrower than the aorta, a sign of pulmonary stenosis.

great arteries results in a single vessel imaged at the three-vessel-trachea view, typically the aorta. Turning the transducer to get an oblique view allows the demonstration of both vessels arising from the right ventricle with the pulmonary artery coursing under the aorta.

Color Doppler

Color Doppler helps in demonstrating unidirectional shunting across the VSD from the left to the right ventricle and in visualizing blood flow from the right ventricle into both the aorta

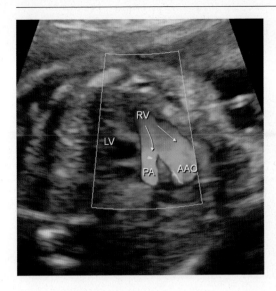

Figure 19-6. Color Doppler in an oblique view of the chest in a fetus with double outlet right ventricle. On two-dimensional ultrasound, the suspected cardiac malformation was transposition of great vessels, ventricular septal defect, and pulmonary stenosis. Color Doppler clearly demonstrates the origin of both great vessels from the right ventricle (RV) (*arrows*). The pulmonary artery (PA) appears narrower than the ascending aorta (AAO) with no color turbulence, a sign of mild pulmonary stenosis, LV, left ventricle.

and the pulmonary artery (Fig. 19-6). Color Doppler can also help demonstrate the presence of outflow stenosis or atresia by showing turbulent (Fig. 19-7) or reverse flow in the corresponding vessel. The anatomic relationship of the great arteries can also be better defined by color Doppler.

Early Gestation

DORV can be diagnosed in early gestation (11 to 14 weeks) in the presence of an abnormal four-chamber view or an abnormal three-vessel-trachea view with discrepant vessel size. A thickened nuchal translucency may lead to a more comprehensive anatomic evaluation of the fetus where DORV with associated extracardiac abnormalities may be found. DORV, however, is difficult to diagnose in early gestation when isolated or when the four-chamber view appears normal. Figure 19-8 demonstrates DORV in a fetus at 14 weeks' gestation.

Three-dimensional Ultrasound

Three-dimensional ultrasound can be used with tomography imaging to demonstrate various DORV findings in one display (14). Three-dimensional (3-D) rendering, using surface, minimum (transparent), inversion, or color mode, can demonstrate the type of spatial arrangements of the great arteries (Figs. 19-9 and 19-10). Longitudinal volume calculation of the left ventricle during pregnancy may be an interesting application. Three-dimensional imaging may help in better defining the anatomic relationship of the VSD to the great arteries in the future.

Associated Cardiac and Extracardiac Findings

Associated cardiac findings are common and include a full spectrum of cardiac lesions. Pulmonary stenosis is the most common associated malformation and occurs in about 70% of cases (15). Various cardiac malformations at the level of the atrioventricular valves, atrial and ventricular septae, and great vessels have been reported with DORV including mitral atresia, a cleft anterior mitral leaflet, atrial septal defects, atrioventricular septal defects, subaortic stenosis, aortic coarctation, right aortic arch, persistent left superior vena cava, and anomalous pulmonary venous return, among others. Varying degrees of left ventricular hypoplasia are present primarily based on the level of left ventricular obstruction. DORV can be part of left or right isomerism, and this combination increases the likelihood of associated venous anomalies (16). In isomerism, DORV may be combined with an unbalanced atrioventricular septal defect or with a double inlet single ventricle with commonly associated pulmonary obstruction. DORV can be also found in complex corrected transposition, where the right ventricle is left-sided.

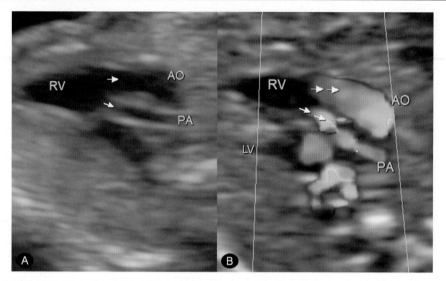

Figure 19-7. Two-dimensional **(A)** and color Doppler **(B)** ultrasound in a fetus with double out-let right ventricle and critical pulmonary stenosis. On two-dimensional ultrasound (A), both great vessels are shown to arise from the right ventricle (RV) with the aorta (AO) to the right and ante-rior to the hypoplastic pulmonary artery (PA). On color Doppler (B), forward flow is demonstrated in the AO and PA with turbulent flow across the hypoplastic PA, a sign of severe PA stenosis; LV, left ventricle.

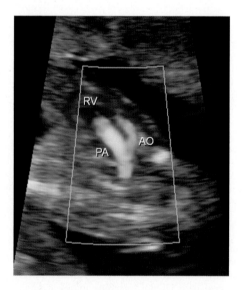

Figure 19-8. Double outlet right ventricle in a fetus at 14 weeks' gestation demonstrated with color Doppler. The aorta (AO) and pulmo-nary artery (PA) are both seen to arise from the right ventricle (RV).

Extracardiac anomalies are very common in fetuses with DORV and are nonspecific for organ systems (17). Chromosomal abnormalities are frequently found in the range of 12% to 40% in fetuses with DORV and primarily include trisomies 18 and 13 and 22q11 deletion (4,18,19). The association of DORV with anomalies of the atrioventricular valves increases the risk for numerical chromosomal abnormalities, and the association of DORV with a cono-truncal anomaly increases the risk for the 22q11 deletion. The association of DORV with iso-merism practically excludes the presence of chromosomal abnormalities (18).

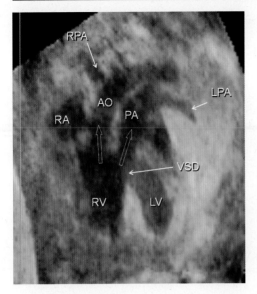

Figure 19-9. Three-dimensional ultrasound in minimum transparent mode in a fetus with double outlet right ventricle (anatomic specimen of this fetus shown in Fig. 19-2). Both the aorta (AO) and pulmonary arteries (PA) are shown to arise from the right ventricle (RV) in a side-by-side orientation. The ventricular septal defect (VSD) is subpulmonic, and it connects the small left ventricle (LV) with the dilated RV. The bifurcation of the PA into the right (RPA) and left pulmonary arteries (LPA) is also seen. RA, right atrium.

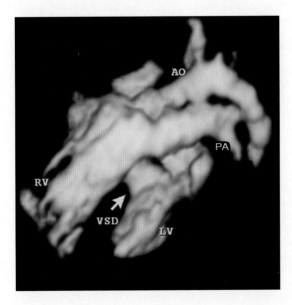

Figure 19-10. Three-dimensional ultrasound in inversion mode in a fetus with double outlet right ventricle demonstrating both aorta (AO) and pulmonary arteries (PA) arising from the right ventricle (RV) in a side-by-side orientation. The lumens of the left (LV) and right ventricles are connected with the ventricular septal defect (VSD) (*arrow*).

Differential Diagnosis

Tetralogy of Fallot and transposition of the great arteries are the two main differential diagnoses for DORV. The prognosis and surgical approach, however, are more dependent on the anatomic description of the lesion rather than its exact terminology or classification. Common arterial trunk is also part of the differential diagnosis, especially when DORV is associated with hypoplasia of one of the outflow tracts. Since the great vessels appear parallel in most DORV cases, transposition of the great arteries is the most common referral diagnosis for fetuses with DORV (13).

TABLE 19-3	Cardiac Anatomic Findings in Double Outlet Right Ventricle and Their Impact on Prognosis	
Cardiac findings	Good prognosis	Poor prognosis
Aortic arch	Normal-sized aortic arch	Tubular aortic arch hypoplasia
Pulmonary artery	Patent pulmonary artery	Pulmonary atresia
Ventricle	Normal-sized ventricles	Hypoplastic left ventricle
		Single ventricle anatomy
Atrioventricular valve anatomy	Normal formed atrioventricular valves	Mitral atresia
		Atrioventricular septal defect
Situs	Normal situs	Situs ambiguous

The authors prefer to use the term *malposition* of the great vessels rather than transposition when complex anomalies are found in combination with parallel orientation of the great arteries.

Prognosis and Outcome

The intrauterine course of a fetus with DORV is usually uneventful, unless it is complicated by atrioventricular valve insufficiency or left isomerism with heart block, which may lead to cardiac failure, hydrops, and in utero demise. The overall prognosis for fetuses with DORV is generally poor, not only related to the primary lesion but also depending on the associated abnormalities (17). Pregnancy termination is reported between 31% and 55% in prenatal series, and survival is reported in 30% to 60% of fetuses (11,17). An overall survival rate of 10% is reported in one fetal series when pregnancy termination and follow-up beyond the neonatal period are included (17). This poor prognosis is related to the associated extracardiac and chromosomal abnormalities and isomerism, commonly found prenatally (17). Table 19-3 lists cardiac abnormalities commonly associated with poor prognosis in fetuses with DORV.

Significant improvement in survival has been reported for DORV neonates operated on recently due to refinement in surgical techniques and postsurgical management. Recent data suggest a surgical mortality of 4% to 8% for repair in the neonatal period (20), and long-term follow-up exceeding 90% has been reported for DORV with subaortic VSD (21). Overall neonatal prognosis, however, is dependent on associated cardiac and extracardiac abnormalities.

■ KEY POINTS: DOUBLE OUTLET RIGHT VENTRICLE

- DORV is a type of ventriculoarterial connection in which both great vessels arise either entirely or predominantly from the right ventricle.
- Several types exist, differing with regard to the spatial relationship of the great arteries, the location of the ventricular septal defect, and the presence or absence of outflow obstruction.
- Four types of spatial relationships of the aorta to the pulmonary artery and four anatomic locations for ventricular septal defects in DORV have been described.
- The four-chamber view is usually normal in the first and second trimesters.
- The five-chamber view is abnormal, as it shows the ventricular septal defect and the origin of both great arteries from the anterior chamber (right ventricle).
- The presence of outflow tract obstruction in DORV is best assessed by size discrepancy of the great vessels rather than Doppler flow measurements.
- Associated cardiac findings are common and include a full spectrum of cardiac lesions, including right and left isomerism.
- Pulmonary stenosis is the most common associated malformation and occurs in about 70% of cases.
- Chromosomal abnormalities are frequently found in the range of 12% to 40% in fetuses with DORV and primarily include trisomies 18 and 13 and 22q11 deletion.
- Tetralogy of Fallot and transposition of the great arteries are the two main differential diagnoses for DORV.
- The overall prognosis for fetuses with DORV is generally poor.
- Neonatal outcome has significantly improved in recent series.

References

1. Walters HL, Mavroudis C, Tchervenkov CI, et al. Congenital Heart Surgery Nomenclature and Database Project: double outlet right ventricle. *Ann Thorac Surg* 2000;69:249–263.
2. Sridaromont S, Feldt RH, Ritter DG, et al. Double-outlet right ventricle: hemodynamic and anatomic correlations. *Am J Cardiol* 1976;38:85–94.
3. Mitchell SC, Korones SB, Berendes HW. Congenital heart disease in 56,109 births: incidence and natural history. *Circulation* 1971;43:323–332.
4. Allan LD, Sharland GK, Milburn A, et al. Prospective diagnosis of 1,006 consecutive cases of congenital heart disease in the fetus. *J Am Coll Cardiol* 1994;23(6):1452–1458.
5. Paladini D, Rustico M, Todros T, et al. Conotruncal anomalies in prenatal life. *Ultrasound Obstet Gynecol* 1996;8(4):241–246.
6. Tometzki AJ, Suda K, Kohl T, et al. Accuracy of prenatal echocardiographic diagnosis and prognosis of fetuses with conotruncal anomalies. *J Am Coll Cardiol* 1999;33(6):1696–1701.
7. Chaoui R, Kalache KD, Heling KS, et al. Absent or hypoplastic thymus on ultrasound: a marker for deletion 22q11.2 in fetal cardiac defects. *Ultrasound Obstet Gynecol* 2002;20(6):546–552.
8. Kim N, Friedberg MK, Silverman NH. Diagnosis and prognosis of fetuses with double outlet right ventricle. *Prenat Diagn* 2006;26(8):740–745.
9. Sivanandam S, Glickstein JS, Printz BF, et al. Prenatal diagnosis of conotruncal malformations: diagnostic accuracy, outcome, chromosomal abnormalities, and extracardiac anomalies. *Am J Perinatol* 2006;23(4):241–245.
10. Smith RS, Comstock CH, Kirk JS, et al. Double-outlet right ventricle: an antenatal diagnostic dilemma. *Ultrasound Obstet Gynecol* 1999;14(5):315–319.
11. Hornberger L. Double outlet right ventricle. In: L Allan, L Hornberger, G Sharland, eds. *Textbook of fetal cardiology.* London: Greenwich Medical Media, 2000;274–287.
12. Ferencz C, Rubin JD, McCarter RJ, et al. Maternal diabetes and cardiovascular malformations: predominance of double outlet right ventricle and truncus arteriosus. *Teratology* 1990;41:319–326.
13. Allan LD. Sonographic detection of parallel great arteries in the fetus. *AJR Am J Roentgenol* 1997;168(5):1283–1286.
14. Paladini D, Vassallo M, Sglavo G, et al. The role of spatio-temporal image correlation (STIC) with tomographic ultrasound imaging (TUI) in the sequential analysis of fetal congenital heart disease. *Ultrasound Obstet Gynecol* 2006;27(5):555–561.
15. Bradley TJ, Karamlou T, Kulik A, et al. Determinants of repair type, reintervention and mortality in 393 children with double-outlet right ventricle. *J Thorac Cardiovasc Surg* 2007;134:967–973.
16. Berg C, Geipel A, Kamil D, et al. The syndrome of right isomerism—prenatal diagnosis and outcome. *Ultraschall Med* 2006;27(3):225–233.
17. Gedikbasi A, Oztarhan K, Gul A, et al. Diagnosis and prognosis in double-outlet right ventricle. *Am J Perinatol* 2008;25(7):427–434.
18. Obler D, Juraszek AL, Smoot LB, et al. Double outlet right ventricle: aetiologies and associations. *J Med Genet* 2008;45(8):481–497.
19. Chaoui R, Korner H, Bommer C, et al. [Prenatal diagnosis of heart defects and associated chromosomal aberrations]. *Ultraschall Med* 1999;20(5):177–184.
20. Allen HD, Driscoll DJ, Shaddy RE, et al., eds. *Moss and Adams' heart disease in infants, children and adolescents.* Baltimore, MD: Williams & Wilkins, 1995;1119–1120.
21. Kirklin JW, Pacifico AD, Blackstone EH, et al. Current risks and protocols for operations for double-outlet right ventricle. *J Thorac Cardiovasc Surg* 1986;92:913–993.

COMPLETE TRANSPOSITION OF THE GREAT ARTERIES

Definition, Spectrum of Disease, and Incidence

Complete transposition of the great arteries (TGA) is a common cardiac malformation, with atrioventricular concordance and ventriculoarterial discordance. This implies a normal connection between the atria and ventricles; the right atrium is connected to the right ventricle through the tricuspid valve and the left atrium is connected to the left ventricle through the mitral valve, but there is a switched connection of the great vessels, the pulmonary artery arising from the left ventricle and the aorta arising from the right ventricle. Both great arteries display a parallel course, with the aorta anterior and to the right of the pulmonary artery (Fig. 20-1), hence the term D-TGA (D = "dexter"). D-TGA is a relatively frequent cardiac anomaly occurring in 5% to 7% of all congenital cardiac malformations, with an incidence of 0.315 cases per 1000 live births and a 2:1 male preponderance (1,2). D-TGA can be an isolated cardiac malformation, termed simple D-TGA, or complex, when associated with other cardiac anomalies. Ventricular septal defects and pulmonary stenosis (left ventricular tract outflow obstruction) are common associations with D-TGA and may be present either alone or in combination in up to 30% to 40% of cases (3,4). Associated extracardiac malformations are rare.

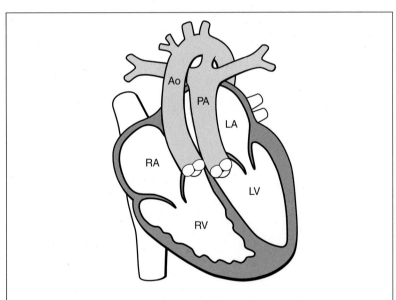

- Normal four-chamber anatomy, with atrioventricular concordance
- Aorta (Ao) arising from the right ventricle (RV)
- Pulmonary artery (PA) arising from the left ventricle (LV)
- Parallel course of great vessels with aorta anteriorly and to the right of the pulmonary artery

Figure 20-1. Complete transposition of the great arteries (D-TGA). RA, right atrium; LA, left atrium.

Prenatal diagnosis of D-TGA is still a challenge. Prenatal screening policy for congenital heart disease, which primarily focuses on the four-chamber view alone, will undoubtedly fail in detecting TGA. Prenatal screening for congenital heart disease at a population level reports detection rates of 3% to 17% for simple TGA (5–7). The detection rate of TGA increased from 12.5% to 72.5% during a period of rapid progress and increased access to prenatal diagnosis in a population-based study (8). Given an associated decrease in neonatal morbidity and mortality in prenatally detected TGA, assessment of the great vessels as part of the extended basic cardiac examination of the fetus should be performed when feasibly achievable (8–10). Figure 20-2 shows an anatomic fetal specimen of a heart with TGA.

Ultrasound Findings

Gray Scale

The four-chamber view is typically normal in fetuses with D-TGA (Fig. 20-3A), except for an associated ventricular septal defect. Visualization of the five-chamber view will show the pulmonary artery arising from the left ventricle and bifurcating, shortly after its origin, into two branches: right and left pulmonary arteries (Fig. 20-3B). The aorta is noted to arise from the right ventricle in an anterior and parallel course to the pulmonary artery. This parallel orientation of the great arteries in D-TGA is best obtained in an oblique plane of the heart, spatially oriented from the right shoulder to the left hip of the fetus (Fig. 20-4A,B). A transverse view in the upper thorax will show, instead of the three-vessel-trachea view in most cases, a single large vessel (the transverse aortic arch) with a superior vena cava to its right (Fig. 20-5A,B). The large vessel noted in the three-vessel-trachea view is the aorta, which is positioned anteriorly and superiorly to the pulmonary artery. The short-axis view at the level of the great vessels shows both the aorta and pulmonary artery as circular structures adjacent to each other (Fig. 20-6B) instead of their normal orientation (longitudinal pulmonary artery wrapping around a circular aorta) (Fig. 20-6A). On longitudinal views, the aortic arch is seen arising from the anterior right ventricle, giving rise to head and neck vessels and assuming a

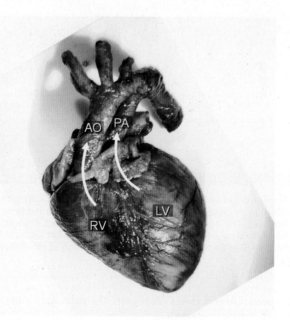

Figure 20-2. Anatomic specimen of a fetal heart with D-transposition of the great arteries. Note the aorta (AO) arising from the right ventricle (RV), anterior and parallel to the pulmonary artery (PA), which arises from the left ventricle (LV). Compare with an anatomic specimen of a normal heart in Figure 4-4.

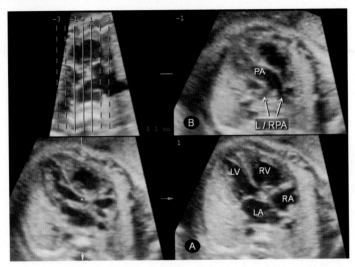

Figure 20-3. The four-chamber view **(A)** appears normal with atrioventricular concordance in a fetus with transposition of great arteries. The five-chamber view **(B)** demonstrates the pulmonary artery (PA) arising from the posterior (left) ventricle. Note the bifurcation of the pulmonary artery into the left and right pulmonary arteries (L/RPA). These images were obtained from a three-dimensional volume. RV, right ventricle; LA, left atrium; RA, right atrium; LV, left ventricle.

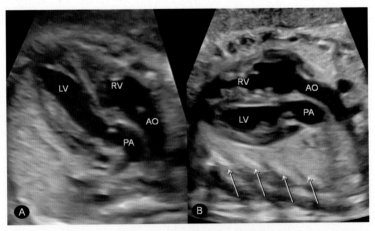

Figure 20-4. Parallel origin of the great vessels in two fetuses **(A,B)** with transposition of the great arteries shown in an oblique plane of the heart, spatially oriented from the right shoulder to the left hip of the fetus. The aorta (AO) arises more anteriorly from the right ventricle (RV) and is to the right of the pulmonary artery (PA), which arises from the left ventricle (LV). The oblique orientation of these planes is demonstrated by the cross section of ribs (*arrows*) in the outer perimeter of the chest.

"hockey stick" orientation as it curves posteriorly. The pulmonary artery assumes the "candy cane" orientation in longitudinal views.

Color Doppler
Color Doppler can be helpful in diagnosing D-TGA but is not necessary (11). Color Doppler helps in demonstrating the parallel course of the great vessels (Fig. 20-7). Visualization of an

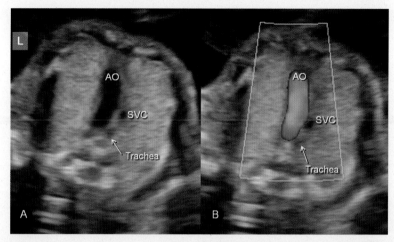

Figure 20-5. The three-vessel-trachea view in gray scale **(A)** and color Doppler **(B)** in a fetus with transposition of the great arteries demonstrating the aorta (AO) as a single large vessel with the superior vena cava (SVC) to its right. Color Doppler in B confirms antegrade flow in the AO. The pulmonary artery is generally located in an inferior position to the AO and thus is not visible in the three-vessel-trachea view. L, left.

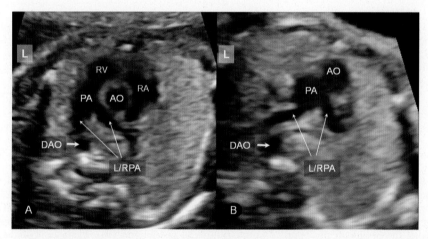

Figure 20-6. Short-axis views in a normal fetus **(A)** and in a fetus with complete transposition of the great arteries (TGA) **(B)**. In the normal fetus (A), the short-axis view shows a longitudinal view of the pulmonary artery (PA) wrapping around a cross section of the aorta (AO). The AO is inferior to the PA, which bifurcates into the left and right pulmonary arteries (L/RPA). In the fetus with TGA (B), both great vessels are seen in a cross-sectional orientation with the AO anterior to the PA. DAO, descending aorta; RV, right ventricle; RA, right atrium; L, left.

associated ventricular septal defect (Fig. 20-7B), confirming patency of the foramen ovale and assessing left ventricular outflow (pulmonary artery), can be enhanced by color Doppler. In early gestation, color Doppler can help in demonstrating the crossing of the great vessels in normal conditions or their parallel course in D-TGA.

Early Gestation
D-TGA can be diagnosed at the 11- to 14-week ultrasound, but its recognition is more difficult than in the second trimester, as reported in one series of targeted fetal echocardiography

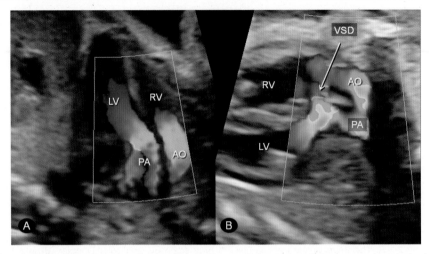

Figure 20-7. Color Doppler demonstrating the parallel course of the great vessels in two fetuses **(A, B)** with transposition of the great arteries shown in an oblique plane of the chest. In B, color Doppler helps in confirming the presence of a ventricular septal defect (VSD) (*arrow*). RV, right ventricle; LV, left ventricle; AO, aorta; PA, pulmonary artery.

at 11 to 14 weeks where D-TGA was missed in most cases (12). An enlarged nuchal translucency in the setting of normal fetal chromosomes can be a marker for the presence of D-TGA (13). The three-vessel-trachea view, with its finding of a single great vessel, may be helpful in early gestation (Fig. 20-8A). By rotating the transducer to view an oblique plane of the chest, the parallel course of the vessels can be demonstrated (Fig. 20-8B).

Three-dimensional Ultrasound

Various reports, focusing on rotations along different axes and color display of rendered volumes, emphasize the role of three-dimensional ultrasound in the diagnosis of D-TGA (14–17). Tomographic ultrasound imaging (Fig. 20-9), glass body mode (Fig. 20-10), inversion mode (Fig. 20-11A), B flow (Fig. 20-11B), and other three-dimensional–rendered displays have the ability to enhance visualization of the spatial relationship of the great vessels as they arise from their respective cardiac chambers. The use of the reconstructed *en face* view with color Doppler imaging of the four cardiac valves in three-dimensional volumes of fetuses with TGA can demonstrate the different types of spatial relationships of the arterial trunks, which may predict the likelihood of abnormal coronary arterial distribution (18). Evaluation of three-dimensional–automated software on volumes of fetuses with TGA demonstrated the abnormality in ventricular-arterial connections in all fetuses (19).

Associated Cardiac and Extracardiac Findings

Ventricular septal defects (VSDs) and pulmonary stenosis (left ventricular outflow obstruction) are the two most common associated cardiac findings in D-TGA. VSDs are common and occur in about 40% of cases and are typically perimembranous but can be located anywhere in the septum (20). Pulmonary stenosis coexists with a VSD in D-TGA patients in about 30% of cases, and the stenosis is usually more severe and complex than in D-TGA with intact ventricular septum (20). Abnormal course and bifurcation of coronary arteries are found in patients with a D-TGA, and its prevalence is more than 50% when the great vessels are side by side or when the aorta is posterior and to the right of the pulmonary artery (21,22). Other associated cardiac anomalies are rare and can involve the atrioventricular valves, the aortic arch, and great vessels.

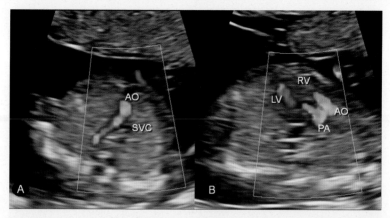

Figure 20-8. Color Doppler ultrasound at the three-vessel-trachea view **(A)** and an oblique view of the chest **(B)** at 14 weeks' gestation in a fetus with transposition of the great arteries (TGA). The three-vessel-trachea view (A) demonstrates a single large vessel (aorta, AO), which gives a clue to the presence of TGA. TGA is then confirmed in the oblique view of the chest (B) by demonstrating the parallel course of the great vessels. PA-, pulmonary artery; SVC, superior vena cava; LV, left ventricle; RV, right ventricle.

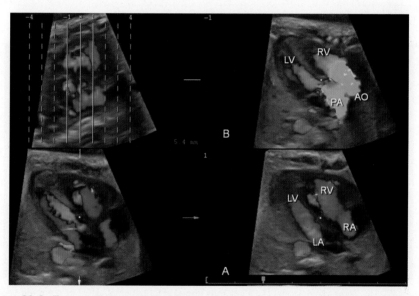

Figure 20-9. Tomographic mode display of a three-dimensional color spatio-temporal image correlation (STIC) volume showing the normal four-chamber appearance **(A)** and the typical parallel course of the great arteries **(B)** in a fetus with transposition of the great arteries. RV, right ventricle; LV, left ventricle; RA, right atrium; LA, left atrium; AO, aorta; PA, pulmonary artery.

Extracardiac anomalies may be present, but rare and numerical chromosomal aberrations are practically absent in D-TGA. Microdeletion of 22q11 could be present and should be ruled out, especially when extracardiac malformations or a complex D-TGA is present. Situs abnormalities can be present, such as abdominal situs inversus, and depending on the venoatrial connection, a balanced circulation may be found. Among the few associated extracardiac anomalies in D-TGA, the authors report one ear anomaly, one cleft lip, and one wide cleft lip and palate.

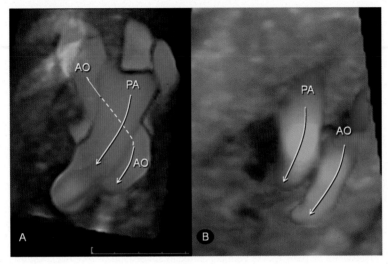

Figure 20-10. Glass body mode rendering of a cranial view of the great vessels in a normal fetus **(A)** and in a fetus with a transposition of the great arteries **(B).** The normal and parallel crossing of the great vessels are demonstrated in A and B, respectively. AO, aorta; PA, pulmonary artery.

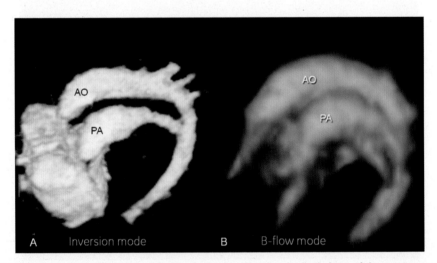

Figure 20-11. Three-dimensional (3-D) volumes showing longitudinal views of the great vessels from the left side in two fetuses with complete transposition of the great vessels. **Plane A** is obtained from a 3-D static volume rendered in inversion mode, and **plane B** is obtained from a B-flow spatio-temporal image correlation (STIC) volume. Both planes (A and B) demonstrate the parallel course of the great vessels very clearly. PA, pulmonary artery; AO, aorta.

Differential Diagnosis

Double outlet right ventricle and corrected TGA are the two most common cardiac anomalies in the differential diagnosis of D-TGA as they all share the absence of "cross-over" of the great vessels. Differentiating D-TGA from congenitally corrected TGA is explained in the next section.

False-positive diagnosis of TGA may occur at the level of the three-vessel-trachea view if the novice examiner assumes a parallel course of the vessels as they are imaged side by side at this level. The display of a parallel course of the great vessels in the diagnosis of TGA should include the ventricles, the semilunar valves, and the ventricular septum separating the great vessels.

Prognosis and Outcome

D-TGA is well tolerated in utero. Prenatal follow-up examination with color Doppler should focus on the presence or absence of a VSD and on the subsequent development of pulmonary stenosis, which is not commonly detected in the second trimester. Furthermore, flow assessment with color and spectral Doppler, at the level of the foramen ovale and ductus arteriosus, should be given close attention closer to term. Premature closure or narrowing of the foramen ovale and/or the ductus arteriosus is associated with worsening neonatal outcome and may require emergency postnatal procedures (23,24).

Prognosis of a neonate with D-TGA is excellent provided the child is born at a tertiary institution with pediatric cardiology intensive services (6,9). Prenatal detection of D-TGA and/or neonatal treatment before cyanosis appears to improve outcome (6,9). The effect of prenatal diagnosis on the outcome of D-TGA is still controversial, however, and recent studies did not find an enhanced outcome with prenatal diagnosis (25,26).

Prostaglandin infusion to maintain patency of the ductus arteriosus and a balloon atrial septostomy is usually required in order to enhance oxygenation and preparation for corrective surgery. An emergency balloon septostomy may be required within hours after birth in some cases of obstructed foramen flow, hence the importance of delivery at a center equipped to perform these procedures (9,23,24). Corrective surgery currently involves an arterial switch operation, where the aorta and pulmonary artery are transacted above the semilunar valves and switched with reimplantation of the coronary circulation.

▉ KEY POINTS: COMPLETE TRANSPOSITION OF GREAT ARTERIES

- ▪ There is atrioventricular concordance and ventriculoarterial discordance in D-TGA.
- ▪ Both great arteries display a parallel course, with the aorta more commonly anterior and to the right of the pulmonary artery.
- ▪ The four-chamber view is typically normal in fetuses with D-TGA, except for an associated ventricular septal defect.
- ▪ Visualization of the five-chamber view will show the pulmonary artery arising from the left ventricle and bifurcating, shortly after its origin, into two branches: right and left pulmonary arteries.
- ▪ The three-vessel-trachea view will demonstrate, in most cases, a single large vessel (aorta) with a superior vena cava to its right.
- ▪ The short-axis view at the level of the great vessels shows both the aorta and pulmonary artery as circular structures adjacent to each other.
- ▪ Ventricular septal defects and pulmonary stenosis are the two most common associated cardiac findings.
- ▪ Ventricular septal defects occur in about 40% of cases and are typically perimembranous.
- ▪ Pulmonary stenosis coexists with a ventricular septal defect in about 30% of cases.
- ▪ Extracardiac anomalies may be present, but rare and numerical chromosomal aberrations are practically absent.
- ▪ Premature closure or narrowing of the foramen ovale and/or the ductus arteriosus is associated with worsening neonatal outcome and may require emergency postnatal procedures.
- ▪ Prognosis is excellent when detected prenatally and the child is born at a tertiary center.

CONGENITALLY CORRECTED TRANSPOSITION OF THE GREAT ARTERIES

Definition, Spectrum of Disease, and Incidence

Congenitally corrected transposition of the great arteries (cc-TGA), previously called l-TGA for levo-TGA, is a rare cardiac anomaly characterized by atrioventricular and ventriculoarterial discordance. In this condition the morphologic right atrium is connected to the morphologic left ventricle by the mitral valve and the morphologic left atrium is connected to the morphologic right ventricle by the tricuspid valve (Fig. 20-12). The great vessels are also transposed and discordantly connected to the ventricles; the pulmonary artery is connected to the morphologic left ventricle and the aorta is connected to the morphologic right ventricle. The aorta is thus located anteriorly and to the left of the pulmonary artery. Discordance at both the atrioventricular and ventriculoarterial levels results in hemodynamic compensation where the systemic venous blood leads to the pulmonary artery and the pulmonary venous blood leads to the aorta.

Cc-TGA occurs in about 20% of all TGA cases, has a prevalence of 0.03 per 1000 live births, and accounts for less than 1% of congenital heart disease (27–29). As is the case in D-TGA, cc-TGA is seen more commonly in males. Cc-TGA has a recurrence risk of approximately 2% in first-degree relatives (30) and is thought to result from abnormal left-looping of the bulboventricular cardiac tube during embryogenesis (31). The spectrum of disease is wide and cc-TGA is isolated in only 9% to 16% of cases (32,33). Associated cardiac anomalies are the norm and most commonly include ventricular septal defects, pulmonary outflow obstruction, tricuspid valve abnormalities, dextrocardia/mesocardia, and rhythm disturbances (32–38) (Table 20-1).

Ultrasound Findings

Gray Scale

Identifying normal situs and the position of the heart in the chest are initial steps in the prenatal evaluation of the heart. Situs inversus is noted in 5% of cc-TGA cases (39) and dextrocardia/mesocardia is present in about 25% of cc-TGA cases (40). The diagnosis of cc-TGA is primarily based on the recognition of atrioventricular discordance, which can be noted if a

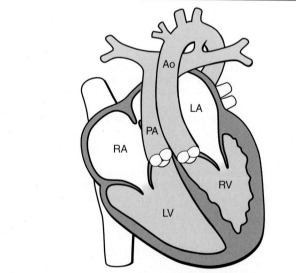

- Abnormal four-chamber anatomy with atrioventricular discordance
- Right atrium (RA) abnormally connected through the mitral valve to the left ventricle (LV)
- Left atrium (LA) abnormally connected through the tricuspid valve to the right ventricle (RV)
- Aorta (Ao) arising from the morphologic right ventricle (RV)
- Pulmonary artery (PA) arising from the morphologic left ventricle (LV)
- Parallel course of great vessels, with an anterior aorta to the left of pulmonary artery

Figure 20-12. Congenitally corrected transposition of the great arteries (cc-TGA).

TABLE 20-1	Congenitally Corrected Transposition of Great Arteries: Associated Intracardiac Anomalies in Fetal and Pediatric Series	
Cardiac anomaly	**Fetal series (%)**	**Pediatric series (%)**
None	13	9–16
Ventricular septal defect	70	70–84
Pulmonary obstruction	40	30–50
Tricuspid valve anomalies	33	14–56
Dextrocardia/mesocardia	17	25
Ventricular hypoplasia	17	NA
Complete atrioventricular block	13	12–33
Aortic arch abnormalities	10	13
Re-entry tachycardia	7	6

(Modified from Paladini D, Volpe P, Marasini M, et al. Diagnosis, characterization and outcome of congenitally corrected transposition of the great arteries in the fetus: a multicenter series of 30 cases. *Ultrasound Obstet Gynecol* 2006;27:281–285, with permission.)

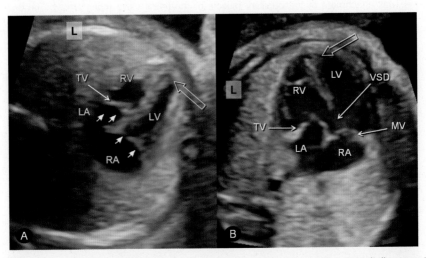

Figure 20-13. Abnormal apical four-chamber views in two fetuses with congenitally corrected transposition showing the typical discordance of the atrioventricular connections. In both fetuses the atria are in normal positions but the left ventricle (LV) and the mitral valve (MV) are on the right side connected to the right atrium (RA), while the more apically inserted tricuspid valve (TV) and its corresponding right ventricle (RV) are on the left side, connected to the left atrium (LA). Note that the apex of the heart (*open arrow*) is formed by the right-sided left ventricle. A ventricular septal defect (VSD), a common association, is noted in **B.** L, left.

sequential segmental evaluation of the fetal heart is followed (see Chapter 4). Recognizing the anatomic characteristics of the cardiac chambers is critical in the ability to identify atrioventricular discordance (see Chapter 5). The four-chamber view allows the assessment of typical ventricular morphology (Fig. 20-13). The morphologic right ventricle in cc-TGA is found posterior on the left side connected to the left atrium and is characterized by a prominent moderator band, an apical attachment of the atrioventricular valve, chordal attachment of the atrioventricular valve directly to the wall, irregularity of the endocardial surface, and a more triangular shape (Fig. 20-14). The morphologic left ventricle in cc-TGA is found anterior on the right side connected to the right atrium and showing a typical smooth surface, a more

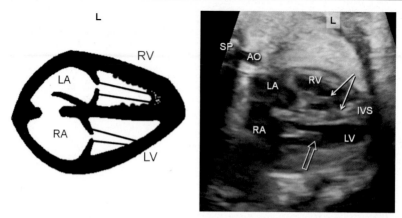

Figure 20-14. Axial view of the four chambers in a fetus with a corrected transposition of the great arteries illustrating the characteristic atrioventricular discordance. The right ventricle (RV) is left-sided and connected to the left atrium (LA). The RV is recognized by the apical insertion of the chordae tendineae of the tricuspid valve to the right ventricular wall and apex of the heart (*two arrows*). The left ventricle (LV) is attached to the right atrium (RA). The LV is recognized by the free wall attachment of the papillary muscle of the mitral valve (*open arrow*). The drawing highlights the anatomic characteristics of the ventricles. Compare with the normal finding in Figure 5-6. SP, spine; AO, aorta; IVS, interventricular septum; L, left.

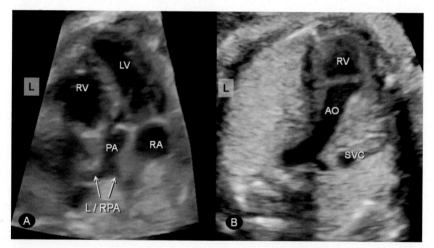

Figure 20-15. Apical views of the outflow tracts in corrected transposition of the great arteries. **A:** The pulmonary artery (PA) arising from the morphologic left ventricle (LV) is identified by its bifurcation into right and left pulmonary arteries (L/RPA) (*arrows*). Note a narrow PA in A, a sign of associated pulmonary stenosis. **B:** The aorta (AO) is seen to arise from the morphologic right ventricle (RV). Note the course of the AO to the left hemithorax in corrected transposition in comparison to complete transposition, where it courses to the right hemithorax. SVC, superior vena cava; RA, right atrium; L, left.

elongated appearance, and apex forming (Figs. 20-13 and 20-14). Assessment of the outflow tracts shows the pulmonary artery arising from the right-sided morphologic left ventricle and the aorta arising from the left-sided morphologic right ventricle in a parallel course with the aorta anterior and to the left of the pulmonary artery (Figs. 20-15 and 20-16). Interestingly, the pulmonary artery arising from the right-sided ventricle has a course to the left side

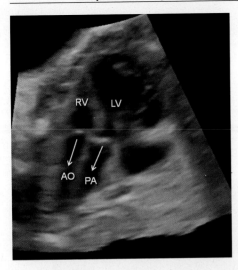

Figure 20-16. Longitudinal view of the great arteries in corrected transposition showing the parallel course of the great arteries with the aorta (AO) anterior to the pulmonary artery (PA). RV, right ventricle; LV, left ventricle.

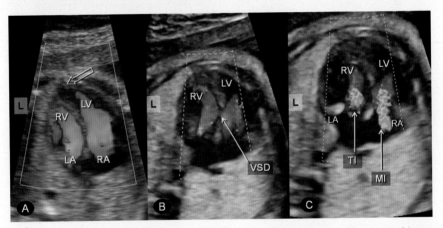

Figure 20-17. Color Doppler at the four-chamber view in three fetuses with corrected transposition demonstrating regular filling of the right (RV) and left ventricle (LV) with the cardiac apex primarily formed by the right-sided LV (*open arrow*) in **plane A,** the commonly associated ventricular septal defect (VSD) in **plane B,** and mitral (MI) and tricuspid insufficiency (TI) in **plane C.** LA, left atrium; RA, right atrium; L, left.

(Fig. 20-15), and it is often difficult to identify the anteriorly positioned aorta with its course also to the left unless a longitudinal view is attempted (Fig. 20-16). In isolated cases the abnormal anatomy of the great vessels is first recognized and then the comprehensive examination of the heart reveals the abnormality in the four-chamber plane. In cases associated with other intracardiac anomalies, the four-chamber plane will generally appear abnormal and is commonly the primary reason for fetal echocardiography referral in cc-TGA fetuses (32,33).

Color Doppler
Color Doppler (Fig. 20-17) is important for the detection or exclusion of commonly associated intracardiac abnormalities in cc-TGA. The presence of VSD (Fig. 20-17B), pulmonary stenosis, and tricuspid valve regurgitation (Fig. 20-17C) can be noted by color Doppler evaluation. Color Doppler can also help in confirming the parallel course of the great vessels, especially if either the aorta or the pulmonary artery shows severe obstruction.

Early Gestation

The diagnosis can be achieved in early gestation primarily by the detection of the abnormal origin and course of the great vessels, rather than the atrioventricular discordance. Color Doppler is helpful at early gestation in identifying the course of great vessels.

Three-dimensional Ultrasound

Three-dimensional ultrasound in its orthogonal planes or with tomographic display (Fig. 20-18) can be of help in demonstrating the anatomy of the ventricles and atrioventricular valves as well as the origin and course of the great vessels (see also "Three-dimensional Ultrasound" in D-TGA section). Volume rendering can reveal the abnormal four-chamber-view anatomy (Fig. 20-19) as well as the parallel vessels, either by using surface mode or in combination

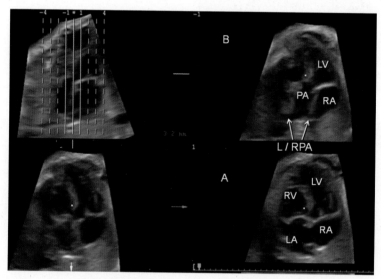

Figure 20-18. Three-dimensional ultrasound of a spatio-temporal image correlation (STIC) volume displayed in tomographic mode in a fetus with corrected transposition. This display shows in one glance the abnormal four-chamber view **(plane A)** in addition to the pulmonary artery (PA) arising from the right-sided left ventricle (LV) with a leftward course **(plane B).** LA, left atrium; L/RPA, left and right pulmonary artery branches; RA, right atrium; RV, right ventricle.

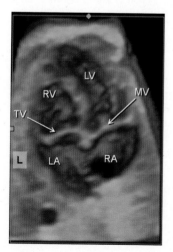

Figure 20-19. Three-dimensional surface rendering in a fetus with a corrected transposition showing the atrioventricular discordance in the four-chamber view. Compare with Figure 20-13A and B. LA, left atrium; LV, left ventricle; MV, mitral valve; RA, right atrium; RV, right ventricle; TV, tricuspid valve, L, left.

with color Doppler, power Doppler, inversion mode, or others. The *en face* view of the atria and great vessel can demonstrate the spatial arrangement of the great vessels with the aorta anterior and to the left of the pulmonary artery (18).

Associated Cardiac and Extracardiac Findings

Associated intracardiac anomalies are common in cc-TGA and are summarized in Table 20-1. Similar to D-TGA, extracardiac malformations are rarely found and chromosomal anomalies are practically absent in cc-TGA. Screening for 22q11 microdeletion is recommended especially when cc-TGA is associated with other cardiac and extracardiac abnormalities.

Differential Diagnosis

Double outlet right ventricle and D-TGA are the two most common cardiac anomalies in the differential diagnosis of cc-TGA as they all share the absence of "cross-over" of the great vessels. Differentiating cc-TGA from D-TGA is summarized in Table 20-2.

The presence of D-TGA, single-ventricle heart, L-malposition arrangement of the great arteries, dextrocardia, mesocardia, or situs inversus should prompt for a sonographic targeted cardiac evaluation for cc-TGA.

Prognosis and Outcome

Fetal course in cc-TGA is general uneventful, unless complicated by severe tricuspid valve dysplasia and regurgitation (Ebstein malformation) or atrioventricular block, which may lead to fetal hydrops and death. Postnatal prognosis is primarily dependent on the associated cardiac findings. Complex cardiac malformations associated with cc-TGA cast a poor prognosis, especially in the presence of single ventricular anatomy, atresia of one of the great vessels, or severe dysplasia of the tricuspid valve (36). Isolated cc-TGA has generally an uneventful postnatal period and requires no immediate treatment (35). Poor long-term prognostic factors include associated Ebstein malformation of the tricuspid valve, degree of tricuspid regurgitation, systemic right ventricular dysfunction, and complete heart block (36,41,42). Heart block is rarely present prenatally but can develop during infancy and childhood, prompting the need

TABLE 20-2	Differentiating Features of Complete and Congenitally Corrected Transposition of the Great Arteries	
	Complete transposition	**Congenitally corrected transposition**
Ventricles	Normal	Inverted
Right ventricle	Anterior on the right	Posterior on the left
Left ventricle	Posterior on the left	Anterior on the right
Tricuspid valve	Normal on the right	On the left, may be insufficient, or displaced into the ventricle as left-sided Ebstein or atretic
Mitral	Normal on the left	On the right
Ventricular septal defect (VSD)	Present in about 40%	Present in about 70%
Pulmonary artery	Pulmonary artery from the left-sided ventricle toward the right thoracic side	Pulmonary artery from the right-sided left ventricle toward the left thoracic side
Aorta	Anterior and to the right side of the pulmonary artery	Anterior and to the left side of the pulmonary artery
Associated cardiac findings	VSD, pulmonary stenosis	VSD, pulmonary stenosis, tricuspid atresia, hypoplastic ventricle, dextrocardia, aortic arch hypoplasia, heart block, etc.

for pacemaker therapy. Heart block in cc-TGA is related to the abnormal position of the atrioventricular node and bundle of His, which are subject to fibrosis (43). In two fetal series, survival rates exceeding 80% were noted following prenatal diagnosis of cc-TGA when pregnancy was continued (32,33). Long-term survival is reported to be more than 90% after 10 years (36).

■ KEY POINTS: CONGENITALLY CORRECTED TRANSPOSITION OF THE GREAT ARTERIES

- Cc-TGA is characterized by atrioventricular and ventriculoarterial discordance.
- The morphologic right atrium is connected with the morphologic left ventricle and the morphologic left atrium is connected with the morphologic right ventricle.
- The pulmonary artery is connected to the morphologic left ventricle and the aorta is connected to the morphologic right ventricle.
- Great vessels are parallel with the aorta commonly located anteriorly and to the left of the pulmonary artery.
- There is hemodynamic compensation where the systemic venous blood leads to the pulmonary artery and the pulmonary venous blood leads to the aorta.
- The four-chamber view is abnormal.
- Associated cardiac abnormalities are the norm.
- Ventricular septal defect, pulmonary obstruction, and tricuspid valve abnormalities are commonly associated with cc-TGA.
- Extracardiac malformations are rare and chromosomal anomalies are practically absent.
- Isolated cc-TGA has generally an uneventful postnatal period and requires no immediate treatment.
- Poor long-term prognostic factors include associated Ebstein malformation of the tricuspid valve, degree of tricuspid regurgitation, systemic right ventricular dysfunction, and complete heart block.
- Survival rates exceeded 80% in prenatally diagnosed cc-TGA when pregnancy was continued.

References

1. Webb GD, McLaughlin PR, Gow RM, et al. Transposition complexes. *Cardiol Clin* 1993;11(4):651–664.
2. Allan LD, Crawford DC, Anderson RH, et al. The spectrum of congenital heart disease detected echocardiographically in prenatal life. *Br Heart J* 1985;54:523–526.
3. Kirklin JW, Barratt-Boyes BG. Complete transposition of the great arteries. In: Kirklin JW, Barratt-Boyes BG, eds. *Cardiac surgery*. New York: Churchill Livingston, 1993;1383–1467.
4. Jex RK, Puga FJ, Julsrud PR, et al. Repair of transposition of the great arteries with intact ventricular septum and left ventricular outflow tract obstruction. *J Thorac Cardiovasc Surg* 1990;100:682–686.
5. Bull C. Current and potential impact of fetal diagnosis on prevalence and spectrum of serious congenital heart disease at term in the UK. British Paediatric Cardiac Association. *Lancet* 1999;354(9186):1242–1247.
6. Blyth M, Howe D, Gnanapragasam J, et al. The hidden mortality of transposition of the great arteries and survival advantage provided by prenatal diagnosis. *BJOG* 2008;115(9):1096–1100.
7. Chew C, Halliday JL, Riley MM, et al. Population-based study of antenatal detection of congenital heart disease by ultrasound examination. *Ultrasound Obstet Gynecol* 2007;29(6):619–624.
8. Khoshnood B, de Vigan C, Vodovar V, et al. Trends in prenatal diagnosis, pregnancy termination, and perinatal mortality of newborns with congenital heart disease in France, 1983–2000: a population-based evaluation. *Pediatrics* 2005;115(1):95–101.
9. Bonnet D, Coltri A, Butera G, et al. Detection of transposition of the great arteries in fetuses reduces neonatal morbidity and mortality. *Circulation* 1999;99(7):916–918.
10. Cardiac screening examination of the fetus: guidelines for performing the 'basic' and 'extended basic' cardiac scan. *Ultrasound Obstet Gynecol* 2006;27(1):107–113.
11. Chaoui R, McEwing R. Three cross-sectional planes for fetal color Doppler echocardiography. *Ultrasound Obstet Gynecol* 2003;21(1):81–93.
12. Becker R, Wegner RD. Detailed screening for fetal anomalies and cardiac defects at the 11–13-week scan. *Ultrasound Obstet Gynecol* 2006;27(6):613–618.
13. Wald NJ, Morris JK, Walker K, et al. Prenatal screening for serious congenital heart defects using nuchal translucency: a meta-analysis. *Prenat Diagn* 2008;28(12):1094–1104.
14. Chaoui R, Hoffmann J, Heling KS. Three-dimensional (3D) and 4D color Doppler fetal echocardiography using spatio-temporal image correlation (STIC). *Ultrasound Obstet Gynecol* 2004;23(6):535–545.
15. Goncalves LF, Espinoza J, Romero R, et al. A systematic approach to prenatal diagnosis of transposition of the great arteries using 4-dimensional ultrasonography with spatiotemporal image correlation. *J Ultrasound Med* 2004;23(9):1225–1231.

16. DeVore GR, Polanco B, Sklansky MS, et al. The 'spin' technique: a new method for examination of the fetal outflow tracts using three-dimensional ultrasound. *Ultrasound Obstet Gynecol* 2004;24(1):72–82.
17. Vinals F, Ascenzo R, Poblete P, et al. Simple approach to prenatal diagnosis of transposition of the great arteries. *Ultrasound Obstet Gynecol* 2006;28(1):22–25.
18. Paladini D, Volpe P, Sglavo G, et al. Transposition of the great arteries in the fetus: assessment of the spatial relationships of the arterial trunks by four-dimensional echocardiography. *Ultrasound Obstet Gynecol* 2008;31(3):271–276.
19. Rizzo G, Capponi A, Cavicchioni O, et al. Application of automated sonography on 4-dimensional volumes of fetuses with transposition of the great arteries. *J Ultrasound Med* 2008;27:771–776.
20. Allen HD, Driscoll DJ, Shaddy RE, et al., eds. *Moss and Adams' heart disease in infants, children and adolescents*, 7th ed. Baltimore: Lippincott Williams & Wilkins, 2007;1044–1045.
21. Massoudy P, Baltalarli A, de Laval MR, et al. Anatomic variability in coronary arterial distribution with regard to the arterial switch procedure. *Circulation* 2002;106:1980–1984.
22. Pasquini L, Sanders SP, Parness IA, et al. Coronary echocardiography in 406 patients with D-loop transposition of the great arteries. *J Am Coll Cardiol* 1994;24:763–768.
23. Jouannic JM, Gavard L, Fermont L, et al. Sensitivity and specificity of prenatal features of physiological shunts to predict neonatal clinical status in transposition of the great arteries. *Circulation* 2004;110(13): 1743–1746.
24. Maeno YV, Kamenir SA, Sinclair B, et al. Prenatal features of ductus arteriosus constriction and restrictive foramen ovale in d-transposition of the great arteries. *Circulation* 1999;99(9):1209–1214.
25. Raboisson MJ, Samson C, Ducreux C, et al. Impact of prenatal diagnosis of transposition of the great arteries on obstetric and early postnatal management. *Eur J Obstet Gynecol Reprod Biol* 2009;142(1):18–22.
26. Kumar RK, Newburger JW, Gauvreau K, et al. Comparison of outcome when hypoplastic left heart syndrome and transposition of the great arteries are diagnosed prenatally versus when diagnosis of these two conditions is made only postnatally. *Am J Cardiol* 1999;83(12):1649–1653.
27. Ferencz C, Rubin JD, McCarter RJ, et al. Congenital heart disease: prevalence at livebirth. The Baltimore-Washington Infant Study. *Am J Epidemiol* 1985;121:31–36.
28. Fyler DC. Report of the New England Regional Infant Cardiac Program. *Pediatrics* 1980;65(suppl):376–461.
29. Samanek M, Voriskova M. Congenital heart disease among 815,569 children born between 1980 and their 15-year survival: a prospective Bohemia survival study. *Pediatr Cardiol* 1999;20:411–417.
30. Becker TA, Van Amber R, Moller JH, et al. Occurrence of cardiac malformations in relatives of children with transposition of the great arteries. *Am J Med Genet* 1996;66(1):28–32.
31. Stending G, Seidl W. Contribution to the development of the heart. Part 2: morphogenesis of congenital heart diseases. *Thorac Cardiovasc Surg* 1981;29:1–16.
32. Sharland G, Tingay R, Jones A, et al. Atrioventricular and ventriculoarterial discordance (congenitally corrected transposition of the great arteries): echocardiographic features, associations, and outcome in 34 fetuses. *Heart* 2005;91(11):1453–1458.
33. Paladini D, Volpe P, Marasini M, et al. Diagnosis, characterization and outcome of congenitally corrected transposition of the great arteries in the fetus: a multicenter series of 30 cases. *Ultrasound Obstet Gynecol* 2006;27:281–285.
34. Freedom RM, Dyck JD. Congenitally corrected transposition of the great arteries. In: Emmanouilides, GC, Reimenschneider TA, Allen HD, et al., eds. *Heart disease in infants, children, and adolescents including the fetus and young adult*, 5th ed. Baltimore: Williams & Wilkins, 1995;1225–1242.
35. McEwing RL, Chaoui R. Congenitally corrected transposition of the great arteries: clues for prenatal diagnosis. *Ultrasound Obstet Gynecol* 2004;23(1):68–72.
36. Rutledge JM, Nihil MR, Fraser CD, et al. Outcome of 121 patients with congenitally corrected transposition of the great arteries. *Pediatr Cardiol* 2002;23:137–145.
37. Presbitero P, Somerville J, Rabajoli F, et al. Corrected transposition of the great arteries without associated defects in adult patients: clinical profile and follow up. *Br Heart J* 1995;74:57–59.
38. Allan L. Atrioventricular discordance. In: Allan L, Hornberger L, Sharland G, eds. *Textbook of fetal cardiology*. London: Greenwich Medical Media Limited, 2000;183–192.
39. Wtham AC. Double outlet right ventricle: a partial transposition complex. *Am Heart J* 1957;53:928–939.
40. Losekoot TG, Becker AE. Discordant atrioventricular connection and congenitally corrected transposition. In: Anderson RH, Macartney FJ, Shinebourne EA, et al., eds. *Pediatric cardiology*. Edinburgh: Churchill Livingstone, 1987;867–888.
41. Graham TP Jr, Bernard YD, Mellen BG, et al. Long term outcome in congenitally corrected transposition of the great arteries: a muti-institutional study. *J Am Coll Cardiol* 2000;36:255–261.
42. Hraska V, Duncan BW, Mayer JE Jr, et al. Long-term outcome of surgically treated patients with corrected transposition of the great arteries. *J Thorac Cardiovasc Surg* 2005;129:182–191.
43. Hosseinpour A-R, McCarthy KP, Griselli M, et al. Congenitally corrected transposition: size of the pulmonary trunk and septal malalignment. *Ann Thorac Surg* 2004;77:2163–2166.

INTRODUCTION

It is generally acknowledged that anomalies of aortic arch branching are best understood when basic embryology of the aortic arch is reviewed. The hypothetical double aortic arch theory, suggested by Edwards (1), provides an explanation for various aortic arch abnormalities (2–4). This theory is based on the presence of double aortic arch in the embryo, where the ascending aorta splits into a right and a left aortic arch, which merge to form the descending aorta, anatomically located in a central position, anterior to the spine (Fig. 21-1). A complete vascular ring, surrounding the trachea and esophagus, is thus formed by the left and right arches. The left and right aortic arches give rise to two vessels each; the left and right common carotid and subclavian arteries, respectively (Fig. 21-1). In addition, the left and right pulmonary arteries are connected to the left and right aortic arch, respectively, by a left and right ductus arteriosus in the region of the subclavian arteries (Fig. 21-1). Normal and abnormal development of the aortic arch branching is thus related to which site of the left or right aortic arch regresses or persists during embryonic development (3,4). Common aortic arch abnormalities encountered on prenatal ultrasound are discussed in this chapter.

EMBRYOLOGIC FINDINGS

Embryologic events that result in various anatomic orientations of the aortic arch and its branches are hereby presented.

A: Normal (Left-sided) Aortic Arch

The regression of the right aortic arch segment distal to the origin of the right subclavian artery results in a left aortic arch (normal anatomy) (Fig. 21-1A). The right subclavian and right common carotid arteries merge to form the right brachiocephalic (or innominate) artery. The left ductus arteriosus persists whereas the right ductus arteriosus regresses.

B: Left-sided Aortic Arch With Aberrant Right Subclavian Artery

This anomaly results from partial regression of the right aortic arch between the origin of the right common carotid artery and the right subclavian artery (Fig. 21-1B). This leads to the presence of a left-sided aortic arch with the following arising vessels: the right common carotid artery as the first branch, the left common carotid artery as the second branch, the left subclavian artery as the third branch, and an aberrant right subclavian artery as the last branch (Fig. 21-1B). The course of the right subclavian artery is posterior to the esophagus and trachea toward the right arm. The left ductus arteriosus persists, whereas the right ductus arteriosus regresses.

C: Right-sided Aortic Arch With Mirror Image Branching

This is a mirror image version of the normal left-sided aortic arch. In this anomaly, the left aortic arch distal to the origin of the left subclavian artery regresses, resulting in a right aortic arch (Fig. 21-1C). The left subclavian and the common carotid arteries merge to form the left brachiocephalic (innominate) artery, which arises as the first branch off the right aortic arch followed by the right common carotid artery and the right subclavian artery (Fig. 21-1C). In almost all cases, the right ductus arteriosus persists, whereas the left ductus arteriosus regresses. This condition is often found in association with other congenital heart defects.

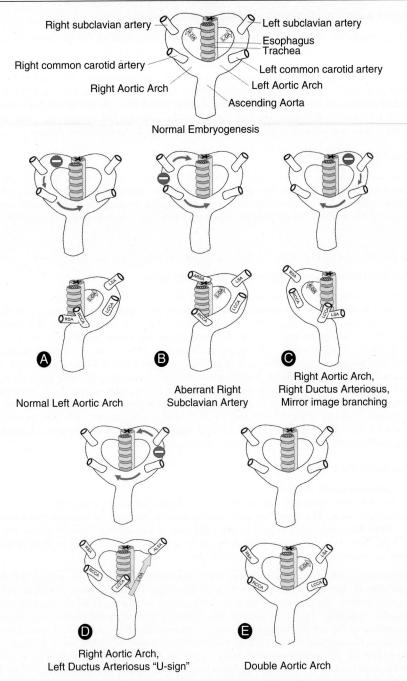

Figure 21-1. Explanation for various aortic arch abnormalities. During embryogenesis (top drawing) a double aortic arch exists made by the left and right aortic arch, which forms a complete vascular ring surrounding the trachea and esophagus. The left and right aortic arches give rise to two vessels each; the left (LCCA) and right (RCCA) common carotid and left (LSA) and right (RSA) subclavian arteries, respectively. In addition, a left (L-DA) and right (R-DA) ductus arteriosus exist in the region of the subclavian arteries. Normal and abnormal development of the aortic arch branching is thus related to which site of the left or right aortic arch regresses or persists during embryonic development. **A:** Normal development. **B:** Left aortic arch with aberrant right subclavian artery. **C:** Right aortic arch with mirror image branching. **D:** Right aortic arch with left ductus arteriosus. **E:** Double aortic arch. See text for details.

D: Right Aortic Arch With Left Ductus Arteriosus

In this anomaly, the left aortic arch regresses between the origin of the left common carotid artery and the left subclavian artery (Fig. 21-1D). The left ductus arteriosus persists in the region of the left subclavian artery, whereas the right ductus arteriosus regresses. This leads to the presence of a right-sided aortic arch and a vascular ring surrounding the trachea from the left side as well (Fig. 21-1D). The following vessels arise from the aorta: first the left common carotid artery, second the right common carotid artery, third the right subclavian, and fourth an aberrant left subclavian artery. On rare occasions the aberrant left subclavian arises directly from the descending aorta through an arterial conduit called Kommerell diverticulum (5).

E: Double Aortic Arch

This anomaly results from persistence of right and left aortic arches (Fig. 21-1E). The left ductus arteriosus persists, whereas the right ductus arteriosus regresses. Each aortic arch gives rise to a subclavian and a common carotid artery. The double aortic arch forms a tight vascular ring around the trachea and esophagus, which may need surgical intervention postnatally.

RIGHT AORTIC ARCH AND DOUBLE AORTIC ARCH

Definition, Spectrum of Disease, and Incidence

In normal conditions, the left aortic arch crosses the left bronchus in the upper chest. Right aortic arch is defined by the aortic arch that crosses the right bronchus instead of the left bronchus. In fetal echocardiography, a right aortic arch is diagnosed when the transverse aortic arch is located to the right of the trachea on transverse imaging of the chest (6) (Fig. 21-2B–D). A right aortic arch occurs in about 1 in 1000 of the general population (6), but the prevalence of right aortic arch is probably higher when associated cases with other cardiac anomalies are considered. A right aortic arch is associated with three main subgroups of arch abnormalities; right aortic arch with a right ductus (see section C in Embryologic Findings [Figs. 21-1C and 21-2B]); right aortic arch with left-sided ductus (see section D in Embryologic Findings [Figs. 21-1D and 21-2C]); and double aortic arch (see section E in Embryologic Findings [Figs. 21-1E and 21-2D]). Right aortic arch can be part of a complex cardiac malformation, but can often also be an isolated finding (7).

Ultrasound Findings

Gray Scale and Color Doppler

In the four-chamber view, the descending aorta is more centrally located anterior to the spine in right aortic arch. The detection and classification is achieved in the three-vessel-trachea view, where the aorta has a course to the right side of the trachea (instead to the left) (see Fig. 21-2). Three subgroups of a right arch can be generally differentiated by fetal echocardiography in combination with color Doppler (7,8):

1. **Right aortic arch with a right ductus arteriosus (right V-sign):** In this group, the ductus arteriosus is right sided (see section C in Embryologic Findings). Both the aorta and pulmonary arteries merge together in a V-configuration on the right of the trachea with no vascular rings (Fig. 21-3). We refer to this anatomic finding as the right V-sign in contradistinction to the left V configuration seen in normal anatomy. Because in most cases this condition is associated with a cardiac malformation, mainly a "conotruncal anomaly," it is often difficult to demonstrate the exact course of the ductus arteriosus. The brachiocephalic vessels arise in mirror image branching to the normal left aortic arch. Color Doppler is helpful in the demonstration of the course of the vessels.

2. **Right aortic arch with left ductus arteriosus (U-sign):** The aortic arch is right sided and the pulmonary trunk and ductus arteriosus are to the left of the trachea (see section D in Embryologic Findings). In this condition the trachea is seen as an echogenic structure between the transverse aortic arch (right) and the ductus arteriosus (left) (Fig. 21-4). These vessels surround the trachea in a U-configuration, called the "U-sign" (6,9). It is considered a loose "vascular ring" in comparison to the tight vascular ring seen with double aortic

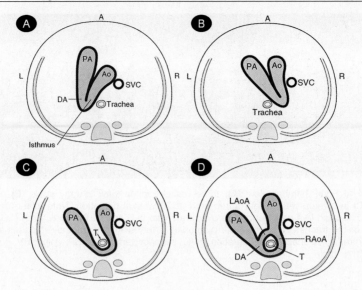

Figure 21-2. Schematics of the three-vessel-trachea view in a normal fetus where the transverse aortic arch (Ao) and isthmus merge with the pulmonary artery (PA) and ductus arteriosus (DA) into the descending aorta in a "V-shape" configuration to the left of the trachea **(A)** and a right-sided aortic arch with a right-sided DA in a "V-shape" configuration to the right side of the trachea **(B)**. In B, the most common branching of the brachiocephalic vessels is a "mirror branching" to that in A (see text for details). **C:** A right aortic arch with the transverse aortic arch to the right side of the trachea (T); the DA is left-sided and the connection of aortic and ductal arches constitutes a vascular ring around the trachea in a "U-shape" configuration. **D:** A rare subform of right aortic arch (RAoA) with a left DA forming a double aortic arch with the transverse aortic arch bifurcating into a right and a left aortic arch (LAoA) surrounding the trachea and esophagus. L, left; R, right; SVC, superior vena cava.

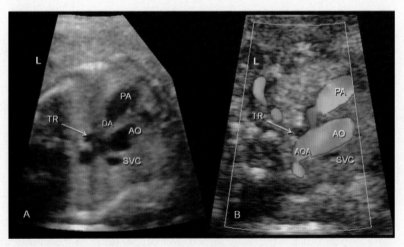

Figure 21-3. Gray scale **(A)** and color Doppler **(B)** at the three-vessel-trachea view in a fetus with right aortic arch (AOA) with right ductus arteriosus (DA). Note that both aortic and ductal arches are pointing to the right side of the trachea (TR). 22q11 microdeletion was confirmed postnatally. PA, pulmonary artery; AO, aorta; SVC, superior vena cava; L, left.

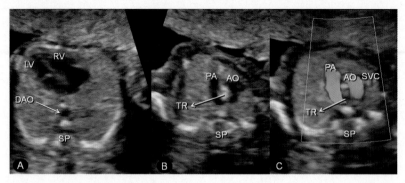

Figure 21-4. Four-chamber view **(A)**, three-vessel-trachea view in gray scale **(B)**, and color Doppler **(C)** in a fetus with a right aortic arch at 18 weeks' gestation. Note in the descending aorta (DAO) located in a central position over the spine. In B and C, the aortic arch (AO) is to the right side of the trachea (TR), while the pulmonary artery (PA) and ductus arteriosus are to the left. This forms a "U-shape" configuration. SVC, superior vena cava; SP, spine; RV, right ventricle; LV, left ventricle.

arch. This condition is commonly an isolated finding in the majority of cases with rare cardiac or extracardiac associated malformations (7). Color Doppler can easily demonstrate the U-sign (Fig. 21-5B) (9) and in almost all cases, the aberrant course of the left subclavian artery, arising from the region of the junction of the ductus arteriosus with the descending aorta called Kommerell diverticulum (5).

3. **Double aortic arch:** The aortic arch has a course to the right side of the trachea but bifurcates directly at the level of the trachea to have one arch to the right and one to the left in the Greek letter "lambda" (λ) configuration (Fig. 21-6) (10). Behind the trachea both arches fuse into the descending aorta which has a course directly central and anterior to the spine. The esophagus and trachea are entrapped between the right and left aortic arches. Generally the left arch is narrower than the right and in some conditions hypoplastic. Generally, the ductus arteriosus has a left side course and connects with the left arch or descending aorta. Two vessels arise from each aortic arch, a left and a right common

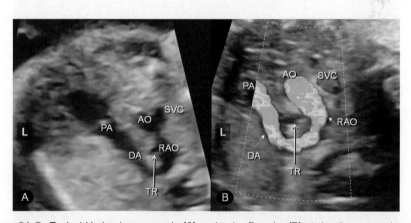

Figure 21-5. Typical U-sign in gray scale **(A)** and color Doppler **(B)** at the three-vessel-trachea view plane demonstrating a right-sided aortic arch (RAO) to the right side of the trachea (TR) and a left-sided ductus arteriosus (DA). This plane raises suspicion of a right aortic arch but does not allow clear differentiation between a right and a double aortic arch. (See Figs. 21-6 and 21-7 for details.) SVC, superior vena cava; PA, pulmonary artery; AO, aorta; L, left.

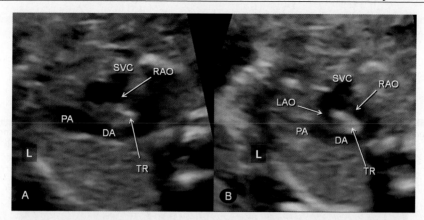

Figure 21-6. Three-vessel-trachea view in a fetus with double aortic arch. In **plane A**, a right aortic arch (RAO) with left ductus arteriosus (DA) (U-sign) is initially suspected. When a more cranial plane is obtained **(B)**, the bifurcation of the aortic arch into a right and left aortic arch (LAO) is recognized. Diagnostic accuracy is increased by using color Doppler (see Fig. 21-7). PA, pulmonary artery; TR, trachea; SVC, superior vena cava; L, left.

carotid and subclavian artery. Color Doppler is helpful in the demonstration of the lambda bifurcation in front of the trachea and the course of the vessels (Fig. 21-7). A longitudinal view of the trachea can show in most cases a compression at the anatomic level of the double aortic arch.

Early Gestation

The diagnosis of a right aortic arch is possible in early gestation at 11 to 14 weeks and is enabled by the use of color Doppler at the three-vessel-trachea view (11). It is commonly suspected on transabdominal scanning when the relationship of the transverse aortic and ductal

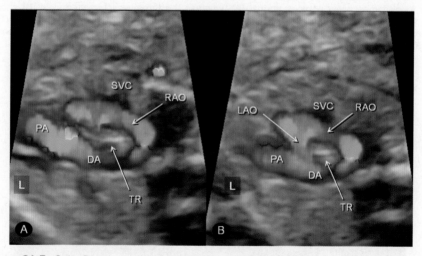

Figure 21-7. Color Doppler applied to the same case shown in Figure 21-6. A right aortic arch (RAO) with a left ductus arteriosus (DA) is first suspected in **A** and when a more cranial plane is obtained **(B)**, the double aortic arch is recognized. The trachea (TR), which is slightly compressed, is encircled by the branches of the right and left (LAO) aortic arches, forming a tight vascular ring. SVC, superior vena cava; PA, pulmonary artery; L, left.

arches is evaluated. Transvaginal scanning can help in confirming the diagnosis. In recent years, we were able to diagnose right-sided aortic arch with its three subgroups in early gestation. Differentiating between the U-sign right aortic arch and the double aortic arch (lambda sign) may be difficult in early gestation. Figures 21-8 and 21-9 show right aortic arch cases diagnosed in early gestation.

Three-dimensional Ultrasound

Tomographic ultrasound imaging display can be of help in fetuses with right aortic arch in demonstrating anatomic findings in various planes. Three-dimensional rendering may show the spatial relationship of the right arch and the corresponding associated finding such as

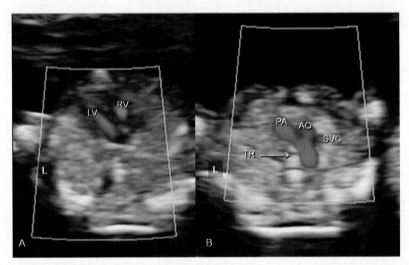

Figure 21-8. Detection of a right aortic arch in early gestation is facilitated by color Doppler. The four-chamber view appears normal **(A)**, whereas the three-vessel-trachea view **(B)** shows the "V-shaped" configuration of the arches with a course to the right side of the trachea (TR). L, left; PA, pulmonary artery; AO, aorta; RV, right ventricle; LV, left ventricle; SVC, superior vena cava.

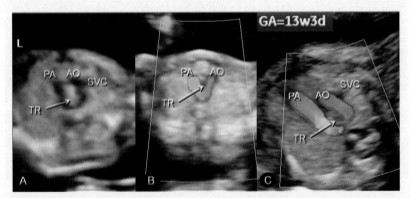

Figure 21-9. Right aortic arch with a left ductus (U-sign) detected on two-dimensional ultrasound at 13 weeks' gestation in transabdominal scanning **(A)** and confirmed by color Doppler **(B)**. The transvaginal approach in combination with color Doppler improves visualization of this abnormality **(C)**. PA, pulmonary artery; AO, aorta; SVC, superior vena cava; TR, trachea; L, left.

double arch, V-sign, or U-sign (5,10). This rendering can be achieved by color Doppler (10); power Doppler (5); B-flow mode; or inversion mode (Figs. 21-10 and 21-11).

Associated Cardiac and Extracardiac Findings

Even if the right aortic arch appears as an isolated finding on ultrasound, fetal chromosomal karyotyping should be offered to rule out chromosomal aberrations, primarily trisomy 21 and 22q11 microdeletion (7,12). Associated intracardiac anomalies are more common when the aorta and ductus arteriosus are on the right (V-sign) than with double aortic arch or with the U-sign right aortic arch (7). Typical cardiac anomalies observed with a right aortic arch are tetralogy of Fallot, pulmonary atresia with ventricular septal defect, common arterial trunk, absent pulmonary valve, tricuspid atresia, and double outlet right ventricle (7,12). The presence of a right aortic arch in association with a conotruncal anomaly increases the risk for

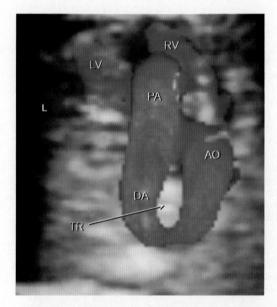

Figure 21-10. Three-dimensional ultrasound using spatio-temporal image correlation and color Doppler in a glass-body mode in a fetus with a right aortic arch (AO) and left ductus arteriosus (DA) in a "U-shaped" configuration. The view is from the upper thorax showing the U-sign in color Doppler surrounding the trachea (TR) with the four-chamber view seen in the background. RV, right ventricle; LV, left ventricle; L, left.

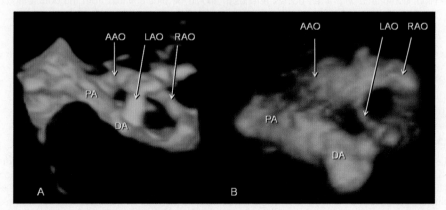

Figure 21-11. A: Double aortic arch using inversion mode in a spatio-temporal image correlation volume showing the bifurcation of the arch into a right (RAO) and a left (LAO) aortic arch with a left ductus arteriosus (DA). **B:** B-flow in a fetus with a double aortic arch and a hypoplastic left arch. The left ductus arteriosus is large. AAO, ascending aorta; PA, pulmonary artery.

the 22q11 microdeletion (7,12,13). Associated extracardiac malformations can be found but no typical malformation is reported.

Differential Diagnosis

A right aortic arch should not be confused with a right-sided aorta in cases of isomerism or situs inversus. In right aortic arch, the arch is right sided to the trachea but the abdominal aorta is left sided, unlike cases of isomerism or situs inversus. The most difficult challenge is the differentiation between a right aortic arch with a U-sign, which can be isolated with no impact on neonatal outcome, and double aortic arch with a tight vascular ring around the trachea and the esophagus, which needs surgical treatment postnatally. The difficulty resides in differentiating a narrow left aortic arch in double aortic arch from the left common carotid artery in U-sign right aortic arch, as both have the same anatomic course.

Prognosis and Outcome

Double aortic arch causes pressure on the trachea, which may cause stridor in the neonatal period. Delivery at a tertiary center is recommended, and intervention should be planned before symptoms occur or before the pressure on the trachea causes tracheomalacia. A right aortic arch with a left ductus arteriosus creates a loose vascular ring, which may cause tracheal compression in rare cases. Parents should be informed of such possibility as the need for surgery to remove the ligamentum arteriosum (closed ductus arteriosus) may be necessary on rare occasions. Ductal closure may also involve the aberrant left subclavian artery in these conditions, which may lead to reduced perfusion of the left arm. A stent may need to be placed in order to rescue the closing vessel (14). A right aortic arch with a right ductus is an isolated finding and has no impact on prognosis.

■ KEY POINTS: RIGHT AND DOUBLE AORTIC ARCH

- ■ Right aortic arch is best detected in the three-vessel-trachea view in the fetus.
- ■ In right aortic arch, the transverse arch is to the right of the trachea in cross-sectional planes.
- ■ Right aortic arch can be associated with a right ductus arteriosus and no ring around the trachea. In this condition cardiac anomalies are commonly seen in more than 90% of cases.
- ■ Right aortic arch can be associated with a left ductus arteriosus (so-called U-sign) with a loose vascular ring around the trachea.
- ■ Right aortic arch with a left ductus arteriosus should be differentiated from the double aortic arch.
- ■ In double aortic arch, the aortic arch splits into a right and a left arch to encircle the trachea and esophagus. Both arches merge to form the descending aorta.
- ■ Right aortic arch malformations are associated with chromosomal aneuploidy such as trisomy 21 and 22q11 microdeletion.

ABERRANT RIGHT SUBCLAVIAN ARTERY

Definition, Spectrum of Disease, and Incidence

Left aortic arch with an aberrant right subclavian artery (ARSA) is the most common abnormality or variant of the aortic arch occurring in 0.5% to 1.4% of the normal population (15–17). Whereas under normal conditions the left aortic arch gives rise to three vessels, in this condition four vessels arise from the aortic arch in the following sequence from proximal to distal: the right common carotid artery, the left common carotid artery, the left subclavian artery, and the aberrant right subclavian artery (18,19). The aberrant right subclavian artery arises from the distal portion of the aortic arch and courses from the left side of the upper chest, behind the esophagus and the trachea, to the right upper arm (Fig. 21-12). This

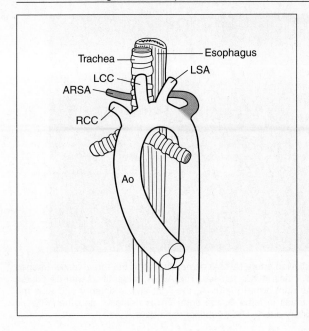

Figure 21-12. Aberrant right subclavian artery; note its course posterior to the trachea and esophagus toward the right arm. Ao, aorta; RCC, right common carotid; LCC, left common carotid; LSA, left subclavian artery; ARSA, aberrant right subclavian artery.

aberrant vessel is also called retroesophageal right subclavian artery. Lusorian artery is another term that was used in the past for the aberrant right subclavian artery. The embryologic origin of the aberrant right subclavian artery is discussed earlier, in section B of Embryologic Findings.

Ultrasound Findings

Gray Scale and Color Doppler

ARSA is a common finding and may be considered a normal variant. Imaging the ARSA is not typically achieved on two-dimensional gray scale but rather on color Doppler when an aberrant right subclavian artery is suspected. The three-vessel-trachea view is most optimal for the diagnosis where the ARSA is demonstrated from the junction of the aortic arch and ductus arteriosus with a course behind the trachea toward the right clavicle and shoulder. The ARSA is shown by lowering the color velocities to the range of 10 to 15 cm/sec (Fig. 21-13) (18,19). When ARSA is suspected, its presence should be confirmed by demonstrating arterial flow on pulsed Doppler.

Early Gestation

ARSA can be demonstrated in early gestation at 11 to 14 weeks' scan (20), and the ability to image the ARSA is significantly enhanced when transvaginal fetal ultrasound is performed (Fig. 21-14).

Three-dimensional Ultrasound

In our experience three-dimensional ultrasound is of help in the multiplanar display, which allows for the retrieval of the ideal plane demonstrating the course of ARSA. In most cases, however, color Doppler is sufficient for the diagnosis. Applying postprocessing algorithms such as glass body mode or B-flow may help in identifying an ARSA (Fig. 21-15).

Associated Cardiac and Extracardiac Findings

The association of ARSA with trisomy 21 has been reported in the pediatric literature (2,21). The first observation of ARSA in fetuses with trisomy 21 was first reported by Chaoui et al. (18).

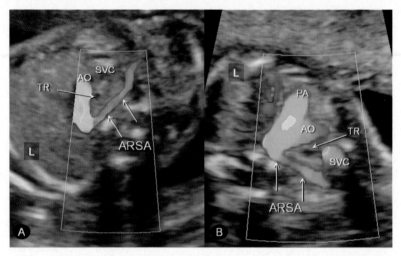

Figure 21-13. Aberrant right subclavian artery (ARSA) demonstrated in the three-vessel-trachea view with color Doppler in low velocities in two fetuses. The ARSA is identified with its course behind the trachea (TR) toward the right arm. In fetus **A,** the right arm is anterior and thus the course of the ARSA is in *red*, whereas in fetus **B,** the right arm is posterior and the ARSA is seen in *blue*. AO, aorta; PA, pulmonary artery; SVC, superior vena cava; L, left.

An association in the range of 14% to 20% of ARSA with trisomy 21 fetuses was recently reported (19,22). In most detected cases, additional trisomy 21 markers are noted on ultrasound such as echogenic intracardiac focus, absent nasal bone, and others. ARSA can also be found in other aneuploidies (23).

In a study involving 4102 pathologic specimens of congenital heart disease, ARSA was identified in 128 cases of which 11 cases were isolated and 117 cases were associated with cardiac anomalies, primarily conotruncal malformations (15). The combination of ARSA with a conotruncal anomaly increases the risk for 22q11 microdeletion (13).

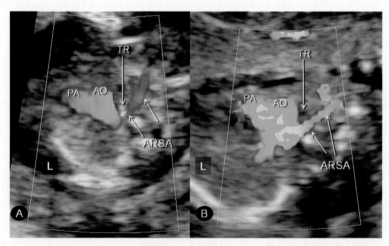

Figure 21-14. Aberrant right subclavian artery (ARSA) in a 13 weeks' fetus **(A)** noted during the nuchal translucency measurement and in fetus **B,** ARSA was diagnosed at 16 weeks' gestation. AO, aorta; PA, pulmonary artery; TR, trachea; L, left.

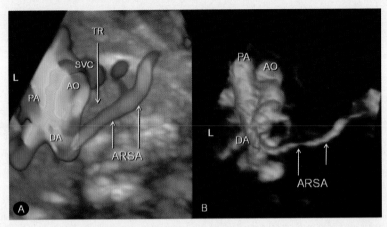

Figure 21-15. A: Three-dimensional ultrasound in glass-body mode of a spatio-temporal image correlation volume demonstrating the course of the aberrant right subclavian artery (ARSA) behind the trachea (TR). **B:** B-flow demonstrates the three-vessel-view with an ARSA showing its course. In B-flow mode, the trachea is not visualized. AO, aorta; PA, pulmonary artery; DA, ductus arteriosus; SVC, superior vena cava; L, left.

Differential Diagnosis

The azygos vein, which courses behind the trachea before it enters the superior vena cava, can be confused with ARSA. Spectral Doppler can help differentiate ARSA from an azygos vein by demonstrating an arterial Doppler pattern.

Prognosis and Outcome

In most cases ARSA is considered a normal variant and results in a normal postnatal course. On rare occasions, ARSA can cause pressure on the esophagus, resulting in dysphagia. When transesophageal echocardiography or gastroscopy is performed on patients with ARSA, care should be exercised in order to avoid pressure of the ARSA, which may cause decreased right arm perfusion.

■ KEY POINTS: ABERRANT RIGHT SUBCLAVIAN ARTERY

- Aberrant right subclavian artery (ARSA) is best detected by using color Doppler in the three-vessel-trachea view.
- ARSA typically courses behind the trachea and the esophagus from the left posterior thoracic side to the right arm.
- ARSA is a frequent condition, seen in about 1.5% of the general population and is considered a normal variant.
- ARSA is commonly associated with trisomy 21 (14% to 20%) and other chromosomal anomalies.
- ARSA, when associated with other cardiac malformations, increases the risk for chromosomal aneuploidies, especially 22q11 microdeletion and trisomy 21.

References

1. Edwards JE. Malformation of the aortic arch system manifested as 'vascular rings.' *Lab Invest* 1953;2:56–75.
2. Weinberg PM. Aortic arch anomalies. In: Allen HD, Clark EB, Gutgesell HP, et al., eds. *Moss and Adams' congenital heart disease in infants, children and adolescents.* Philadelphia: Lippincott Williams & Wilkins, 2001:707–735.
3. Yoo SJ, Min JY, Lee YH, et al. Sonographic diagnosis of aortic arch anomalies. *Ultrasound Obstet Gynecol* 2003;22:535–546.
4. Yoo SJ, Bradley T, Jaeggi E. Aortic arch anomalies. In: Yagel S, Silvermann N, Gembruch U, eds. *Fetal cardiology.* London: Martin Dunitz, 2003;329–342.

5. Chaoui R, Schneider BES, Kalache KD. Right aortic arch with vascular ring and aberrant left subclavian artery: prenatal diagnosis assisted by three-dimensional power Doppler ultrasound. *Ultrasound Obstet Gynecol* 2003;22:661–663.
6. Achiron R, Rotstein Z, Heggesh J, et al. Anomalies of the fetal aortic arch: a novel sonographic approach to in-utero diagnosis. *Ultrasound Obstet Gynecol* 2002;20:553–557.
7. Berg G, Bender F, Soukup M, et al. Right aortic arch detected in fetal life. *Ultrasound Obstet Gynecol* 2006;28:882–889.
8. Jeanty P, Chaoui R, Tihonenko I, et al. A review of findings in fetal cardiac section drawings. Part 3: the 3-vessel-trachea view and variants. *J Ultrasound Med* 2008;27(1):109–117.
9. Chaoui R, McEwing R. Three cross-sectional planes for fetal color Doppler echocardiography. *Ultrasound Obstet Gynecol* 2003;21(1):81–93.
10. Chaoui R, Hoffmann J, Heling KS. Three-dimensional (3D) and 4D color Doppler fetal echocardiography using spatio-temporal image correlation (STIC). *Ultrasound Obstet Gynecol* 2004;23:535–545.
11. Bronshtein M, Lorber A, Berant M, et al. Sonographic diagnosis of fetal vascular rings in early pregnancy. *Am J Cardiol* 1998;81(1):101–103.
12. Zidere V, Tsapakis G, Huggon D, et al. Right aortic arch in the fetus. *Ultrasound Obstet Gynecol* 2006;28:876–881.
13. Rauch R, Rauch A, Koch A, et al. Laterality of the aortic arch anomalies of the subclavian artery—reliable indicators for 22q11.2 deletion syndrome? *Eur J Pediatr* 2004;163:642–645.
14. Tschirch E, Chaoui R, Wauer RR, et al. Perinatal management of right aortic arch with aberrant left subclavian artery associated with critical stenosis of the subclavian artery in a newborn. *Ultrasound Obstet Gynecol* 2005;25(3):296–298.
15. Zapata H, Edwards JE, Titus JL. Aberrant right subclavian artery with left aortic arch—associated cardiac anomalies. *Pediatr Cardiol* 1993;14(3):159–161.
16. Chaoui R, Thiel G, Heling KS. Prevalence of an aberrant right subclavian artery (ARSA) in normal fetuses: a new soft marker for trisomy 21 risk assessment. *Ultrasound Obstet Gynecol* 2005;26:256.
17. Zalel Y, Achiron R, Yagel S, et al. Fetal aberrant right subclavian artery in normal and Down syndrome fetuses. *Ultrasound Obstet Gynecol* 2008;31:25–29.
18. Chaoui R, Heling KS, Sarioglu N, et al. Aberrant right subclavian artery as a new cardiac sign in second- and third-trimester fetuses with Down syndrome. *Am J Obstet Gynecol* 2005;192:257–263.
19. Chaoui R, Rake A, Heling KS. Aortic arch with four vessels: aberrant right subclavian artery. *Ultrasound Obstet Gynecol* 2008;31(1):115–117.
20. Borenstein M, Cavoretto P, Allan L, et al. Aberrant right subclavian artery at 11+0 to 13+6 weeks of gestation in chromosomally normal and abnormal fetuses. *Ultrasound Obstet Gynecol* 2008;31(1):20–24.
21. Goldstein WB. Aberrant right subclavian artery in mongolism. *Am J Roentgenol Radium Ther Nucl Med* 1965;95:131–134.
22. Vibert-Guigue C, Fredouille C, Gricorescu R, et al. Données foetopathologiques sur une serie de fœtus trisomique 21. *Rev Prat Gynecol Obstet* 2006;103:35–40.
23. Chaoui R, Thiel G, Heling KS. Prevalence of an aberrant right subclavian artery (ARSA) in fetuses with chromosomal aberrations. *Ultrasound Obstet Gynecol* 2006;28:414.

FETAL HETEROTAXY WITH LEFT ATRIAL ISOMERISM AND RIGHT ATRIAL ISOMERISM

Definition, Terminology, and Incidence

The embryologic development of abdominal and thoracic structures follows a spatially controlled and coordinated manner leading to well-defined right-sided and left-sided anatomic positions within the body. Right-sided structures include a major part of the liver, the inferior and superior vena cava, the right atrium with its appendage, and a trilobed right lung with an eparterial bronchus (see Table 4-1). Left-sided structures include the stomach, the spleen, the left atrium with its appendage, the pulmonary veins, and a bilobed left lung with a hyparterial bronchus (see Table 4-1). Normal development and positioning of abdominal and thoracic organs is referred to as *situs solitus* (*solitus* means common) for the visceral arrangement, and *levocardia* (heart on the left side) for the thoracic arrangement of organs (1–3). *Situs inversus* refers to a mirror-image arrangement of the visceral and thoracic structures to that of situs solitus. Any arrangement of visceral and/or thoracic organs other than situs solitus or situs inversus is referred to as *situs ambiguous* (unknown or complex situs). Situs ambiguous, unlike situs solitus or inversus, is often associated with various anomalies including anomalies of the spleen, either as asplenia or polysplenia. The term *cardiosplenic syndrome* was first used to describe situs ambiguous associated with anomalies of the spleen. Since the spleen is not always abnormal in situs ambiguous and cannot be reliably used for classification, the term *heterotaxy syndrome* has been suggested (1,2). Heterotaxy syndrome (in Greek, *heteros* means different and *taxis* means arrangement) is a general term that is used to describe the complete spectrum of abnormal organ arrangement including conditions such as asplenia and polysplenia. Since many pathologists observed that the subgroups of asplenia and polysplenia are better classified by describing the atrial morphology, the term *right and left atrial isomerism* (in Greek, *iso* means same and *meros* means turn) has been suggested and used (4) (Fig. 22-1A–C). Heterotaxy of the abdominal organs involves an irregular arrangement of the nonpaired solitary organs. Heterotaxy of the thoracic organs is characterized by a rather symmetric arrangement of the otherwise asymmetric structures including the atria and lungs (3), thus allowing a classification into two main groups: bilateral right-sidedness, also called right atrial isomerism (asplenia, Ivemark syndrome), and bilateral left sidedness, also called left atrial isomerism (polysplenia).

Heterotaxy syndrome is found in between 2.2% and 4.2% of infants with congenital heart disease (5,6). In fetal series, left isomerism is more common than right isomerism. In postnatal series, right isomerism is more common owing to an increased incidence of in utero demise of fetuses with left isomerism due to complete heart block and hydrops (3). Fetal heterotaxy has an increased risk of recurrence in subsequent pregnancies, and that risk has been reported in up to 10% in some series (7). A genetic etiology for heterotaxy recurrence that may include autosomal dominant, autosomal recessive, X-linked, and single gene disorder has been suggested (8–10). Recurrence of heterotaxy in families is not limited to the specific anomaly but may involve the full spectrum including right or left isomerism and situs inversus.

Prenatal Diagnosis of Heterotaxy Associated with Right and Left Atrial Isomerism

Suspecting the presence of isomerism in the fetus may be easy when careful examination of the chest and abdomen is performed, but the accurate classification into right or left isomerism remains challenging as there are no typical pathognomonic cardiac malformations for these anomalies. The identification of the right or left atrial appendage on prenatal ultrasound may be possible in some conditions (11) (Fig. 22-2) but cannot be reliably used for

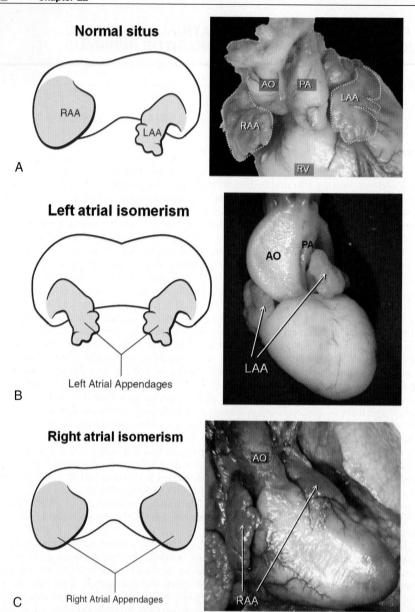

Figure 22-1. A: Anterior view of an anatomic specimen and a drawing of a normal fetal heart demonstrating the right atrial appendage (RAA) with its broad pyramidal shape and its wide junction with the right atrium, and the left atrial appendage (LAA) with its fingerlike hook shape and its narrow junction with the left atrium. **B:** Anterior view of an anatomic specimen and a drawing of a fetal heart with left atrial isomerism demonstrating two morphologic left atrial appendages with their typical fingerlike hook shape and narrow junction with the atria. The dilated aorta (AO) and narrow pulmonary artery (PA) are part of associated cardiac malformation. **C:** Anterior view of an anatomic specimen and a drawing of a fetal heart with right atrial isomerism demonstrating two morphologic right atrial appendages with their typical broad pyramidal shape and wide junction with the atria. The single vessel arising from the heart is a dilated aorta as part of associated cardiac malformation. RV, right ventricle.

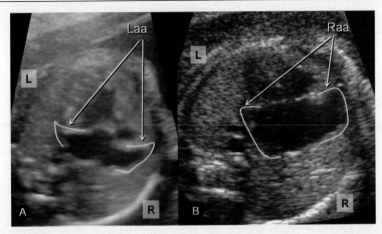

Figure 22-2. Apical four-chamber views of two fetuses with left **(A)** and right **(B)** atrial isomerism. Note the fingerlike hook shape of the bilaterally symmetric left atrial appendages (Laa) in A and the broad pyramidal shape of the bilaterally symmetric right atrial appendages (Raa) in B. It is rather difficult to recognize atrial morphology on ultrasound examination, and the diagnosis should be performed by other ultrasound features. L, left; R, right.

classification (3). One of the most reliable signs remains the evaluation of vessel arrangement in the upper abdomen as is commonly used in postnatal echocardiography (12). In general, a reliable diagnosis of right or left isomerism can be attained by assessing vessel arrangement in the upper abdomen in combination with intrathoracic findings. The main impact on outcome, however, is primarily dependent on the specific cardiac malformation rather than the actual classification. According to the authors' experience, there are three common ways in which fetal isomerism is suspected and confirmed:

1. Fetal heart and stomach on opposing sides of the body, leading to the suspicion of situs abnormality and thus directing targeted ultrasound examinations of the chest and abdomen (Fig. 22-3)

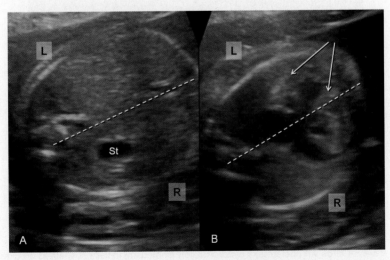

Figure 22-3. A fetus with heterotaxy syndrome initially suspected on ultrasound examination when the stomach (St) is noted in the upper right abdomen **(A)** and the heart in the left side of the chest **(B).** The myocardium is thickened (*arrows*) with a common atrioventricular valve. L, left; R, right.

2. The presence of complex cardiac malformation on an ultrasound examination, prompting a targeted segmental evaluation of the fetal situs and heart

3. The presence of complete heart block or other fetal arrhythmia with or without fetal hydrops on an ultrasound examination, which leads to a targeted evaluation of cardiac and abdominal anatomy (Fig. 22-4)

The main prenatal ultrasound features for left and right isomerism are presented in the following sections.

Ultrasound Findings in Left Atrial Isomerism (Polysplenia)

Left atrial isomerism is associated with the presence of "double" left-sided structures with the underdevelopment or absence of right-sided structures. One of the most common associations with left isomerism is the absence of the intrahepatic part of the inferior vena cava, a finding that is present in 80% to 90% of cases (2,3). The inferior vena cava is interrupted at its suprarenal part and connects with the azygos (or hemiazygos) venous system, which drains the abdominal venous blood to the heart. The azygos (or hemiazygos) vein is then dilated with its typical course side by side and slightly posterior to the descending aorta along the spine. The dilated azygos passes through the diaphragm and typically drains into the superior vena cava or less commonly to a persistent left superior vena cava in the upper chest (1). This condition, termed *interruption of the inferior vena cava with azygos continuation*, can be detected as a "double vessel" sign in a cross section of the upper abdomen (12,13) (Fig. 22-5) or in a four-chamber view behind the heart (Fig. 22-6) (14). A parasagittal view of the abdomen and chest can also demonstrate the azygos vein posterior to the descending aorta (Fig. 22-7), and color Doppler can demonstrate the azygos vein draining into the superior vena cava in the three-vessel view (Fig. 22-8) and in a sagittal view of the chest. The hepatic veins may connect directly into the right atrium in the absence of an inferior vena cava.

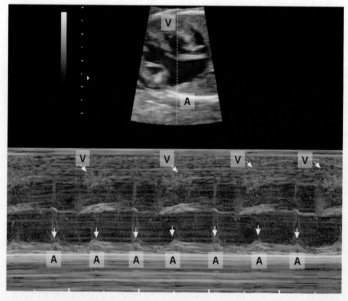

Figure 22-4. A fetus with heterotaxy syndrome (left isomerism) initially suspected on ultrasound examination by the presence of heart block and congenital heart disease (atrioventricular septal defect). M-mode ultrasound shows a regular atrial (A) rhythm (*vertical arrows*) and a slow ventricular (V) rhythm (*oblique arrows*).

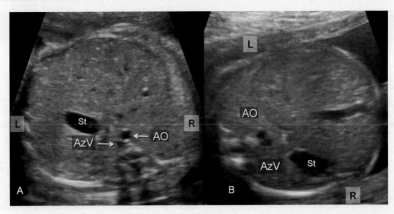

Figure 22-5. Left atrial isomerism in two fetuses showing different positions of the stomach (St) in the abdomen: left-sided stomach in **A** and right-sided stomach in **B.** The position of the stomach in the abdomen is not of diagnostic importance in heterotaxy syndrome. The presence of a dilated azygos vein (AzV) (double vessels in front of the spine) in both fetuses suggests the diagnosis of left atrial isomerism. AO, descending aorta; St, stomach; L, left; R, right.

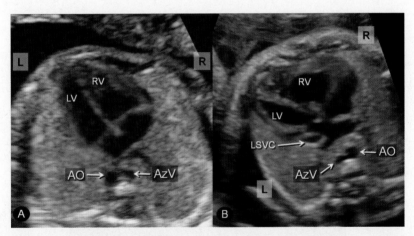

Figure 22-6. Four-chamber views in two fetuses: one with normal cardiac anatomy **(A)** and the other one with complex cardiac malformation **(B).** Note the presence of double vessels in front of the spine in both fetuses (the azygos vein [AzV] and the descending aorta [AO]), which suggests interrupted inferior vena cava and left isomerism in both fetuses. Cardiac malformation in B includes discrepancy of left and right ventricular width due to aortic coarctation and a persistent left superior vena cava (LSVC). L, left; R, right; RV, right ventricle; LV, left ventricle.

Another feature of left isomerism is the absence of the morphologic right atrium with its sinus node. This can lead in many conditions to bradyarrhythmia, commonly as complete heart block, seen in 40% to 70% of cases (2,3,15). The combination of complete heart block with a complex cardiac anomaly, especially in an interrupted vena cava with azygos continuation, is typical for the presence of left atrial isomerism (1). The presence of complete heart block with a complex cardiac malformation may often lead to cardiac failure and fetal hydrops (Fig. 22-9B) in more than 30% of cases (3,15) and is responsible for the high rate of in utero demise in these fetuses.

Other abnormalities in left isomerism include a right-sided stomach, atresia of the upper gastrointestinal tract such as duodenal or jejunal atresia, a symmetric left-sided or midline

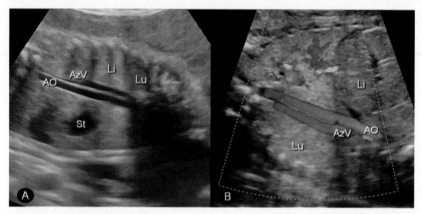

Figure 22-7. Coronal planes of the chest and abdomen in two fetuses with left atrial isomerism and interrupted inferior vena cava showing the azygos vein (AzV) running parallel and posterior to the descending aorta (AO). Color Doppler in **B** shows reverse direction of blood flow in the azygos vein (toward the heart) to that in the aorta (away from the heart). St, stomach; Li, liver; Lu, lung.

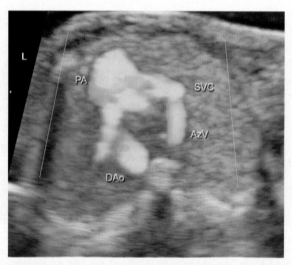

Figure 22-8. Three-vessel view of a fetus with left isomerism, interrupted vena cava, and azygos vein (AzV) continuation. Note the drainage of the azygos vein into the superior vena cava (SVC) demonstrated in this view. PA, pulmonary artery; DAo, descending aorta.

liver, and, rarely, absence of the gallbladder. The presence of multiple spleens (polysplenia) has been reported in up to 96% of infants with left isomerism (3,7), but antenatal diagnosis of polysplenia is not reliable on ultrasound. The presence of a splenic artery on color Doppler prenatally, however (Fig. 22-9), can confirm the presence of one or multiple spleens, which may help in classifying the abnormality as left atrial isomerism (16).

The left atrial appendage, which can be identified near the pulmonary trunk in normal conditions, is narrow and hook shaped (Fig. 22-1A). In left atrial isomerism, both atria are morphologically left with their corresponding appendages and can be seen in a plane slightly cranial to the four-chamber view (Fig. 22-1B). The cardiac axis is often to the left or to the middle of the chest and occasionally dextroversion is found. Interestingly, intracardiac

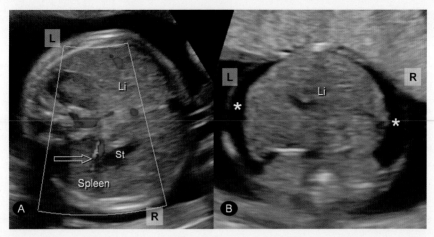

Figure 22-9. Two fetuses with suspected left atrial isomerism. Color Doppler at the level of the abdominal circumference in fetus **A** with a right-sided stomach (St) shows the splenic artery and vein (*open arrow*), which confirms the presence of one or multiple spleens and thus rules out asplenia. The fetus in **B** has left isomerism with heart block and fetal hydrops. Note the symmetric liver (Li) in the transverse view of the upper abdomen and the presence of ascites (*asterisk*), which is a poor prognostic sign. L, left; R, right.

malformations may be absent in left isomerism, which is rarely the case in right isomerism. When a cardiac anomaly is present, it is generally of a biventricular type, and most commonly (50%) an unbalanced atrioventricular septal defect (AVSD) (2) (see Chapter 15). In AVSD associated with complete heart block, the myocardium may be hypertrophied with cardiomegaly (3). The origin of the great vessels is generally concordant and double outlet right ventricle can occur in combination with a ventricular septal defect or AVSD. The aorta and pulmonary trunk may show outflow tract obstruction (aortic coarctation, pulmonary stenosis, and atresia). Left superior vena cava is found in 50% to 60% of the cases (see Chapter 23), and an abnormal pulmonary venous connection at the cardiac level is occasionally seen but not as frequently as in right isomerism (2). Table 22-1 summarizes anatomic findings of left atrial isomerism, right atrial isomerism, and situs inversus.

Ultrasound Findings in Right Atrial Isomerism (Asplenia)

Right atrial isomerism is associated with the presence of "double" right-sided structures with the underdevelopment or absence of left-sided structures. The upper abdomen is often characterized by a large liver in a more central position with a left-sided or right-sided stomach. Typically in right atrial isomerism, the position of the inferior vena cava is anterior and on the same side of the descending aorta, both being either on the left or right side of the spine (12), a condition termed juxtaposition of the aorta and inferior vena cava (Fig. 22-10). Autopsy studies noted an absent spleen (asplenia) in 74% of cases of right isomerism (3), and in the absence of a spleen, the authors observed the stomach to be displaced posteriorly in the abdomen with an absence of a splenic artery on color Doppler (16). Bowel malrotation and atresia may occur due to a symmetric liver and nonfixation of the gastrointestinal tract. Herniation of a midline-positioned stomach into the thoracic cavity occurs in up to 25% of right isomerism and can be noted on ultrasound in the third trimester of pregnancy (1,2,17).

The cardiac axis is often to the right but can be to the left or midline, and dextroversion is more common in right than left atrial isomerism. Intracardiac anomalies are present in nearly all cases of right isomerism and are generally more severe than those found in left isomerism (Fig. 22-11) (18). There is no pathognomonic cardiac anomaly for right isomerism, but the association with an unbalanced AVSD is present in up to 80% to 90% of cases with one-chamber dominance, detected as a univentricular atrioventricular connection (2,3,19) (Fig. 22-11). Abnormal ventriculoarterial connections (double outlet ventricle, malposition of

TABLE 22-1	Likely Findings in Fetuses with Left Atrial Isomerism, Right Atrial Isomerism, and Situs Inversus

	Left atrial isomerism	Right atrial isomerism	Situs inversus
Visceral findings			
Liver	Symmetric, commonly left-sided	Symmetric, large, midline or right-sided	Left-sided
Aorta and IVC	Azygos continuity with IVC interruption	Juxtaposition of aorta and IVC either on right or left side	Aorta right and posterior, IVC left and anterior
Gastrointestinal	Stomach commonly right-sided, can be on the left side. Upper gastrointestinal obstruction	Stomach can be in the middle or right- or left-sided. Hiatus hernia with stomach in lower thorax can occur	Stomach on the right
Spleen[a]	Polysplenia	Asplenia	Normal spleen, right-sided
Thoracic findings			
Bronchus[a]	Long bronchus, hyparterial in both lungs	Short bronchus, eparterial in both lungs	Left bronchus hyparterial and right bronchus eparterial
Lung[a]	Both bilobed	Both trilobed	Right lung bilobed, left lung trilobed
Atrium[a]	Two left atrial appendages hook shaped with a narrow junction	Two right atrial appendages pyramidal shaped with a broad junction	Right atrial appendage hook shaped and left atrial appendage pyramidal shaped
Atrioventricular connection	Commonly biventricular connection	Commonly univentricular connection	Normal
Atrioventricular septal defect	In 80%–90% of cases, commonly unbalanced	In 40%–50% of cases, often unbalanced	Absent
Ventriculoarterial connection	Commonly concordant. Left- or right-sided outflow obstruction may occur	Commonly discordant. Pulmonary atresia or stenosis is common	Concordant
Abnormal pulmonary venous connection	Occasional	Common	Absent
Left superior vena cava	Common finding	Common finding	Rare
Bradycardia, heart block	Common finding	Absent	Absent
Hydrops and in utero demise	Common finding	Absent	Absent

IVC, inferior vena cava
[a]Difficult to detect on prenatal ultrasound.

the great arteries) associated with pulmonary stenosis or atresia are more commonly seen in right isomerism. One of the most complex cardiac malformations in right isomerism is the presence of partial or total abnormal pulmonary venous connection (TAPVC) (see Chapter 23), due to the absence of the anatomic left atrium where the pulmonary veins normally connect (Fig. 22-12). In one series of right isomerism, supracardiac TAPVC was observed in 30%, infradiaphragmatic in 25%, cardiac in 30%, and mixed in 15% (3). The presence of TAPVC, which can be overlooked prenatally, is associated with a worse prognosis (19,20).

The right atrium is defined by the presence of the right atrial appendage, which is wide, has a pyramidal shape, and has a broad junction with the right atrium (Fig. 22-1A). In right atrial isomerism, both atria are morphologically right with their corresponding appendages as

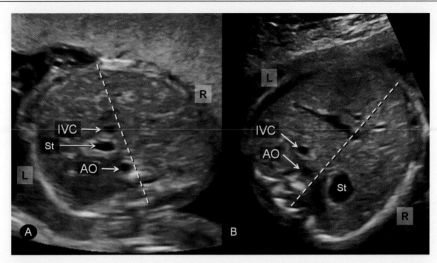

Figure 22-10. Right atrial isomerism in two fetuses showing different positions of the stomach (St), left-sided (or rather midline) in **A** and right-sided in **B.** The stomach position is therefore not of diagnostic help in heterotaxy syndromes. An important pathognomonic sign of right isomerism is the juxtaposition (both vessels on the same side) of inferior vena cava (IVC) and aorta (AO), which is demonstrated in both fetuses. L, left; R, right.

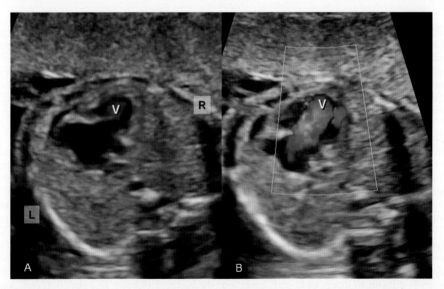

Figure 22-11. Complex cardiac anomaly as "single ventricle" (V) and dextrocardia on two-dimensional **(A)** and color Doppler **(B)** ultrasound in a fetus with right isomerism. Right isomerism is associated with more severe cardiac anomalies, typically univentricular, than left isomerism. L, left; R, right.

can be seen on ultrasound examination (11), albeit with difficulty (Fig. 22-1C). Right isomerism is also associated with the presence of a left persistent superior vena cava in up to 60% of the cases, and the left superior vena cava may enter the left-sided atrium directly (3). Table 22-1 summarizes anatomic findings in left atrial isomerism, right atrial isomerism, and situs inversus.

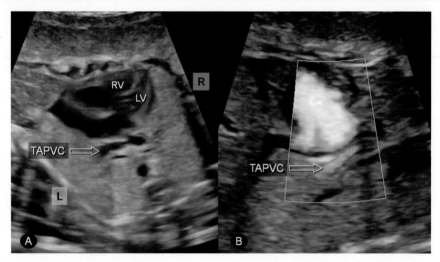

Figure 22-12. Dextrocardia, unbalanced atrioventricular septal defect, and total anomalous pulmonary venous connection (TAPVC) in a fetus with right atrial isomerism. **A:** Note the presence of a confluent vessel (*open arrow*) as a collecting vein behind the posterior atrium consistent with TAPVC, a common association with right isomerism. **B:** Color Doppler shows antegrade flow in the confluent vein with absent connection to the atrium. L, left; R, right; RV, right ventricle; LV, left ventricle.

Color Doppler

Color Doppler can help in the diagnosis of cardiac malformation and vessel arrangements, which may help in the differentiation of right or left atrial isomerism. This includes assessment of venous connections, great vessel relationship and patency, atrioventricular valve regurgitation, and others, as described in related chapters (see Chapters 15, 17, 19, 20, and 23). Furthermore, the use of color Doppler may help in the identification of a spleen when a splenic artery is seen (16).

Early Gestation

Right and left isomerism can be detected in early gestation, at the 11- to 14-week ultrasound, owing to a thickened nuchal translucency in combination with cardiac anomaly or when hydrops with complete heart block is noted (3,21). Abnormal situs on ultrasound may represent the first clue to the presence of right or left isomerism in early gestation (Fig. 22-13). The presence of complete heart block in early gestation should raise suspicion for left atrial isomerism, since Sjögren antibodies are rarely the cause of bradyarrhythmias in early pregnancy. The detection of AVSD and single ventricle is feasible in early gestation, and the suspicion of such an anomaly, especially in combination with a right-sided stomach, should suggest the presence of heterotaxy. The arrangement of the abdominal vessels either as juxtaposition of the aorta and inferior vena cava or as interruption of the inferior vena cava with azygos continuity is difficult to diagnose at early gestation; the addition of color Doppler, however, may assist in the diagnosis. The assessment of pulmonary venous connections is possible but rather difficult, and such an early diagnosis of abnormal pulmonary venous connection has not been reported to date.

Three-dimensional Ultrasound

Rendering of the interrupted inferior vena cava with azygos continuation in a three-dimensional volume has been reported using inversion mode with power Doppler or glass body mode (22) (Fig. 22-14A). Surface rendering may play a role in identifying atrial morphology by demonstrating the shape of the atrial appendage. Furthermore, the relationship of the various heart and stomach positions in the chest and abdomen, respectively, can be achieved with the minimum mode (Fig. 22-14B).

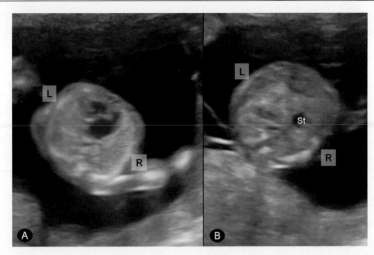

Figure 22-13. A fetus at 14 weeks' gestation with isomerism detected due to the discrepant positions of the heart **(A)** and stomach (St) **(B)**. A cardiac anomaly is recognizable in the four-chamber view in A. L, left; R, right.

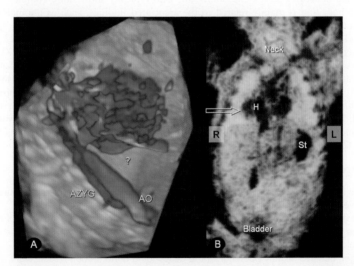

Figure 22-14. **A:** Three-dimensional ultrasound in glass body mode of a parasagittal view in a fetus with left isomerism and interrupted inferior vena cava with azygos continuity. The aorta (AO) and azygos vein (AZYG) are side by side, with different flow direction. The inferior vena cava is not identified (location marked by the "?" sign). **B:** Another fetus with isomerism demonstrating in transparent minimum mode the anterior-posterior projection with a discordant position of the heart (H) (*open arrow*) in the right chest and stomach (St) in the upper left abdomen. L, left; R, right.

Associated Cardiac and Extracardiac Findings

Associated cardiac malformations are numerous and have been described in detail earlier in this chapter (Table 22-1). Associated extracardiac anomalies primarily involve the abdominal cavity with various gastrointestinal anomalies such as bowel atresia or bowel malrotation

(23). The nonfixation of the stomach may lead to its herniation into the thorax. The most severe extracardiac malformation, observed in left isomerism, is extrahepatic biliary atresia with the absence of the gallbladder. The authors, however, have not observed this condition on prenatal ultrasound. Anomalies of the face, brain, or limbs can occur but are not typical. Interestingly, chromosomal aberrations such as trisomies are nearly absent in this group, and occasionally other chromosomal aberrations such as disomies or 22q11 microdeletion have been reported.

Differential Diagnosis

Differential diagnosis of isomerism includes situs inversus with dextrocardia or situs inversus with levocardia. The detection of AVSD with isomerism requires its differentiation from isolated AVSD given wide differences in chromosomal aneuploidy risks. Another challenging differential diagnosis to isomerism is dextrocardia with corrected transposition in rare association with heart block.

Prognosis and Outcome

The prognosis of right and left isomerism detected in the fetus is generally poor, owing to the severity of the cases detected antenatally. Fetuses with left isomerism and heart block are at risk for in utero death following the development of hydrops (24). On the other hand, newborns with left isomerism and a mild form of cardiac anomaly have an excellent prognosis. In such mild conditions, visualization of the gallbladder will rule out associated biliary atresia (25).

Outcome of fetuses with right isomerism, who typically show more complex anomalies, is generally poor and is mainly related to the associated findings, such as anomalous pulmonary venous connection, pulmonary atresia, or single ventricle anatomy (24). In a study involving 71 fetuses with heterotaxy, including 48 with left atrial isomerism and 23 with right atrial isomerism, 46 (32 with left isomerism and 14 with right isomerism) out of 71 (65%) of the mothers chose to continue the pregnancy (24). Fetal left isomerism was associated with a mortality rate of 31%, and 3 out of the 14 with right isomerism were alive at 48 months' follow-up (24). In addition, right isomerism with asplenia is associated with an increased risk for infection in postnatal life. Survival of actively managed children with left isomerism is typically significantly better than for those with right isomerism (26). Most neonates with left isomerism undergo successful biventricular cardiac surgery, unlike their counterparts with right isomerism (26).

▓ KEY POINTS: LEFT ATRIAL ISOMERISM

■ Left atrial isomerism is associated with the presence of "double" left-sided structures with the underdevelopment or absence of right-sided structures.
■ Absence of the intrahepatic part of the inferior vena cava occurs in 80% to 90% of cases.
■ When the inferior vena cava is interrupted, the azygos venous system drains the abdominal venous blood to the heart.
■ The azygos courses slightly posterior to the descending aorta (double vessel sign).
■ Complete heart block occurs in 40% to 70% of cases.
■ The presence of multiple spleens (polysplenia) has been reported in the majority of infants.
■ Left superior vena cava is found in 50% to 60% of cases.

▓ KEY POINTS: RIGHT ATRIAL ISOMERISM

■ Right atrial isomerism is associated with the presence of "double" right-sided structures with the underdevelopment or absence of left-sided structures.
■ Juxtaposition of the aorta and inferior vena cava occurs in right atrial isomerism.
■ Absent spleen (asplenia) is seen in 74% of cases.
■ Herniation of a midline-positioned stomach into the thoracic cavity occurs in up to 25% of cases.
■ Intracardiac anomalies are present in nearly all cases and are more severe than in left atrial isomerism.

- There is a common association with abnormal pulmonary venous connection.
- Left superior vena cava persists in up to 60% of cases.
- Prognosis is generally worse than that of left atrial isomerism.

SITUS INVERSUS

Definition, Spectrum of disease, and Incidence

Situs inversus is defined as a mirror-image arrangement of the thoracic and abdominal organs to situs solitus (normal anatomy). Partial situs inversus can be either limited to the abdominal organs and is generally called *situs inversus with levocardia* or limited to the chest and is called *dextrocardia*. An increased incidence of cardiac anomalies, in the order of 0.3% to 5%, is found in fetuses and newborns with situs inversus (27). Cardiac anomalies in situs inversus, however, occur in a much lower frequency than in left or right atrial isomerism and do not involve the venoatrial connections. Situs inversus is also commonly associated with Kartagener syndrome, an autosomal dominant disease with primary ciliary dyskinesia, which results in recurrent respiratory infections and reduced fertility in adult life (28,29). About 50% of patients with Kartagener syndrome have situs inversus (28,29).

The true incidence of situs inversus is unknown, but it can range from between 1 in 2500 and 1 in 20,000 live births (2). Situs inversus commonly remains undetected in life until it is diagnosed by imaging of a physical examination for unrelated reasons.

Ultrasound Findings

Determining fetal situs should be part of every ultrasound examination performed in the second and third trimester of pregnancy, and the technical aspects of situs determination on ultrasound are explained in detail in Chapter 4. In situs inversus, the liver and inferior vena cava are on the left side of the fetus, and the stomach, descending aorta, and heart are on the right side (Fig. 22-15). The heart axis points to the right anterior thorax, a condition called dextrocardia, and since the inferior vena cava and the right atrium are concordant, the right atrium and ventricle are on the left anterior aspect of the chest, and the left atrium and ventricle are on the right posterior aspect of the chest.

Color Doppler
Color Doppler may be of help when structural anomalies are suspected and to accurately visualize the venous connections.

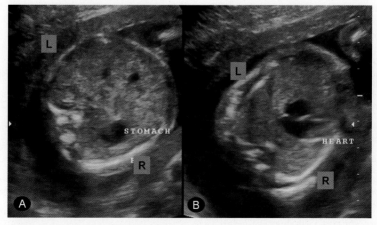

Figure 22-15. Situs inversus in a fetus with stomach **(A)** and heart **(B)** on the right side and no additional cardiac or venous anomalies. L, left; R, right.

Early Gestation

Partial and complete situs inversus can be detected in early gestation. The transvaginal approach to determining fetal situs may be challenging given the difficulty inherent in endovaginal probe orientation. Suspected situs abnormalities should be confirmed at a later gestation.

Three-dimensional Ultrasound

Three-dimensional ultrasound may be of help in documenting the concordance or discordance of heart chambers and upper abdominal structures in a volume data set. In addition, the projection in minimum mode can be used to show the relationship of the heart and stomach in a single view.

Associated Cardiac and Extracardiac Findings

Associated cardiac anomalies with situs inversus include ventricular septal defect, tetralogy of Fallot, double outlet right ventricle, and complete or corrected transposition of the arteries. Extracardiac malformations are not typically found in situs inversus, but an association exists with Kartagener syndrome as highlighted earlier in this chapter.

Differential Diagnosis

Differential diagnosis for situs inversus includes right and left isomerism. Another differential diagnosis is normal anatomy mistaken for situs inversus due to wrong orientation of the ultrasound probe or inexperience of the operator during the ultrasound examination. Differentiating dextrocardia from situs inversus is discussed in Chapter 4.

Prognosis and Outcome

Prognosis is related to the associated cardiac and extracardiac findings. Isolated situs inversus cases have an excellent prognosis with an uneventful prenatal and postnatal course. The association with Kartagener syndrome, which can be diagnosed postnatally, will have long-term implications with regard to recurrent pulmonary infections and infertility.

▨ KEY POINTS: SITUS INVERSUS

■ Situs inversus is defined as a mirror-image arrangement of the thoracic and abdominal organs to situs solitus (normal anatomy).

■ Partial situs inversus can involve the abdominal organs, called situs inversus with levocardia, or the heart, called dextrocardia.

■ An increased incidence of cardiac anomalies is found in fetuses and newborns with situs inversus.

■ Situs inversus is also commonly associated with Kartagener syndrome.

■ Determining fetal situs should be part of every ultrasound examination performed in the second and third trimester of pregnancy.

■ Prognosis is related to the associated cardiac and extracardiac findings.

References

1. Chaoui R. Cardiac malpositions and syndromes with right or left atrial isomerism. In: Yagel S, Silvermann N, Gembruch U, eds. *Fetal cardiology.* London, New York: Martin Dunitz, 2003;173–182.
2. Yoo SJ, Friedberg MK, Jaeggi E. Abnormal visceral and atrial situs and congenital heart disease. In: Yagel S, Silvermann N, Gembruch U, eds. *Fetal cardiology,* 2nd ed. London, New York: Martin Dunitz, 2003;265–280.
3. Sharland GK, Cook A. Heterotaxy syndromes/isomerism of the atrial appendages. In: Allan L, Hornberger LK, Sharland GK, eds. *Textbook of fetal cardiology.* London: Greenwich Medical Media Limited, 2000;333–346.
4. Sapire DW, Ho SY, Anderson RH, et al. Diagnosis and significance of atrial isomerism. *Am J Cardiol* 1986;58(3):342–346.
5. Ferencz C, Rubin JD, Loffredo CA, et al. *The epidemiology of congenital heart disease: the Baltimore–Washington Infant Study 1981–1989. Perspectives in pediatric cardiology,* Vol. 4. Mount Kisco, NY: Futura Publishing, 1993.
6. Fyler DC, Buckley LP, Hellenbrand WE, et al. Report of the New England Regional Infant Cardiac Programme. *Pediatrics* 1980;65(suppl):376–461.
7. Allan LD, Crawford DC, Chitta SK, et al. The familial recurrence of congenital heart disease in a prospective series of mothers referred for fetal echocardiography. *Am J Cardiol* 1986;58:334–337.

8. Bowers PN, Martina M, Yost HJ. The genes of left-right development and heterotaxia. *Semin Perinatol* 1996;20:577–588.
9. Zhu L, Belmont JW, Ware SM. Genetics of human heterotaxias. *Eur J Hum Genet* 2006;14:17–25.
10. Morelli SH, Young L, Reid B, et al. Clinical analysis of families with heart, midline and laterality defects. *Am J Med Genet* 2001;101:388–392.
11. Berg C, Geipel A, Kohl T, et al. Fetal echocardiographic evaluation of atrial morphology and the prediction of laterality in cases of heterotaxy syndromes. *Ultrasound Obstet Gynecol* 2005;26:538–545.
12. Huhta J, Smallhorn JF, Macartney FJ. Two-dimensional echocardiographic diagnosis of situs. *Br Heart J* 1982;48:97–108.
13. Sheley RC, Nyberg DA, Kapur R. Azygous continuation of the interrupted inferior vena cava: a clue to prenatal diagnosis of the cardiosplenic syndromes. *J Ultrasound Med* 1995;14:381–387.
14. Berg C, Georgiadis M, Geipel A, et al. The area behind the heart in the four-chamber view and the quest for congenital heart defects. *Ultrasound Obstet Gynecol* 2007;30(5):721–727.
15. Berg C, Geipel A, Kamil D, et al. The syndrome of left isomerism: sonographic findings and outcome in prenatally diagnosed cases. *J Ultrasound Med* 2005;24:921–931.
16. Abuhamad AZ, Robinson JN, Bogdan D, et al. Color Doppler of the splenic artery in the prenatal diagnosis of heterotaxic syndromes. *Am J Perinatol* 1999;16(9):469–473.
17. Wang JK, Chang MH, Li YW, et al. Association of hiatus hernia with asplenia syndrome. *Eur J Pediatr* 1993;152:418–420.
18. Freedom RM, Jaeggi ET, Lim JS, et al. Hearts with isomerism of the right atrial appendages—one of the worst forms of disease in 2005. *Cardiol Young* 2005;15:554–567.
19. Berg C, Geipel A, Kamil D, et al. The syndrome of right isomerism—prenatal diagnosis and outcome. *Ultraschall Med* 2006;27:225–233.
20. Batukan C, Schwabe M, Heling KS, et al. Prenatal diagnosis of right atrial isomerism (asplenia syndrome): case report. *Ultraschall Med* 2005;26:234–238.
21. Baschat A, Gembruch U, Knöpfle G, et al. First trimester heart block: a marker for cardiac anomaly. *Ultrasound Obstet Gynecol* 1999;14:311–314.
22. Espinoza J, Concalves LF, Lee W, et al. A novel method to improve prenatal diagnosis of abnormal systemic venous connections using three- and four-dimensional ultrasonography and 'inversion mode'. *Ultrasound Obstet Gynecol* 2005;25:428–434.
23. Ticho BS, Goldstein AM, Van Praagh R. Extracardiac anomalies in the heterotaxy syndromes with focus on anomalies of midline-associated structures. *Am J Cardiol* 2000;85:729–734.
24. Taketazu M, Lougheed J, Yoo SJ, et al. Spectrum of cardiovascular disease, accuracy of diagnosis, and outcome in fetal heterotaxy syndrome. *Am J Cardiol* 2006;97:720–724.
25. Carmi R, Magee CA, Neill CA, et al. Extrahepatic biliary atresia and associated anomalies: etiologic heterogeneity suggested by distinctive patterns of associations. *Am J Med Genet* 1993;45:683–693.
26. Lim JSL, McCrindle BW, Smallhorn JF, et al. Clinical features, management, and outcome of children with fetal and postnatal diagnoses of isomerism syndromes. *Circulation* 2005;112:2454–2461.
27. De Vore GS, Sarti DA, Siassi B, et al. Prenatal diagnosis of cardiovascular malformations in the fetus with situs inversus viscerum during the second trimester of pregnancy. *J Clin Ultrasound* 1986;14:454–457.
28. Bush A, Cole P, Hariri M, et al. Primary ciliary dyskinesia: diagnosis and standards of care. *Eur Respir J* 1998;12:982–988.
29. Holzmann D, Ott PM, Felix H. Diagnostic approach to primary ciliary dyskinesia: a review. *Eur J Pediatr* 2000;159(1–2):95–98.

ANOMALIES OF SYSTEMIC AND PULMONARY VENOUS CONNECTIONS

INTRODUCTION

Anomalies of systemic and pulmonary venous connections can occur as isolated anomalies or as part of simple (atrial septal defect) or complex cardiac malformations (heterotaxy syndrome). Prenatal detection of venous anomalies increased in the last several years facilitated by the advent of high-resolution gray-scale and color Doppler ultrasound. Systemic venous malformations include anomalies of the inferior and superior vena cava and coronary sinus. Persistent left superior vena cava, which is presented in this chapter, and interruption of the inferior vena cava with azygos continuation (see Chapter 22) are two systemic venous malformations commonly found in fetal and postnatal series. Other systemic venous malformations including absence of the right superior vena cava (1) and unroofed coronary sinus are rare conditions and are not discussed in this chapter. Anomalies of the fetal abdominal veins, such as the ductus venosus or the umbilical vein (2,3) are beyond the scope of this book. Anomalies of the pulmonary venous system including total or partial anomalous connections are discussed in this chapter.

PERSISTENT LEFT SUPERIOR VENA CAVA

Definition, Spectrum of Disease, and Incidence

In the embryo, the involution of the left superior vena cava, which becomes the ligament of Marshall, follows the development of the left innominate vein at the seventh week of gestation (4). Persistent left superior vena cava (LSVC) is thought to result from failure of the left anterior and common cardinal veins to involute (4). The persistent LSVC, or simply called LSVC, starts at the junction of the left jugular and subclavian veins, runs anterior to the aortic arch and left pulmonary artery and on the lateral border of the left atrium. LSVC joins the coronary sinus in the posterior left atrioventricular groove (Fig. 23-1) and drains into the right atrium in 92% of cases or into the left atrium in the remainder of cases when the coronary sinus is partially or completely unroofed (5). LSVC is the most common variant of the thoracic venous system and is reported in about 0.3% to 0.5% of the population (6–8). LSVC coexists with congenital heart disease in up to 5% to 9% of infants and up to 9% of fetuses with cardiac malformations (6–9). Cardiac malformations commonly associated with LSVC include heterotaxy syndrome, left ventricular tract obstructive defects, and conotruncal malformations (9–12). The right superior vena cava can also be absent in association with LSVC (13,14).

Ultrasound Findings

Gray Scale

The diagnosis of a LSVC may be easy to make if the operator is aware of the anatomic course of the LSVC and its diagnostic planes in the chest. Identifying a LSVC can be achieved in three transverse planes and in one longitudinal plane (Fig. 23-2A); a plane just inferior to the four-chamber view (Fig. 23-2B); the four-chamber view (Fig. 23-3); the three-vessel-trachea view (Fig. 23-4); and a left parasagittal view (Fig. 23-5). In the four-chamber view, LSVC can be identified in cross section at the left border of the left atrium (Fig. 23-3). In a plane slightly posterior to the four-chamber view, a dilated coronary sinus can be noted in the region of the mitral valve (Fig. 23-2B) (12). Under normal conditions, the coronary sinus has a diameter of 1 to 3 mm, courses perpendicular to the interatrial septum, and opens into the posterior wall of the right atrium. In the presence of a LSVC with or without associated cardiac abnormality, the coronary sinus is dilated and measures between 3 and 7 mm

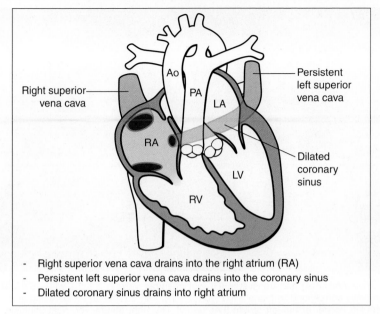

- Right superior vena cava drains into the right atrium (RA)
- Persistent left superior vena cava drains into the coronary sinus
- Dilated coronary sinus drains into right atrium

Figure 23-1. Persistent left superior vena cava. RV, right ventricle; LV, left ventricle; LA, left atrium; PA, pulmonary artery; Ao, aorta.

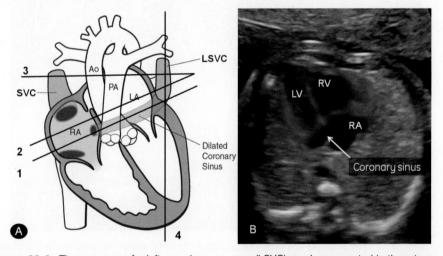

Figure 23-2. The presence of a left superior vena cava (LSVC) can be suspected in three transverse planes as shown in **A** (planes 1, 2, and 3) and confirmed in a parasagittal plane (plane 4). **B:** Corresponds to plane 1 in A. Plane 1 is a plane that is inferior to the four-chamber view and demonstrates a dilated coronary sinus which is the common site of draining of the LSVC. Compare with Figure 5-2 which demonstrates a normal coronary sinus. Plane 2 correspond to the four-chamber view, plane 3 is at the level of the three-vessel-trachea view, and plane 4 is a parasagittal view (see text for details). RA, right atrium; LA, left atrium; RV, right ventricle; LV, left ventricle; PA, pulmonary artery; Ao, aorta; SVC, superior vena cava.

in diameter (Fig. 23-2B) (12). In the three-vessel-trachea view, the LSVC is seen as a fourth vessel located left to the pulmonary artery (Figs. 23-4 and 23-6) (11). Finally, a left parasagittal plane of the thorax and neck can demonstrate the LSVC draining into the coronary sinus (Fig. 23-5).

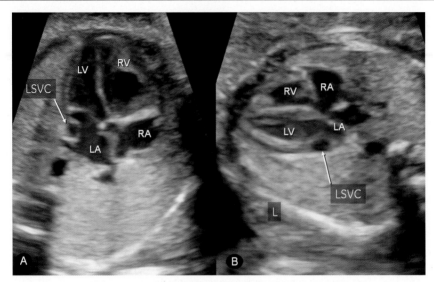

Figure 23-3. Apical **(A)** and transverse **(B)** four-chamber view in a fetus with LSVC. The four-chamber views correspond to plane 2 in Figure 23-2A. The LSVC can be identified in cross section at the left border of the left atrium (LA) (*arrow*). RA, right atrium; RV, right ventricle; LV, left ventricle; L, left.

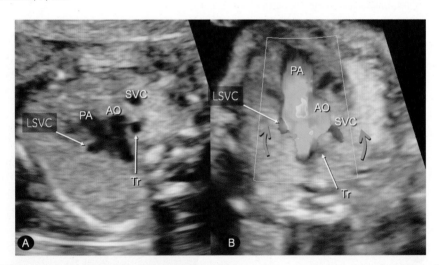

Figure 23-4. Gray scale **(A)** and color Doppler **(B)** at the three-vessel-trachea view in a fetus with left superior vena cava (LSVC). The three-vessel-trachea view corresponds to plane 3 in Figure 23-2A. In this view, which represents the easiest approach to the identification of the LSVC, the LSVC is identified as a fourth vessel on the left side of the pulmonary artery (PA). Color Doppler with low velocities **(B)** can demonstrate blood flow, in the same direction (*red arrows*), in both LSVC and superior vena cava (SVC) on either side of the ductal and aortic arches. AO, aorta; Tr, trachea.

Color Doppler

Color Doppler is not essential for the diagnosis of LSVC but may help in confirming the direction of blood flow toward the heart in the parasagittal plane (Fig. 23-5). Color Doppler applied to the dilated coronary sinus shows blood flow toward the right atrium. Color Doppler can also help in identifying or confirming the absence of a left innominate vein between the left and right superior vena cava.

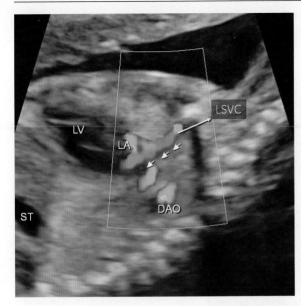

Figure 23-5. Left parasagittal plane in color Doppler confirming the presence of left superior vena cava (LSVC). This plane corresponds to plane 4 in Figure 23-2A. The LSVC course is recognized on color Doppler, which confirms blood flow direction from the head and left arm toward the heart as downstream flow (*small arrows*). ST, stomach; LV, left ventricle; DAO, descending aorta.

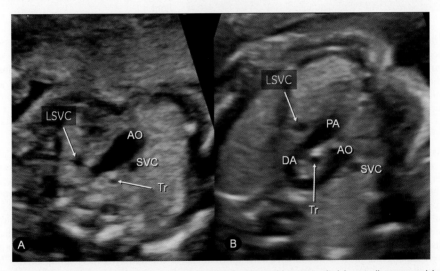

Figure 23-6. Three-vessel-trachea views in two fetuses with congenital heart disease and left superior vena cava (LSVC). Fetus **A** has tricuspid atresia with ventricular septal defect and pulmonary stenosis (not shown in this plane). A dilated transverse aortic arch is visualized surrounded by a right (SVC) and LSVC. Fetus **B** has a right aortic arch, a left ductus arteriosus with the U-sign (see Chapter 21) surrounding the trachea. A right (SVC) and LSVC are present as well. AO, aorta; PA, pulmonary artery; DA, ductus arteriosus; Tr, trachea.

Early Gestation

The detection of LSVC is difficult at 11 to 15 weeks' gestation. If LSVC is suspected, the three-vessel-trachea view provides the best option for diagnosis in early gestation (Fig. 23-7). Increased nuchal translucency has been shown in 29% of fetuses with LSVC irrespective of its association with other cardiac malformations or heterotaxy syndrome (9).

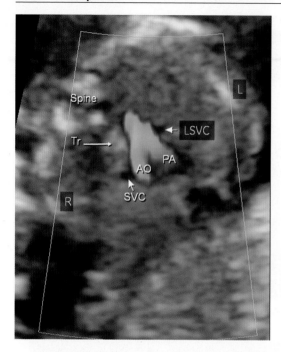

Figure 23-7. Left superior vena cava (LSVC) in a fetus at 15 weeks' gestation shown on color Doppler at the three-vessel-trachea view. Note that color is not seen in the LSVC and the right superior vena cava (SVC) as high-velocity scales were applied during this examination. PA, pulmonary artery; AO, aorta; Tr, trachea; L, left; R, right.

Three-Dimensional Ultrasound

Because LSVC can be demonstrated in different transverse planes, tomographic imaging of three-dimensional volumes can display the LSVC in multiple levels. Surface mode in the four-chamber plane or in the three-vessel view can demonstrate the LSVC as an additional vessel and color Doppler or inversion mode can confirm the anatomic location to the left of the pulmonary artery.

Associated Cardiac and Extracardiac Findings

Associated cardiac malformations are common and primarily include heterotaxy syndrome, left ventricular tract obstructive defects, and conotruncal anomalies (9–12). In two reported fetal series totaling 136 cases of LSVC diagnosed on fetal echocardiography in tertiary centers, absence of associated congenital heart disease was noted in 17 of 136 (12.5%) (9,15). Heterotaxy, which accounted for the most common associated cardiac malformation, occurred in 55 of 136 (40%) of total LSVC cases and in 55 of 119 (46%) of LSVC with associated congenital heart disease (9,15). Atrioventricular septal defects were the most common associated cardiac malformation in the heterotaxy group and ventricular septal defects and coarctation of the aorta were among the most common cardiac malformations in the non-heterotaxy group (9,15). In our experience, LVCS can also be present in fetuses with mesocardia or dextrocardia without heterotaxy. The association of LSVC with partial or total anomalous pulmonary venous connection is often difficult to diagnose. On occasions, the right superior vena cava is absent and the LSVC is the only vein draining systemic venous blood from the upper body (13,14).

Associated extracardiac malformations are common and primarily include abnormalities of the spleen and bowel in fetuses with heterotaxy syndrome (15). Other common extracardiac abnormalities include single umbilical artery and abnormalities of the umbilical venous system (9,15). Chromosomal anomalies such as trisomy 21, 18, and others were reported in 9% of LSVC in one study (15).

Differential Diagnosis

LSVC is commonly missed in the majority of cases especially when isolated. Misdiagnosing a dilated coronary sinus in association with LSVC as an atrial septal defect, atrioventricular septal defect (16) or anomalous pulmonary venous connection (17) is a typical pitfall. Differential diagnosis of LSVC includes the vertical vein in supracardiac pulmonary venous connection (see section in this chapter on total anomalous venous connection). Color Doppler can help differentiate LSVC from the vertical vein as the blood flow is toward the heart in LSVC and in opposite direction in the vertical vein.

Prognosis and Outcome

Pregnancy course of a fetus with LSVC depends on the underlying associated cardiac abnormalities, if any. In "isolated" LSVC attention should be given to the growth of the left ventricle and the aortic isthmus, as coarctation can develop in utero in a fetus with an apparently isolated LSVC. Isolated LSVC does not seem to be associated with clinical problems postnatally. Neonatal echocardiography is, however, recommended to rule out additional findings. When faced with an apparently isolated LSVC prenatally, we inform the parents about the good prognosis, and recommend an echocardiogram postnatally.

■ KEY POINTS: PERSISTENT LEFT SUPERIOR VENA CAVA

- Persistent left superior vena cava (LSVC) is thought to result from failure of the left anterior and common cardinal veins to involute.
- LSVC joins the coronary sinus and drains into the right atrium in 92% of cases or into the left atrium in the remainder of cases.
- Identifying LSVC can be achieved in three transverse planes and in one longitudinal plane; the four-chamber view; a plane just posterior to the four-chamber view; the three-vessel-trachea view; and a left parasagittal view.
- Increased nuchal translucency has been shown in 29% of fetuses with LSVC.
- Heterotaxy accounts for the most common associated cardiac malformation with LSVC.
- Ventricular septal defects and coarctation of the aorta were among the most common associated cardiac malformations in the non-heterotaxy group.
- Chromosomal anomalies were reported in 9% of LSVC in one study.
- Isolated LSVC does not seem to be associated with clinical problems postnatally.

TOTAL AND PARTIAL ANOMALOUS PULMONARY VENOUS CONNECTION

Definition, Spectrum of Disease, and Incidence

Four pulmonary veins, a right and left superior and inferior pair, drain into the posterior wall of the left atrium of the fetus under normal conditions (Fig. 23-8A). Total anomalous pulmonary venous connection (TAPVC) is a condition in which all the pulmonary veins drain either directly or indirectly into the right atrium (Fig. 23-8B–D) (18). Partial anomalous pulmonary venous connection (PAPVC) is characterized by the direct or indirect anomalous drainage of one, two, or three of the four pulmonary veins into the right atrium (18). Other synonyms that are used include anomalous venous drainage or return which lead to other abbreviations such as TAPVD/PAPVD or TAPVR/PAPVR. According to the anatomic site of the anomalous connection, four types of TAPVC exist (Fig. 23-8): Type I, supracardiac (Fig. 23-8B); Type II, cardiac (Fig. 23-8C); Type III, infracardiac (Fig. 23-8D); and Type IV, mixed pattern. Supracardiac anomalous pulmonary connection is the most common and accounts for about 45% of cases (19,20). Obstruction to pulmonary venous return is a fairly common association in TAPVC.

Hemodynamic consequence of anomalous pulmonary venous connection is significant to the neonate as various degrees of mixing of pulmonary and systemic blood occurs, which leads to cyanosis. The diagnosis of TAPVC or PAPVC is difficult in the fetus and most cases have been missed prenatally. Recently with improvement in ultrasound technology, few series and case presentations report on the accurate detection of anomalous pulmonary venous connections in the fetus either in isolation or as part of heterotaxy syndrome (21–32). TAPVC accounts for 2% of live births with congenital heart disease and occurs in about 0.9 per

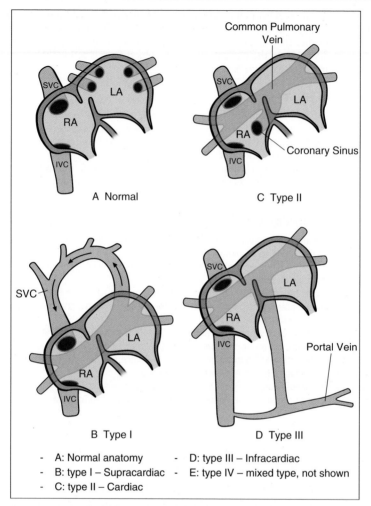

Figure 23-8. Types of total anomalous pulmonary venous connection. LA, left atrium; RA, right atrium; IVC, inferior vena cava; SVC, superior vena cava.

10,000 live births (33,34). TAPVC and PAPVC are commonly found in heterotaxy syndromes, primarily in cases of right isomerism (35) (see Chapter 22).

Ultrasound Findings

Gray Scale

Prenatal ultrasound findings in TAPVC are shown in Table 23-1. The four-chamber view typically shows size discrepancy between the right and left sides of the heart with an enlarged right atrium and ventricle due to increased venous return (Fig. 23-9). The interatrial septum bulges into the left atrium, especially in the third trimester of pregnancy. In many cases, a venous confluence chamber can also be seen behind the left atrium at the four-chamber view plane with no direct connection between the pulmonary veins and the posterior wall of the left atrium (Fig. 23-9). The pulmonary artery may appear enlarged at the three-vessel-trachea view, and a vertical vein can be seen on occasion (25). In TAPVC associated with right or left isomerism, the abnormality at the four-chamber view depends, however, on the underlying cardiac lesion.

TABLE 23-1	Prenatal Ultrasound Findings in Total Anomalous Pulmonary Venous Connections

Enlarged right atrium and right ventricle on four-chamber view
Bulging of interatrial septum into left atrium
Venous confluence chamber behind the left atrium
No direct connection between pulmonary veins and left atrium
Enlarged pulmonary artery in the three-vessel-trachea view
Vertical vein as a fourth vessel in the three-vessel-trachea view

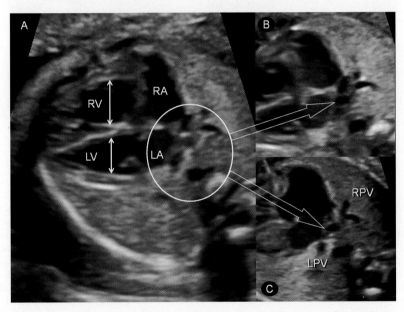

Figure 23-9. Transverse four-chamber view in **A** in a fetus with supracardiac total anomalous pulmonary venous connections (TAPVC) where the posterior region of the left atrium (LA) is enlarged in **B** and **C**. Note the discrepant ventricular size in A with an enlarged right ventricle (RV) due to indirect draining of pulmonary veins into the right atrium (RA). Both right (RPV) and left (LPV) pulmonary veins do not enter the left atrium (LA) (C) but drain into a confluent vein (*open arrows*). The subtype of TAPVC cannot be determined from this view alone. LV, left ventricle.

Color Doppler

Color Doppler is essential for the evaluation of the connections of the pulmonary veins to the left atrium when TAPVC is suspected (Fig. 23-10). Optimal color Doppler presets should be applied, however, in order to avoid a misdiagnosis. Pulsed Doppler interrogation of the pulmonary veins in TAPVC shows a different wave velocity pattern as opposed to the normal connection and this can be of help in diagnosis (23,25,31). A longitudinal view of the pulmonary veins may be helpful in visualizing their normal or abnormal connections to the left atrium (Fig. 23-10). A major concern of TAPVC is the ability to diagnose obstruction to pulmonary venous return prenatally. In our experience, obstruction to pulmonary venous return cannot be accurately predicted prenatally; the presence of continuous nonpulsatile flow in the collecting vein however may be a sign of this condition.

Type I: Supracardiac TAPVC

Type I supracardiac TAPVC is the most common form of anomalous pulmonary venous connection. The four pulmonary veins merge into a confluence posterior to the left atrium and connect via a vertical vein to the left innominate vein (brachiocephalic), which drains into the

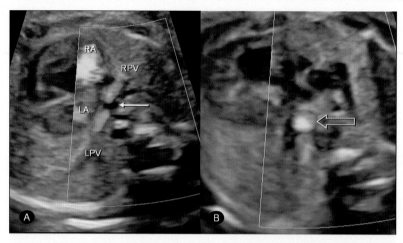

Figure 23-10. Color Doppler of a transverse view of the chest in the fetus shown in Fig. 23-9. Note in **A** that the right (RPV) and left (LPV) pulmonary vein do not enter the left atrium (LA) but rather drain into a confluent vein (*solid arrow*), separated from the LA by a membrane. A slightly cranial orientation, as shown in **B**, demonstrates the confluent vein arising into the upper thorax (*open arrow*). RA, right atrium.

superior vena cava (Fig. 23-8B). This condition can be detected by visualizing the confluence behind the left atrium. At the three-vessel-trachea view plane, a fourth vessel, the vertical vein, can be seen at the same anatomic location as a persistent LSVC (Fig. 23-11). Conversely to persistent LSVC, where blood from the left jugular vein continues via the LSVC toward the heart, blood flow in the vertical vein in supracardiac TAPVC goes the opposite direction, toward the upper thorax (18). Furthermore, the left innominate vein (brachiocephalic) is significantly dilated in TAPVC (Fig. 23-12) when compared to persistent LSVC where the left innominate vein is small or commonly absent. Color Doppler in a longitudinal plane of the

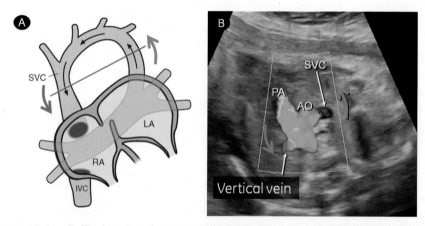

Figure 23-11. A: The blue line shows the level of the transverse ultrasound plane with color Doppler shown in **B** demonstrates the vertical vein and the superior vena cava (SVC) seen on the left and right sides of the pulmonary artery (PA) and aorta (AO), respectively. Blood flows in the vertical vein in opposite direction to that of the SVC conversely and to that of an isolated LSVC (as shown in Fig. 23-4B). Colored arrows show the direction of flow in the SVC and the vertical vein. LA, left atrium; RA, right atrium; IVC, inferior vena cava.

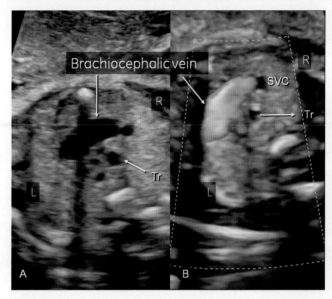

Figure 23-12. Transverse plane in the upper chest at the level of the brachiocephalic (or inno-minate) vein showing a dilated vein **(A)** as it drains the complete lung venous return. Color Dopp-ler **(B)** shows blood flow from left to right, toward the right superior vena cava (SVC). Tr, trachea; L, left; R, right.

chest can demonstrate the pulmonary veins draining into the confluent vein and the tortuous vertical vein (Fig. 23-13). Pulsed Doppler can demonstrate an abnormal pulmonary venous waveform pattern in TAPVC (Fig. 23-14). Another form of supracardiac TAPVC involves a direct connection of the four pulmonary veins to the superior vena cava. The superior vena cava is therefore dilated and this can be seen at the three-vessel-trachea view.

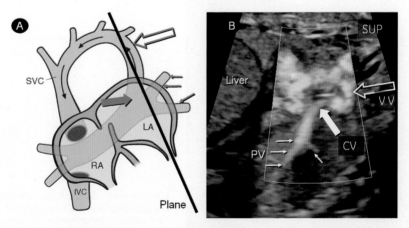

Figure 23-13. A longitudinal view of the chest in color Doppler **(B)** corresponding to the solid line drawn in **A**, is demonstrating the pulmonary veins (PV) (*small arrows*) draining into the con-fluence vein (CV) (*large solid arrow*) which continues as a tortuous vertical vein (VV) (*large open arrow*) into the upper thorax instead of draining into the left atrium (LA). See similar case in Fig. 23-20A. RA, right atrium; IVC, inferior vena cava; SVC, superior vena cava; SUP, superior.

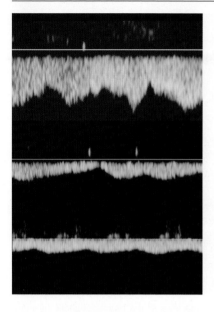

Figure 23-14. Pulsed Doppler waveforms of pulmonary veins, confluent and vertical veins in three fetuses with TAPVC. Note that the Doppler waveforms are abnormal with non-pulsatile continuous flow. Compare with normal pulmonary venous flow shown in Figure 8-25.

Type II: Cardiac TAPVC

In type II cardiac TAPVC, the pulmonary veins connect directly to the coronary sinus, which becomes dilated (Fig. 23-8C), or connect directly into the posterior wall of the right atrium (Fig. 23-15). When the pulmonary veins connect to the coronary sinus, the coronary sinus becomes dilated. A dilated coronary sinus in the absence of a LSVC should raise the suspicion for the presence of TAPVC. The coronary sinus is best demonstrated in a transverse plane inferior to the four-chamber view (Fig. 23-3). Direct connection of the pulmonary veins to the right atrium can be visualized by high-resolution ultrasound on two-dimensional (Fig. 23-15), color, and pulsed Doppler evaluation.

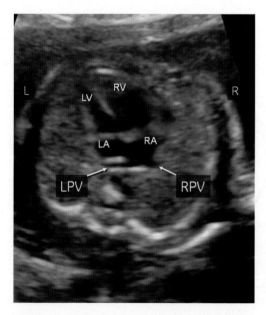

Figure 23-15. Cardiac-type TAPVC shown in a four-chamber view of a fetus with complex cardiac malformations (double outlet right ventricle, ventricular septal defect, and isomerism). Posterior to the left atrium (LA), the right (RPV) and left (LPV) pulmonary veins are seen to drain into the right-sided atrium (RA). LV, left ventricle; RV, right ventricle.

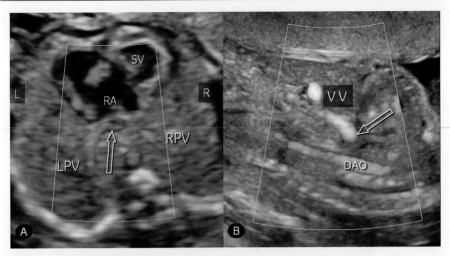

Figure 23-16. Fetus with infracardiac-type III TAPVC. **A:** Color Doppler at the four-chamber view shows the left (LPV) and right (RPV) pulmonary veins draining into a vertical vein (*arrow*). **B:** Longitudinal view of the thorax and abdomen in color Doppler shows the descending aorta (DAO) and a vessel in a parallel course to the DAO (*arrow*) originating from the thorax and draining into the liver. This vessel represents the vertical vein (VV) shown in A (*arrow*). SV, single ventricle; RA, right atrium; L, left; R, right.

Type III: Infracardiac TAPVC

In type III infracardiac TAPVC the four pulmonary veins form a confluence behind the atria (Fig. 23-16A). This confluence is connected to an anomalous descending vein that accompanies the esophagus through the diaphragm and drains into the portal venous system. Obstruction of venous drainage is the rule rather than the exception. The confluence and the descending vein are small and difficult to recognize on routine gray-scale examination (28). Longitudinal view of the chest and upper abdomen on color Doppler may demonstrate a small vessel crossing the diaphragm, entering the liver with cranial to caudal flow direction (Fig. 23-16B). Pulsed Doppler shows a continuous venous flow pattern (31). The authors have diagnosed a total of five fetuses with type III infracardiac TAPVC in the past years, all associated with right isomerism. Figure 23-17 is an anatomic specimen of a fetus with infracardiac TAPVC.

Type IV: Mixed TAPVC

Mixed TAPVC is rare and involves a variety of pulmonary venous drainage where the left pulmonary veins drain to the left innominate vein through a vertical vein and the right pulmonary veins drain into the coronary sinus or directly into the right atrium.

Partial Anomalous Pulmonary Venous Connection (PAPVC) and Scimitar Syndrome

PAPVC is characterized by the direct or indirect anomalous drainage of one, two, or three of the four pulmonary veins into the right atrium (Fig. 23-18). PAPVC is difficult to detect and has been rarely reported prenatally (25). A special association of PAPVC with scimitar syndrome is worth describing as it has been reported prenatally in few studies (25,36).

Scimitar syndrome is the combination of a right lung hypoplasia accompanied by hypoplasia of the right pulmonary artery, and a PAPVC. It is suspected in the four-chamber view due to dextrocardia and hypoplastic right lung (Figs. 23-19 and 4-8D). The right inferior pulmonary vein drains into the inferior vena cava instead of the left atrium, which is best demonstrated in a longitudinal plane (Figs. 23-18 and 23-19). The appearance of the right inferior pulmonary vein on angiography is similar to a saber, hence the name "scimitar." In addition systemic arterial blood flow to the small right lung can be demonstrated as in pulmonary sequestration.

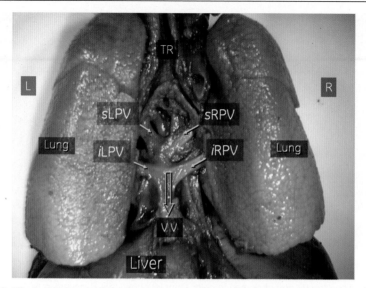

Figure 23-17. Anatomic specimen of a fetus with infracardiac-Type III TAPVC seen from a posterior view. Note the four superior and inferior pulmonary veins draining into a vertical vein (VV) (*open arrow*) with a course toward the liver. The trachea (TR) is open in this specimen. sRPV, superior right pulmonary vein; sLPV, superior left pulmonary vein; iRPV, inferior right pulmonary vein; iLPV, inferior left pulmonary vein; R, right; L, left.

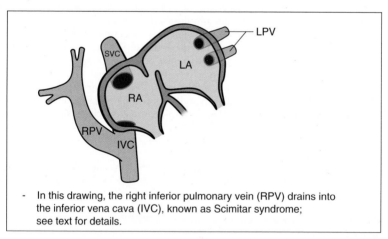

- In this drawing, the right inferior pulmonary vein (RPV) drains into the inferior vena cava (IVC), known as Scimitar syndrome; see text for details.

Figure 23-18. Partial anomalous pulmonary venous connection in Scimitar syndrome. LA, left atrium; SVC, superior vena cava; LPV, left pulmonary vein.

Early Gestation

The diagnosis of TAPVC or PAPVC is difficult to perform in early gestation given the small size of venous connections.

Three-dimensional Ultrasound

Three-dimensional ultrasound combined with tomographic imaging can be used to demonstrate vascular anomalies in different adjacent planes. The combination of color Doppler or B-flow with three-dimensional and projection mode allows a better demonstration of the

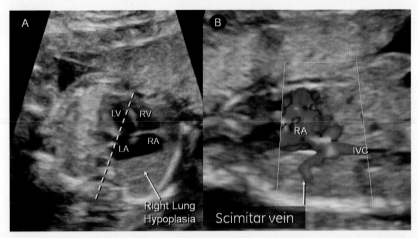

Figure 23-19. A fetus with scimitar syndrome and PAPVC. The four-chamber view **(A)** shows a small right lung (*right lung hypoplasia*) with cardiac dextroposition. Note the position of the heart in the chest in A as the dashed line bisects the chest into two halves. A longitudinal view **(B)** shows the connection of the right pulmonary vein (scimitar vein) with the inferior vena cava (IVC). RV, right ventricle; LV, left ventricle; RA, right atrium; LA, left atrium.

abnormal course of the veins (32,36). Recently the use of three-dimensional ultrasound with B-flow has been used to demonstrate TAPVC in the fetus (32). Figures 23-20 and 23-21 show examples of rendered three-dimensional volumes in fetuses with total or partial pulmonary venous connection abnormalities.

Associated Cardiac and Extracardiac Findings

TAPVC and PAPVC can be isolated but can also occur in association with other cardiac anomalies. One of the most common associated cardiac abnormalities is heterotaxy, primarily

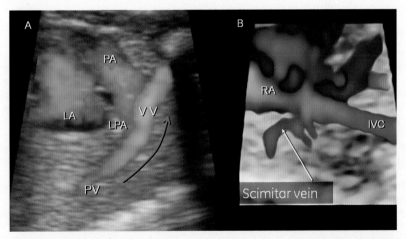

Figure 23-20. Three-dimensional rendering of a chest volume in color Doppler and glass body mode of a fetus with TAPVC (Type I) **(A)** and PAPVC (Scimitar syndrome) **(B)**. Note in A, the course of the pulmonary vein (PV) toward the vertical vein (VV) which connects with the brachiocephalic vein rather than the left atrium (LA). B is the same case shown in Figure 23-19 demonstrating the right pulmonary vein (scimitar vein) as it connects to the inferior vena cava (IVC). LPA, left pulmonary artery; PA, pulmonary artery; RA, right atrium.

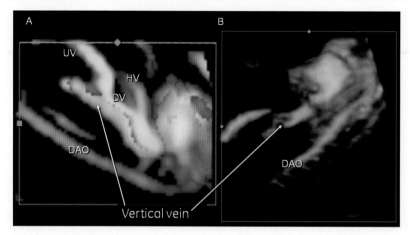

Figure 23-21. Three-dimensional rendering in color Doppler **(A)** and B-Flow **(B)** of a volume of the chest in a fetus with infracardiac type III TAPVC. Note the course of the vertical vein in parallel to the descending aorta (DAO). HV, hepatic vein; DV, ductus venosus; UV, umbilical vein.

right atrial isomerism. Atrial septal defect of the sinus venosus type is associated with TAPVC and PAPVC, but this type of atrial septal defect is not detectable prenatally. Other associated cardiac anomalies include atrioventricular septal defect, single ventricle, coarctation of the aorta, hypoplastic left heart syndrome, and others.

Extracardiac associated anomalies are rare outside of heterotaxy syndrome. In scimitar syndrome the associated right lung hypoplasia is part of the syndrome. Noonan syndrome and cat-eye syndrome can be associated with PAPVC (37,38). Associated chromosomal anomalies are rare.

Differential Diagnosis

Cardiac conditions that result in right-to-left heart size discrepancy should be considered in the differential diagnosis.

Prognosis and Outcome

Prognosis is dependent on the specific type of anomalous venous connection, the presence of pulmonary venous obstruction, and the volume of right-to-left intracardiac shunting. Prenatal series report worse outcomes than neonatal series primarily due to the associated cardiac abnormalities (25). Type III infracardiac TAPVC has a worse prognosis than other types due to a high association with pulmonary venous obstruction. Overall prognosis is good for neonates who survive surgical correction.

■ KEY POINTS: TOTAL AND PARTIAL ANOMALOUS PULMONARY VENOUS CONNECTIONS

- ■ TAPVC is a condition where all the pulmonary veins drain either directly or indirectly into the right atrium.
- ■ PAPVC is characterized by the direct or indirect anomalous drainage of one, two, or three of the four pulmonary veins into the right atrium.
- ■ Four types of TAPVC exist: Type I, supracardiac; Type II, cardiac; Type III, infracardiac; and Type IV, mixed pattern.
- ■ Supracardiac type (Type I) is the most common.
- ■ Obstruction to pulmonary venous return is a common association with TAPVC.
- ■ TAPVC and PAPVC are commonly found in heterotaxy syndromes, primarily in right isomerism.

- The four-chamber view typically shows an enlarged right atrium and ventricle and a venous confluence chamber behind the left atrium in TAPVC.
- The three-vessel-trachea view shows a dilated pulmonary artery and a vertical vein as a fourth vessel.
- In Type I, supracardiac TAPVC, pulmonary veins connect to a confluence behind the left atrium, which drains to a vertical vein connected to the left innominate vein.
- In Type II, cardiac TAPVC, pulmonary veins connect to the coronary sinus or directly to the posterior wall of the right ventricle.
- In Type III, infracardiac TAPVC, pulmonary veins connect to a vertical vein which crosses the diaphragm and connects into the hepatic veins.
- A special association of PAPVC with scimitar syndrome exists.
- Prognosis is dependent on the specific type of anomalous venous connection, the presence of pulmonary venous obstruction, and the volume of right-to-left intracardiac shunting.

References

1. Romer S, Opgen-Rhein B, Chaoui R, et al. Bilateral agenesis of the superior vena cava associated with congenital hydrothorax. *Ultrasound Obstet Gynecol* 2006;28(6):842–844.
2. Berg C, Kamil D, Geipel A, et al. Absence of ductus venosus-importance of umbilical venous drainage site. *Ultrasound Obstet Gynecol* 2006;28(3):275–281.
3. Hille H, Chaoui R, Renz S, et al. Distended azygos and hemiazygos vein without interrupted inferior vena cava in a case of agenesis of the ductus venosus. *Ultrasound Obstet Gynecol* 2008;31(5):589–591.
4. Streeter GL. Developmental horizons in human embryos: description of age group XV, XVI, XVII, XVIII, third issue. *Contrib Embryol Canegie Inst* 1948;32:145–146.
5. Hughes C, Rumore P. Anomalous pulmonary veins. *Arch Pathol* 1944;37:364–366.
6. Cha EM, Khoury GH. Persistent left superior vena cava. Radiologic and clinical significance. *Radiology* 1972;103(2):375–381.
7. Nsah EN, Moore GW, Hutchins GM. Pathogenesis of persistent left superior vena cava with a coronary sinus connection. *Pediatr Pathol* 1991;11(2):261–269.
8. Biffi M, Boriani G, Frabetti L, et al. Left superior vena cava persistence in patients undergoing pacemaker or cardioverter-defibrillator implantation: a 10-year experience. *Chest* 2001;120(1):139–144.
9. Galindo A, Gutierrez-Larraya F, Escribano D, et al. Clinical significance of persistent left superior vena cava diagnosed in fetal life. *Ultrasound Obstet Gynecol* 2007;30(2):152–161.
10. Pasquini L, Fichera A, Tan T, et al. Left superior caval vein: a powerful indicator of fetal coarctation. *Heart* 2005;91(4):539–540.
11. Yoo SJ, Lee YH, Kim ES, et al. Three-vessel view of the fetal upper mediastinum: an easy means of detecting abnormalities of the ventricular outflow tracts and great arteries during obstetric screening. *Ultrasound Obstet Gynecol* 1997;9(3):173–182.
12. Chaoui R, Heling KS, Kalache KD. Caliber of the coronary sinus in fetuses with cardiac defects with and without left persistent superior vena cava and in growth-restricted fetuses with heart-sparing effect. *Prenat Diagn* 2003;23:552–557.
13. Pasquini L, Belmar C, Seale A, et al. Prenatal diagnosis of absent right and persistent left superior vena cava. *Prenat Diagn* 2006;26(8):700–702.
14. Freund M, Stoutenbeek P, ter Heide H, et al. "Tobacco pipe" sign in the fetus: patent left superior vena cava with absent right superior vena cava. *Ultrasound Obstet Gynecol* 2008;32(4):593–594.
15. Berg C, Knuppel M, Geipel A, et al. Prenatal diagnosis of persistent left superior vena cava and its associated congenital anomalies. *Ultrasound Obstet Gynecol* 2006;27(3):274–280.
16. Park JK, Taylor DK, Skeels M, et al. Dilated coronary sinus in the fetus: misinterpretation as an atrioventricular canal defect. *Ultrasound Obstet Gynecol* 1997;10(2):126–129.
17. Papa M, Camesasca C, Santoro F, et al. Fetal echocardiography in detecting anomalous pulmonary venous connection: four false positive cases. *Br Heart J* 1995;73(4):355–358.
18. Chaoui R, Lenz F, Heling KS. Doppler examination of the fetal pulmonary venous circulation. In: Maulik D, eds. *Doppler ultrasound in obstetrics and gynecology.* Heidelberg: Springer Verlag, 2003:451–463.
19. Borroughs JT, Edwards JE. Total anomalous pulmonary venous connection. *Am Heart J* 1960;59:913–931.
20. Karamlou T, Gurofsky R, Al Sukhni E, et al. Factors associated with mortality and reoperation in 377 children with total anomalous pulmonary venous connection. *Pediatr Cardiol* 2007;115:1591–1598.
21. DiSessa TG, Emerson DS, Felker RE, et al. Anomalous systemic and pulmonary venous pathways diagnosed in utero by ultrasound. *J Ultrasound Med* 1990;9:311–317.
22. Wessels MW, Frohn-Mulder IM, Cromme-Dijkhuis AH, et al. In utero diagnosis of infra-diaphragmatic total anomalous pulmonary venous return. *Ultrasound Obstet Gynecol* 1996;8:206–209.
23. Feller PB, Allan LD. Abnormal pulmonary venous return diagnosed prenatally by pulsed Doppler flow imaging. *Ultrasound Obstet Gynecol* 1997;9:347–349.
24. Allan LD, Sharland GK. The echocardiographic diagnosis of totally anomalous pulmonary venous connection in the fetus. *Heart* 2001;85:433–437.
25. Valsangiacomo ER, Hornberger LK, Barrea C, et al. Partial and total anomalous pulmonary venous connection in the fetus: two-dimensional and Doppler echocardiographic findings. *Ultrasound Obstet Gynecol* 2003;22:257–263.

26. Boopathy VS, Rao AR, Padmashree G, et al. Prenatal diagnosis of total anomalous pulmonary venous connection to the portal vein associated with right atrial isomerism. *Ultrasound Obstet Gynecol* 2003;21:393–396.

27. Patel CR, Lane JR, Spector ML, et al. Totally anomalous pulmonary venous connection and complex congenital heart disease: Prenatal echocardiographic diagnosis and prognosis. *J Ultrasound Med* 2005;24:1191–1198.

28. Batukan C, Schwabe M, Heling KS, et al. Prenatal diagnosis of right atrial isomerism (asplenia-syndrome): case report. *Ultraschall Med* 2005;26:234–238.

29. Inamura N, Kado Y, Kita T, et al. Fetal echocardiographic imaging of total anomalous pulmonary venous connection. *Pediatr Cardiol* 2006;27:391–392.

30. Law KM, Leung KY, Tang MH, et al. Prenatal two- and three-dimensional sonographic diagnosis of total anomalous pulmonary venous connection. *Ultrasound Obstet Gynecol* 2007;30:788–789.

31. Lenz F, Chaoui R. Changes in pulmonary venous Doppler parameters in fetal cardiac defects. *Ultrasound Obstet Gynecol* 2006;28:63–70.

32. Volpe P, Campobasso G, De Robertis V, et al. Two- and four-dimensional echocardiography with B-flow imaging and spatiotemporal image correlation in prenatal diagnosis of isolated total anomalous pulmonary venous connection. *Ultrasound Obstet Gynecol* 2007;30:830–837.

33. Ferencz C, Rubin JD, Loffredo CA, et al. *The epidemiology of congenital heart disease: the Baltimore–Washington Infant Study 1981–1989. Perspectives in pediatric cardiology*, Vol 4. Mount Kisco, NY: Futura Publishing, 1993.

34. Grabitz RG, Joffres MR, Collins-Nakai RL. Congenital heart disease: Incidence in the first year of life. Alberta Heritage Pediatric Cardiology Program. *Am J Epidemiol* 1988;128:381–388.

35. Berg C, Geipel A, Kamil D, et al. The syndrome of right isomerism—prenatal diagnosis and outcome. *Ultraschall Med* 2006;27(3):225–233.

36. Michailidis GD, Simpson JM, Tulloh RM, et al. Retrospective prenatal diagnosis of scimitar syndrome aided by three- dimensional power Doppler imaging. *Ultrasound Obstet Gynecol* 2001;17(5):449–452.

37. Noonan JA. Syndromes associated with cardiac defects. In: Engle MA, ed. *Pediatric cardiovascular disease.* Philadelphia: FA Davis, 1981:97–116.

38. Volpe P, Buonadonna AL, Campobasso G, et al. Cat-eye syndrome in a fetus with increased nuchal translucency: three-dimensional ultrasound and echocardiographic evaluation of the fetal phenotype. *Ultrasound Obstet Gynecol* 2004;24:485–487.

DILATED AND HYPERTROPHIC CARDIOMYOPATHIES

Cardiomyopathies are diseases of the myocardium affecting the left, the right, or both ventricles and are commonly associated with abnormal cardiac function. Myocardial changes associated with cardiomyopathy are typically not the result of a structural cardiac malformation.

Generally two types of cardiomyopathies exist: dilated and hypertrophic. In the fetus and neonate, a cardiomyopathy is a very rare event, and the literature presents different causes and prevalence in this population (1). Some form of fetal cardiomyopathy may not be significantly relevant in the postnatal period, and postnatal cardiomyopathy may not develop in the fetus (2). The incidence of cardiomyopathy is less than 1% of all neonates with congenital heart disease.

DILATED CARDIOMYOPATHY

Ultrasound Findings

Dilated cardiomyopathy is generally recognized owing to an enlarged heart with a dilated left ventricle, right ventricle, or commonly both ventricles (Fig. 24-1). Ventricular dilation can be quantified by cardiac measurements (e.g., cardiac width, cardiothoracic ratio) (Fig. 24-2) (3). Ventricular wall contraction is reduced and can be objectively assessed by M-mode measurements demonstrating reduced shortening fraction. Pericardial effusion is usually found (Fig. 24-1). Comprehensive examination of the four-chamber plane and the great vessels usually does not reveal any major structural anomaly, even if occasionally a small ventricular septal defect is found. Color Doppler shows in many cases mild or severe regurgitation of the valve of the affected ventricle(s). The dilation and the insufficiency increase with advancing gestation may result in significant ventricular dysfunction and fetal hydrops. Cardiac failure with hydrops is in some cases the first detected sign leading to the diagnosis (4).

Associated Cardiac and Extracardiac Findings

When a dilated cardiomyopathy is suspected, the big challenge is to find out the underlying cause. A comprehensive ultrasound examination of the fetus is recommended, combined with Doppler investigation of the fetal arteries and precordial veins. A significant number of cases remains "idiopathic." Associated extracardiac findings may give a hint to the possible cause, as in the presence of echogenic foci in the liver or dilated ventricular system in the brain, which may suggest infectious etiologies. Cardiomyopathy in monochorionic twins is generally noted in the recipient twin in twin-twin transfusion syndrome, where the right ventricle is primarily affected (5). Anemia (isoimmunization or parvo-virus) may be the cause of cardiomyopathy with associated hydrops and increased peak velocities in the middle cerebral arteries. The presence of bradycardia with heart block may suggest the presence of maternal autoantibodies (6). Maternal autoantibodies can cause cardiomyopathy without heart block (6). Chromosomal assessment is recommended, including microdeletion 22q11. A family history and genetic counseling may reveal whether a familial inheritance is present. Comprehensive targeted screening of the fetus and placenta with color flow mapping may reveal an unexpected arteriovenous malformation. Follow-up examination may show the presence of intermittent tachycardia, sometimes not present during the first evaluation of the heart. Metabolic diseases are so rare and generally impossible to exclude prenatally if the family history is not informative (1,2,4).

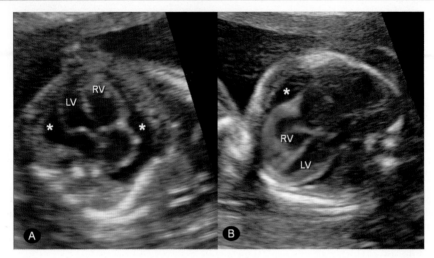

Figure 24-1. Four-chamber view in two fetuses with dilated cardiomyopathies. In fetus **A**, dilated cardiac chambers are noted at 20 weeks' gestation with pericardial effusion (*asterisks*). Work up did not reveal the cause of cardiomyopathy and the fetus developed hydrops and died on subsequent follow-up. Fetus **B** shows dilated cardiomyopathy with echogenic ventricular walls and pericardial effusion (*asterisk*). This fetus was found to have toxoplasmosis infection on work up. LV, left ventricle; RV, right ventricle.

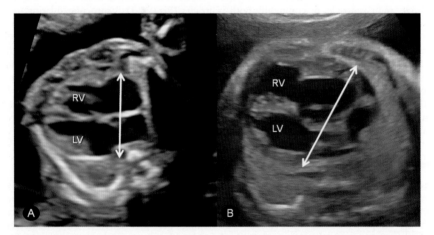

Figure 24-2. Four-chamber view in two fetuses with dilated cardiomyopathies (*arrows*). In fetus **A**, dilated cardiac chambers are noted due to volume overload in aneurysm of the vein of Galen. Fetus **B** has familial cardiomyopathy, which became evident in the third trimester of pregnancy requiring cardiac transplantation after birth. The mother of fetus B had dilated cardiomyopathy and was under treatment when this fetus was diagnosed. LV, left ventricle; RV, right ventricle.

Pitfalls and Differential Diagnosis

Dilated and severe cardiomegaly can be present in association with many conditions and should be considered in the differential diagnosis. Dilated right ventricle is found in Ebstein anomaly and tricuspid dysplasia. Left ventricular endocardiac fibroelastosis with patent but insufficient mitral valve is one of the main differential diagnoses. Bilateral atrioventricular valve insufficiency can be found in myocarditis, volume overload, and other conditions and some of these conditions may lead to cardiomyopathy. Cardiomyopathy may resolve with advancing gestation with normal cardiac function postnatally. A transient fetal infection may be involved when cardiomyopathy resolve prenatally.

HYPERTROPHIC CARDIOMYOPATHY

Ultrasound Findings

Hypertrophic cardiomyopathy is generally recognized owing to an enlarged heart in association with ventricular wall hypertrophy of one or generally both ventricles (1) (Figs. 24-3 and 24-4). The lumen of the affected ventricle(s) can be decreased. A pericardial effusion is usually found (Fig. 24-3). The comprehensive examination of the four-chamber view and the great vessels does not reveal any major structural anomaly correlating with the severity of the finding. An obstruction of the inflow or outflow tract can be found, leading to turbulences on color Doppler and increased velocities measured on pulsed Doppler. Regurgitation of the atrioventricular valves can be found but is not as common as in the dilated type. Ventricular hypertrophy and cardiac compromise increase with advancing gestation and can lead to cardiac failure, hydrops, and in utero death.

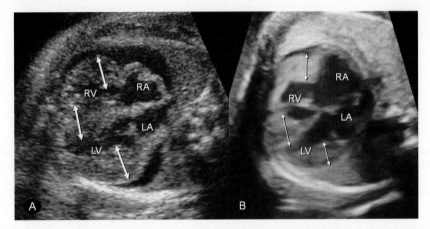

Figure 24-3. Four-chamber view in two fetuses with hypertrophic cardiomyopathies (*arrows*). Fetus **A** has hypertrophic cardiomyopathy with pericardial effusion and thickened myocardial walls as part of carnitine deficiency, which was diagnosed postnatally. Fetus **B** has idiopathic cardiomyopathy. LV, left ventricle; RV, right ventricle; LA, left atrium; RA, right atrium.

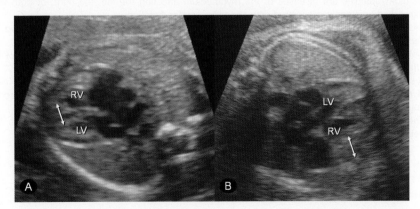

Figure 24-4. Fetus at 22 weeks and 33 weeks with sinus bradycardia and thickened cardiac walls (*arrows*) in association with hypertrophic cardiomyopathy. LV, left ventricle; RV, right ventricle.

Associated Cardiac and Extracardiac Findings

Similarly to dilated cardiomyopathy, identifying the underlying cause of hypertrophic cardio-myopathy can be challenging. A comprehensive examination of the entire fetus can help in detecting additional signs, which may lead to the diagnosis. Storage diseases, which are rare and difficult to diagnose in utero, can be a cause of hypertrophic cardiomyopathy and are associated with hepatomegaly, which results in increased abdominal circumference or changes in liver echogenicity. Many causes of hypertrophic cardiomyopathy remain "idiopathic." The most common condition found in association with a hypertrophic cardiomyopathy is diabetes mellitus, especially with poor glycemic control. This occurs in the last trimester of pregnancy. Another known condition is bilateral renal agenesis or dysplasia with oligohydramnios, lead-ing to a thickening of the myocardium. The pathogenesis is not known but may be due to hypertension either of renal origin or due to pulmonary hypertension with lung hypoplasia. Chromosomal assessment is recommended including microdeletion of 22q11, but other genetic syndromes should also be considered. Noonan syndrome has been reported in associated with hypertrophic cardiomyopathy. A family history and genetic counseling may reveal whether a familial inheritance is present. When consanguinity is present, the occurrence of a storage dis-ease should be sought. Hypertrophic cardiomyopathy can occur in twin-twin transfusion syn-drome especially in the recipient twin, probably due to chronic volume overload.

Pitfalls and Differential Diagnosis

Ventricular hypertrophy can result from stenosis of a semilunar valve or structural cardiac defects. Pulsed Doppler interrogation of the cardiac valves should be part of the work up of cardiomyopathy. Small cardiac tumors such as rhabdomyomas can mimic ventricular hyper-trophy, but high-resolution fetal echocardiography is able to differentiate the echogenic tumor tissue from thickened myocardium.

Prognosis and Outcome of Cardiomyopathies

The prognosis depends on the underlying cause of the cardiomyopathy. It can range from a good prognosis when the cardiomyopathy regresses pre- or postnatally, to very poor when the fetus dies in utero. The risk for in utero or neonatal death increases with the occurrence of hydrops, stiff ventricular cardiac wall, and prematurity. Some fetuses with cardiomyopathy (e.g., familial-type) may require cardiac transplantation postnatally. Because some forms of idiopathic cardiomyopa-thy belong to specific inherited diseases, it is prudent to discuss storing blood and/or fetal tissue with the parents for a later evaluation. Some of these cases show an autosomal recessive disorder, but an autosomal dominant inheritance can be assumed when familiar recurrence is present.

■ KEY POINTS: DILATED AND HYPERTROPHIC CARDIOMYOPATHIES

- Cardiomyopathies are diseases of the myocardium affecting the left, the right, or both ven-tricles and commonly associated with abnormal cardiac function.
- Dilated cardiomyopathy is generally recognized owing to an enlarged heart with a dilated left ventricle, right ventricle, or commonly both ventricles.
- Color Doppler shows in many cases a more or less severe regurgitation of the valve of the affected ventricle(s).
- A significant number of dilated and hypertrophic cardiomyopathy remains "idiopathic."
- Hypertrophic cardiomyopathy is generally recognized owing to an enlarged heart in associa-tion with ventricular wall hypertrophy of one or generally both ventricles.
- The most common condition found in association with a hypertrophic cardiomyopathy is dia-betes mellitus.

HEART TUMORS AND RHABDOMYOMAS

Incidence and Distribution

Heart tumors are generally easy to diagnose prenatally and necessitate an urgent referral to a peri-natal center, due to possible hemodynamic compromise in the fetus. The prevalence of cardiac tumors in fetal series is rare but is more common than in postnatal series. Cardiac tumors were reported to occur in about 2.8% of all fetal cardiac anomalies seen in one center (10).

Cardiac tumors are rhabdomyomas in 80% to 90% of cases (7,9,10,11), but can also be teratoma, fibroma, myxoma, hamartoma, rhabdomyosarcoma, and others. This chapter will primarily focus on rhabdomyomas.

Rhabdomyomas

Echodensity: The diagnosis of a rhadomyoma is achieved by two-dimensional ultrasound, by recognizing an ovale or circular, but well-circumscribed mass, with an echogenic bright density as compared to the echodensity of cardiac walls (Figs. 24-5 and 24-6).

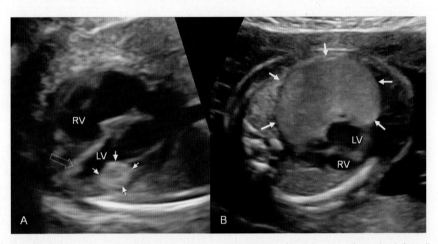

Figure 24-5. **A:** A four-chamber view shows a single tumor (rhabdomyoma) on the left wall of the left ventricle (*arrows*). The open arrow points to a small rhabdomyoma on the septum not initially seen. The fetus in **B** was referred at 22 weeks' gestation for suspected echogenic lungs and cystic lung lesions. Upon echocardiography, the echogenicity was found to be a large rhabdomyoma (*arrows*). Cordocentesis revealed tuberous sclerosis in the fetus. LV, left ventricle; RV, right ventricle.

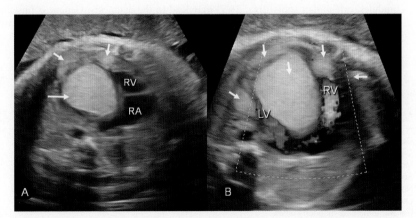

Figure 24-6. Multiple large tumors in a fetus at 35 weeks' gestation **(A)** (*arrows*). Color Doppler shows reduced left (LV) and right (RV) ventricular filling **(B)**. Postnatal course was uneventful, tuberous sclerosis was confirmed in the neonate. LV, left ventricle; RV, right ventricle; RA, right atrium.

Number of tumors and size: Rhabdomyomas can be single, but in most cases are multiple (7–11). Even in cases where a single rhabdomyoma is diagnosed, later evaluation with high-resolution ultrasound may reveal additional rhabdomyomas. Rhabdomyomas can occur within the cardiac walls, the interventricular septum, the cardiac apex, or even the outflow tract conus. The tumor size can vary from 5 to 10 mm to large size such as 40 mm or more (7).

Localization: Rhabdomyomas occur in the septum or the free walls, but can be found in the atria as well. Frequently they protrude into the cardiac lumen and may cause flow obstruction. An exophytic tumor outside the heart is unlikely to be a rhabdomyoma.

Gestational age at detection: Rhabdomyomas develop in utero and are generally detected between 20 and 30 weeks' gestation but not before (10). Early diagnosis at 11 to 14 weeks' gestation has not been reported to date. It appears that rhabdomyomas are under the influence of maternal hormones during pregnancy and as such they tend to grow prenatally and shrink after birth (8).

Complications: It is always interesting to observe that despite the large size of rhabdomyomas and flow obstruction, fetal hemodynamic compromise is rare and is only occasionally observed. Arrhythmias, fetal hydrops, and spontaneous fetal demise have been reported in fetal series, even if it is rather the exception. Interference with the coronary arterial system may cause spontaneous death as well (10).

Association with tuberous sclerosis (Morbus Bourneville-Pringle): Rhabdomyomas are commonly associated with tuberous sclerosis, especially when multiple tumors are noted (10,12,13). Table 24-1 lists the signs of tuberous sclerosis. The spectrum of tuberous sclerosis is wide and the typical facial nodules (Fig. 24-7A), kidneys or brain involvement, or the café-au-lait spots may be absent. When tuberous sclerosis is diagnosed clinically after birth, an association rate of 50% to 80% with rhabdomyomas is possible. Magnetic resonance tomography in pregnancy may support the cardiac diagnosis (14) by demonstrating fetal intracranial lesions, which are found in 40% of the cases (15) (Fig. 24-7B). The absence of brain lesions does not rule out the disease. In recent years, the diagnosis of tuberous sclerosis is achieved by molecular genetic testing for the tuberous sclerosis complex *TSC-1* (Hamartin gene) and *TSC-2* (Tuberin gene) after cordocentesis, chorionic villus sampling or amniocentesis (16). In all consecutive six cases that we have examined recently, the diagnosis of tuberous sclerosis in fetal rhabdomyomas was confirmed by molecular genetic testing. The advantage of this approach is an early diagnosis by chorionic villus sampling with the next pregnancy given an autosomal dominant transmission. Given its autosomal dominant transmission, tuberous sclerosis can be present in the father or the mother with variable expression. A family history of epilepsy, or even chronic headache or subtle skin lesions (nodules, café-au-lait spots) (Fig. 24-7) may lead to the diagnosis. Genetic counselling is recommended for all pregnancies with fetal rhabdomyomas. Figure 24-8 is an anatomic specimen of a fetal heart with rhabdomyomas.

TABLE 24-1	Tuberous Sclerosis

- Genetic disorder with autosomal dominant inheritance and high penetrance
- Caused by mutations in tumors suppressor Hamartin (*TSC-1*) (9q34) and Tuberin (*TSC-2*) (16p13)
- Molecular diagnosis is possible with invasive testing
- Spectrum of tuberous sclerosis complex is variable with a wide clinical spectrum
- Nodules (tubers) as hamartomas in brain, kidneys, and visceral organs are present and may lead to chronic renal failure
- Cardiac tumors as rhabdomyomas
- Seizures
- Mental retardation
- Skin hypopigmentation (café-au-lait spots) and nodules in the skin

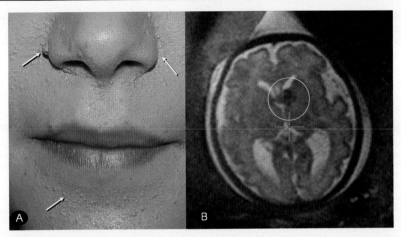

Figure 24-7. The presence of rhabdomyoma(s) in a fetus should raise the suspicion for tuberous sclerosis. In **A**, a pregnant patient shows nasolabial nodules (*arrows*) and was diagnosed with tuberous sclerosis after prenatal ultrasound showed rhabdomyomas in her fetus. Fetal magnetic resonance in **B** shows tuberous nodules in the brain of the fetus (*yellow circle*).

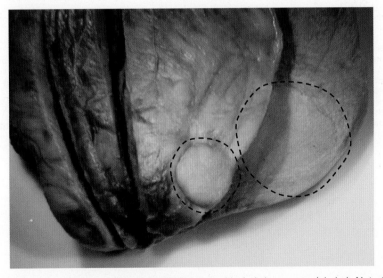

Figure 24-8. An anatomic specimen of a fetal heart with rhabdomyomas (*circles*). Note the uniform color and consistency of the rhabdomyomas when compared to the normal myocardium.

> **Outcome:** Fetal outcome depends on the tumor size, impairment of flow, and occurrence of rhythm disturbances. In general however, rhabdomyomas tend to shrink after birth and an operation is rarely necessary (8). The major problem in neonates and children with this disease is the unpredictable neurologic outcome, especially that some may develop epilepsy and other associated complications.

▓ KEY POINTS: CARDIAC TUMORS

■ Cardiac tumors are rhabdomyomas in 80% to 90% of cases.
■ Rhabdomyomas develop in utero and are generally detected between 20 and 30 weeks' gestation but not before.

- Despite large size, cardiac compression and flow obstruction, fetal hemodynamic compromise is rare with rhabdomyomas.
- Rhabdomyomas are commonly associated with tuberous sclerosis, especially when multiple tumors are noted.
- Fetal intracranial lesions are found in 40% of cases of rhabdomyomas.
- The diagnosis of tuberous sclerosis is now achieved by molecular genetic testing.

References

1. Pedra SR, Smallhorn JF, Ryan G, et al. Fetal cardiomyopathies: pathogenic mechanisms, hemodynamic findings, and clinical outcome. *Circulation* 2002;106(5):585–591.
2. Boldt T, Andersson S, Eronen M. Etiology and outcome of fetuses with functional heart disease. *Acta Obstet Gynecol Scand* 2004;83(6):531–535.
3. Chaoui R, Bollmann R, Goldner B, et al. Fetal cardiomegaly: echocardiographic findings and outcome in 19 cases. *Fetal Diagn Ther* 1994;9(2):92–104.
4. Sivasankaran S, Sharland GK, Simpson JM. Dilated cardiomyopathy presenting during fetal life. *Cardiol Young* 2005;15(4):409–416.
5. Michelfelder E, Gottliebson W, Border W, et al. Early manifestations and spectrum of recipient twin cardiomyopathy in twin–twin transfusion syndrome: relation to Quintero stage. *Ultrasound Obstet Gynecol* 2007;30(7):965–971.
6. Nield LE, Silverman ED, Smallhorn JF, et al. Endocardial fibroelastosis associated with maternal anti-Ro and anti-La antibodies in the absence of atrioventricular block. *J Am Coll Cardiol* 2002;40(4):796–802.
7. D'Addario V, Pinto V, Di Naro E, et al. Prenatal diagnosis and postnatal outcome of cardiac rhabdomyomas. *J Perinat Med* 2002;30(2):170–175.
8. Fesslova V, Villa L, Rizzuti T, et al. Natural history and long-term outcome of cardiac rhabdomyomas detected prenatally. *Prenat Diagn* 2004;24(4):241–248.
9. Geipel A, Krapp M, Germer U, et al. Perinatal diagnosis of cardiac tumors. *Ultrasound Obstet Gynecol* 2001;17:17–21.
10. Allan L. Fetal cardiac tumors. In: Allan L, Hornberger LK, Sharland GK, eds. *Textbook of fetal cardiology.* London: Greenwich Medical Media Limited, 2000;358–365.
11. Holley DG, Martin GR, Brenner JI, et al. Diagnosis and management of fetal cardiac tumors: A multicenter experience and review of published reports. *J Am Coll Cardiol* 1995;26:516–520.
12. Tworetzky W, McElhinney DB, Margossian R, et al. Association between cardiac tumors and tuberous sclerosis in the fetus and neonate. *Am J Cardiol* 2003;92(4):487–489.
13. Bader RS, Chitayat D, Kelly E, et al. Fetal rhabdomyoma: prenatal diagnosis, clinical outcome, and incidence of associated tuberous sclerosis complex. *J Pediatr* 2003;143(5):620–624.
14. Kivelitz DE, Muhler M, Rake A, et al. MRI of cardiac rhabdomyoma in the fetus. *Eur Radiol* 2004;14(8):1513–1516.
15. Muhler MR, Rake A, Schwabe M, et al. Value of fetal cerebral MRI in sonographically proven cardiac rhabdomyoma. *Pediatr Radiol* 2007;37(5):467–474.
16. Milunsky A, Ito M, Maher TA, et al. Prenatal molecular diagnosis of tuberous sclerosis complex. *Am J Obstet Gynecol* 2009;200:321.e1–6.

INTRODUCTION

The prenatal diagnosis of cardiac rhythm abnormalities has been made possible with advancements in ultrasound imaging. M-mode ultrasound in addition to color and pulsed Doppler echocardiography play a significant role in our ability to diagnose complex arrhythmias in the fetus and in monitoring the success of prenatal treatment intervention. The recent addition of tissue Doppler and magnetocardiography to conventional ultrasound will undoubtedly enhance the ability to understand the pathophysiology of fetal rhythm disturbances and to target specific treatment of these conditions.

Fetal cardiac rhythm abnormalities are common and are encountered in about 1% to 2% of pregnancies (1). Irregular fetal cardiac rhythm is the leading cause for referrals to fetal echocardiography centers for rhythm disturbances, and the vast majority of those are benign atrial ectopic beats. Sustained fetal bradyarrhythmias or tachyarrhythmias, which are associated with an increase in neonatal morbidity and mortality, account for less than 10% of referrals (2). This chapter will review the diagnostic modalities currently available for the assessment of fetal rhythm abnormalities and the various types of fetal arrhythmias, as well as their impact on fetal and neonatal outcome and their management.

FETAL RHYTHM ASSESSMENT

M-mode Echocardiography

M-mode (motion mode) echocardiography is obtained by recording ultrasound beam reflections in relation to depth from the transducer and time. The M-mode display is therefore a linear representation of adjacent cardiac structures as a function of time. In clinical practice, a two-dimensional (2-D) image of the fetal heart is first obtained and the M-mode cursor is placed at the desired location within the heart. The linear display of M-mode echocardiography allows for more accurate and reproducible measurements of various cardiac chambers and great vessel diameters. Furthermore, as it detects motion of structures through time, M-mode echocardiography is commonly used in the evaluation of fetal arrhythmias and excursions of various cardiac valves. The M-mode cursor is often placed to intersect an atrium and a ventricle so that the relationship of atrial to ventricular contractions is recorded (Fig. 25-1). The onset and peak of atrial and ventricular contractions are not clearly defined on M-mode, which limits its ability to measure atrioventricular (AV) time intervals, a major limitation of M-mode evaluation of fetal rhythm abnormalities. Furthermore, poor signal quality and suboptimal fetal position are often encountered, which limits the application of M-mode. Incorporating color Doppler into M-mode (Fig. 25-2) and steering of the M-mode beam, which is available in newer ultrasound equipment, allow for enhanced performance.

Pulsed Doppler Echocardiography

Pulsed Doppler echocardiography can provide critical information in the assessment of fetal rhythm abnormalities and is the current preferred method in addition to M-mode echocardiography. Pulsed Doppler allows for the ability to acquire simultaneous signals from atrial and ventricular contractions, which results in the identification of temporal cardiac events and measurement of various time intervals, a required parameter for the classification of various arrhythmias. Information can be provided when the pulsed Doppler gate is placed across the mitral and aortic valves (Fig. 25-3), pulmonary artery and vein (Fig. 25-4), renal artery and vein (Fig. 25-5), or superior vena cava and aorta (Fig. 25-6) (3–5). When the superior vena cava and the aorta are simultaneously interrogated by Doppler, retrograde flow in the superior vena cava marks the beginning of atrial systole, and the onset of aortic forward flow marks the beginning of

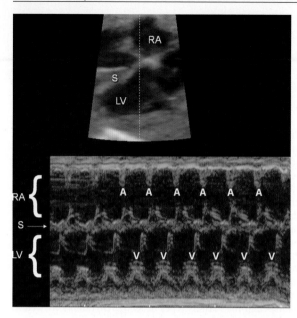

Figure 25-1. M-mode recording of normal sinus rhythm in a fetus. The M-mode cursor line intersects the right atrium (RA), the interventricular septum (S), and the left ventricle (LV). The M-mode recording shows the atrial contractions (A) and the corresponding ventricular contractions (V).

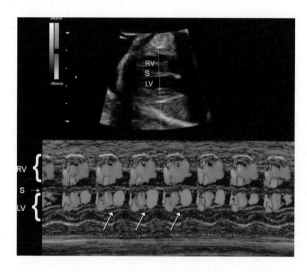

Figure 25-2. Color Doppler M-mode recording of normal sinus rhythm in a fetus. The M-mode cursor line intersects the right ventricle (RV), the interventricular septum (S), and the left ventricle (LV). Given the proximity of LV inflow and outflow, red and blue coloration is noted within the LV (*oblique arrows*).

ventricular systole (Fig. 25-6). The mechanical PR interval can also be evaluated by pulsed Doppler (see below) (6).

Fetal Electrocardiography

Fetal electrocardiography (ECG), derived by abdominal recording of fetal electrical cardiac signals, was reported and introduced about a decade ago. The difficulty of this technique involves the ability to isolate the fetal signals from the overlapping maternal ECG signals. Significant progress is under way, and future technologic improvements in this field will undoubtedly facilitate the use of fetal ECG in the classification of arrhythmias.

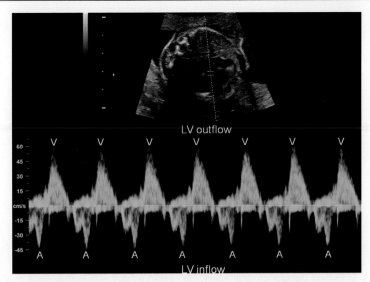

Figure 25-3. Pulsed Doppler of left ventricular (LV) inflow (mitral valve) and outflow (aortic valve) in a fetus with normal sinus rhythm. Atrial contractions (A) are identified by the start of the A wave in the mitral valve and ventricular contractions (V) by the aortic outflow.

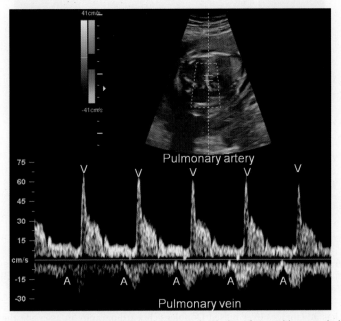

Figure 25-4. Pulsed Doppler of pulmonary artery and vein in a fetus with normal sinus rhythm. Atrial contractions (A) are identified by the start of the A wave in the pulmonary vein Doppler waveform and ventricular contractions (V) by the pulmonary artery flow.

Tissue Doppler Imaging

Tissue Doppler imaging is a new technique that allows direct analysis of segmental wall motion (myocardial velocities) in any area of the fetal heart during the same cardiac cycle (7). This technique, which gives a color-coded map of cardiac structures and their movements

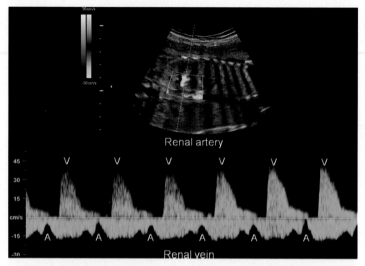

Figure 25-5. Pulsed Doppler of renal artery and vein in a fetus with normal sinus rhythm. Atrial contractions (A) are identified by the start of the A wave in the renal vein Doppler waveform and ventricular contractions (V) by the renal artery flow.

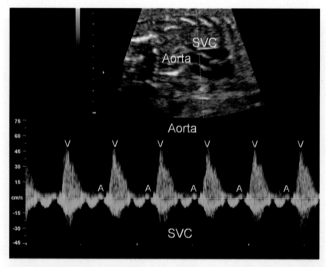

Figure 25-6. Pulsed Doppler of the aorta and superior vena cava (SVC) in a fetus with normal sinus rhythm. Atrial contractions (A) are identified by the retrograde A wave in the SVC and ventricular contractions (V) by the aortic flow.

(Fig. 25-7), has advantages over pulsed Doppler echocardiography in assessing the chronology of atrial and ventricular systolic events. Pulsed Doppler echocardiographic assessment of the AV time interval is indirectly derived from flow measurements, which are influenced by loading condition, intrinsic myocardial properties, heart rate, and propagation speed (8). By sampling atrial and ventricular wall motion, however, tissue Doppler can provide accurate measurements of cardiac intervals and cardiac wall velocities (Fig. 25-8A, B) (8). The narrow availability of tissue Doppler equipment limits the clinical applicability of this technique. By adjusting gain and velocity of color and pulsed Doppler ultrasound, cardiac tissue Doppler imaging can be obtained with standard ultrasound equipment (9). Recommended color

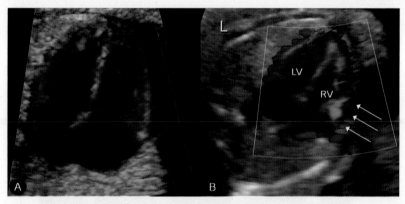

Figure 25-7. Tissue Doppler imaging at the level of the four-chamber view in a normal fetus **(A)** and in a fetus with anemia **(B)**. Note the green coloration of the right ventricle (RV) in fetus B (*arrows*), indicating right ventricular dysfunction. L, left; LV, left ventricle.

Doppler settings for obtaining tissue Doppler on conventional ultrasound equipment are shown in Table 25-1.

Magnetocardiography

Magnetocardiography (MCG) records the magnetic field produced by the electrical activity of the fetal heart and uses signal averaging to generate waveforms that are very similar to those obtained by ECG. Limitations of this technology include its lack of availability in many centers and the need for a magnetically shielded room (10,11). Successful use of this technology in an unshielded environment has been reported (12).

 ## CLASSIFICATION OF ARRHYTHMIAS AND MANAGEMENT OPTIONS

Classification of cardiac arrhythmias in the neonate, the child, and the adult is aided by established criteria primarily by ECG findings. Since such technology is not technically feasible in the fetus, a more practical approach to the classification of fetal arrhythmias is used, which relies on ultrasound-derived technologies such as M-mode, pulsed Doppler, and tissue Doppler. Fetal arrhythmias are classified into three main groups: irregular cardiac rhythm, fetal bradyarrhythmias (below 100 bpm), and fetal tachyarrhythmias (above 180 bpm).

 ## IRREGULAR CARDIAC RHYTHM

Irregular cardiac rhythms are the most common cause of referral for fetal arrhythmia. The majority of fetuses with irregular cardiac rhythms are found to have premature atrial contractions (PACs) (Fig. 25-9). PACs are due to atrial ectopic beats (atrial ectopy), which occur most commonly in the late second trimester of pregnancy through term and are usually benign. PACs can be either conducted or blocked, resulting in an irregular rhythm or a short pause, respectively. PACs are associated with congenital heart disease in up to 1% to 2% of cases (13) and can progress to sustained tachycardia in utero or in the first 3 to 4 weeks of life in up to 2% to 3% of cases (14,15). Risk factors for progression of PACs to tachycardia include low ventricular rate due to multiple blocked atrial ectopic beats and complex ectopy including bigeminy (Fig. 25-10) or trigeminy (Fig. 25-11) (13,16). The presence of PACs in fetuses with evidence of cardiac dysfunction should alert for the possibility of supraventricular tachycardia. Weekly or biweekly assessment of cardiac rhythm by ultrasound or a handheld Doppler device is warranted until PACs resolve or delivery occurs.

On rare occasions, premature beats originate from the ventricle rather than the atrium and are thus termed premature ventricular contractions (PVCs). PVCs are also benign in the majority of cases. Fetal cardiac assessment, however, is warranted when PVCs are encountered.

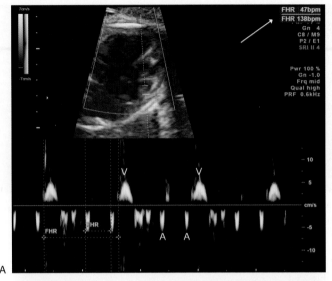

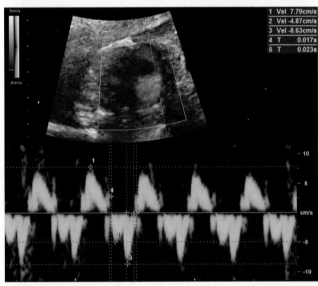

Figure 25-8. A: Tissue Doppler measurement of atrial (A) and ventricular (V) heart rate in a fetus with complete heart block. Note a normal atrial rate of 138 bpm and a ventricular rate of 47 bpm (*arrow*). **B:** Tissue Doppler measurement of longitudinal annular movement velocities in a normal fetus at 20 weeks' gestation.

Differentiating PACs from PVCs can be difficult in the fetus. The demonstration of tricuspid regurgitation on color Doppler or a smaller A wave in the inferior vena cava on pulsed Doppler concurrent with an ectopic beat may suggest a ventricular origin (13).

MANAGEMENT OPTIONS FOR IRREGULAR CARDIAC RHYTHM

No therapy is necessary in the majority of cases with irregular cardiac rhythm when the cause is atrial or with ventricular ectopic beats as most resolve spontaneously. The authors recommend for the mother to stop known or suspected inciting factors such as smoking, excessive

TABLE 25-1	Color and Pulsed Doppler Parameters for Tissue Doppler Obtained on Conventional Ultrasound Equipment

1. Magnify the fetal heart until it occupies 75% of the image.
2. Color box should be adjusted to only cover the heart.
3. Reduce color gain setting until no color signal is noted from blood flow.
4. Reduce pulse repetition frequency (PRF) to detect low-velocity flow.
5. Reduce wall filter to detect low-velocity flow.
6. Adjust parameters to balance between tissue motion detection and frame rate.

(From Tutschek B, Zimmermann T, Buck T, et al. Fetal tissue Doppler echocardiography: detection rates of cardiac structures and quantitative assessment of the fetal heart. *Ultrasound Obstet Gynecol* 2003;21:26–32, with permission.)

caffeine ingestion, and cardiac active drugs (β-mimetics for premature contractions) when possible. Follow-up is suggested on a weekly or biweekly schedule to monitor fetal cardiac rate and rhythm in order to detect progression to fetal tachycardia, which may necessitate fetal therapy. When the fetal irregular beats are sustained until delivery, the authors recommend the performance of an ECG in the neonatal period.

 ## FETAL BRADYARRHYTHMIAS

Fetal bradycardia is defined by a sustained fetal heart rate of less than 100 bpm. Transient episodes of fetal heart rate of less than 100 bpm are usually benign and typically result from increased vagal stimulation in the fetus commonly associated with abdominal pressure by the ultrasound probe. Causes of fetal bradycardia include sinus bradycardia, blocked atrial bigeminy/trigeminy, and high-degree atrioventricular block (17).

Sinus Bradycardia

Sinus bradycardia is rare and may occur in association with sinus node dysfunction, fetal acidemia, congenital long QT syndrome, or congenital abnormalities such as heterotaxy syndromes (18).

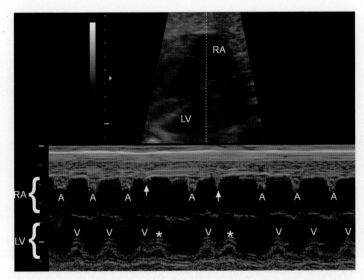

Figure 25-9. M-mode recording of a fetus with conducted premature atrial contractions. The M-mode cursor line intersects the right atrium (RA) and left ventricle (LV). Normal atrial contractions (A) are seen followed by normal ventricular contractions (V). Two premature atrial contractions are shown (*arrows*) followed by two premature ventricular contractions (*asterisk*).

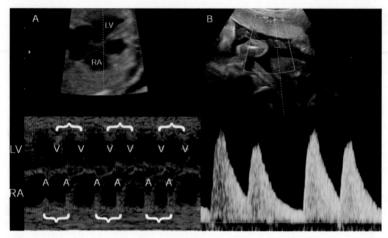

Figure 25-10. M-mode recording **(A)** and pulsed Doppler of the umbilical artery **(B)** in a fetus with bigeminy. The M-mode cursor line intersects the right atrium (RA) and left ventricle (LV). Atrial (A) and ventricular (V) contractions are in doubles (*brackets*) with a longer pause between the double sequence. The bigeminy is also clearly seen in the umbilical artery pulsed Doppler spectrum (B).

Long QT syndrome is suggested in the presence of family history or when intermittent runs of ventricular tachycardia with 2:1 atrioventricular block are noted in this setting (18,19). Characteristics of sinus bradycardia include a one-to-one atrioventricular conduction on echocardiography with a slow atrial rate.

Persistent Atrial Bigeminy or Trigeminy

Persistent atrial bigeminy or trigeminy with blocked premature beats is another cause of fetal bradycardia. Differentiating this type of bradycardia from atrioventricular heart block is

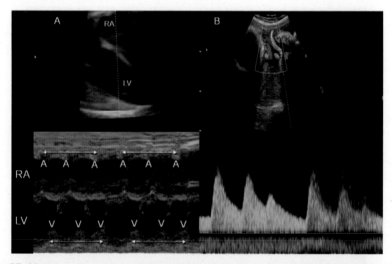

Figure 25-11. M-mode recording **(A)** and pulsed Doppler of the umbilical artery **(B)** in a fetus with trigeminy. The M-mode cursor line intersects the right atrium (RA) and left ventricle (LV). Atrial (A) and ventricular (V) contractions are in triplets (*double-sided arrows*) with a longer pause between the triplet sequence. The trigeminy is also clearly seen in the umbilical artery pulsed Doppler spectrum (B).

critical given a divergent prognosis. In both blocked premature beats and atrioventricular heart block, the atrial rate is higher than the ventricular rate. The time interval between consecutive atrial impulses is relatively constant in atrioventricular block as opposed to a shortened atrial impulse interval on every second or third beat in bigeminy or trigeminy, respectively. Blocked premature beats are typically benign and tend to resolve with increased fetal activity.

Congenital Atrioventricular (AV) Heart Block

Up to 40% of congenital atrioventricular (AV) heart block (CAVB) cases (Fig. 25-12) occur in fetuses with congenital cardiac malformations, especially left atrial isomerism (heterotaxy) (see Chapter 22) or congenitally corrected transposition of the great arteries (see Chapter 20). In the remaining 60% no structural fetal anomaly is found and heart block is almost always caused by a connective tissue disease (immune mediated) of the mother. In most cases, this maternal disease is not known at fetal diagnosis and should be sought. CAVB occurs in about 1 in 11,000 to 1 in 22,000 live births in the general population and in 1% to 2% of live births in pregnancies with anti-SSA/Ro antibodies, with a recurrence risk of 14% to 17% in these pregnancies (20–23). The characteristics of first-degree, second-degree, or third-degree (complete) heart block are presented in Table 25-2.

Pathogenesis of immune-mediated CAVB is thought to result from an inflammatory response and injury to the myocardium and cardiac conduction system in susceptible fetuses, initiated by the circulating maternal antibodies. Cardiac injury in immune-mediated CAVB includes myocardial dysfunction, cardiomyopathy, endocardial fibroelastosis, and conduction abnormalities (24,25). Delayed dilated cardiomyopathy despite successful pacing is seen in up to 11% of children with immune-mediated CAVB (24). CAVB has a high mortality rate, exceeding 70%, when associated with cardiac malformations, whereas a mortality rate of 19% is reported in immune-mediated cases (26).

The mechanical PR interval, measured by Doppler ultrasound, can be used in an attempt to predict the fetus at risk for heart block in pregnancies with anti-SSA antibodies. The mechanical PR interval, which includes the isovolumic contraction phase of the ventricle, is

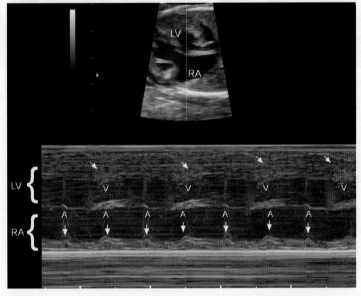

Figure 25-12. M-mode recording of a fetus with complete heart block. The M-mode cursor line intersects the left ventricle (LV) and right atrium (RA). The atrial contractions are shown by straight arrows and occur at a regular and normal rate. The ventricular contractions (V) are shown by oblique arrows and occur at a slower rate, dissociated from the atrial contractions.

TABLE 25-2	Characteristics of First-degree, Second-degree, and Third-degree (Complete) Atrioventricular (AV) Heart Block	
Degree of AV block	AV interval/AV conduction	Heart rate
First degree	Prolonged/AV conduction is 1:1	Normal
Second degree—type 1 (Wenckebach)	Progressive lengthening of AV interval until one impulse is blocked	Commonly irregular
Second degree—type 2 (Mobitz)	Normal AV interval with blocked impulses, commonly 2:1 conduction	Slow, regular
Third degree—complete heart block	Complete interruption of AV conduction, atria and ventricles beat independently	Slow, regular, ventricular rate

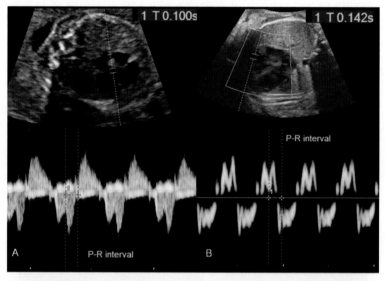

Figure 25-13. PR interval in two normal fetuses. In fetus **A,** the PR interval (0.100 sec) is measured on pulsed Doppler at the mitral-aortic region. In fetus **B**, the PR interval (0.142 sec) is measured on tissue Doppler as shown.

longer than the electric PR interval (27). The normal value for the mechanical PR interval in the fetus is 0.12 ± 0.02 sec when measured from the mitral/aortic valves region (Fig. 25-13A, B) (28). Prolongation of the mechanical PR interval beyond an upper cut-off of 0.14 seconds was noted in 30% of fetuses in pregnancies associated with anti-SSA antibodies (29). Other potential markers include the presence of tricuspid regurgitation, decreased cardiac function, ventricular tachycardia, and fibroelastosis (10,30). Despite these findings, a reliable surveillance test for the prediction of fetuses that will develop heart block in the setting of anti-SSA antibodies does not exist.

MANAGEMENT OPTIONS FOR BRADYARRHYTHMIAS

No fetal therapy is necessary in most cases of sinus bradycardia and blocked atrial ectopic beats. Unfortunately, fetal complete heart block associated with a cardiac malformation cannot be treated in utero, and it has been observed that when the ventricular rate in this setting is less than 50 bpm, an increased association with fetal hydrops is noted (see Chapter 22 on fetal isomerism).

Treatment for pregnancies with immune-mediated heart block with fluorinated steroids such as betamethasone or dexamethasone appears, however, to be effective and has been shown to increase survival at 1 year from 47% to 95% when used systematically (31). Effective treatment is thought to result from the anti-inflammatory effect of fluorinated steroids that cross the placenta. Improvements in conduction abnormalities and cardiac function and, on occasion, resolution of fetal hydrops have been reported. Even in the absence of visible improvement in conduction abnormalities, fluorinated steroids may significantly improve survival of fetuses with complete heart block (31). Guidelines for the in utero treatment of congenital heart block have been established (32). Definitive data, however, on the objective effectiveness of fluorinated steroids from prospective large studies or clinical trials are currently lacking. Repeated doses of steroids have been shown to impair fetal growth and reduce brain weight in animals (33). Patient counseling regarding the risk/benefit of treatment in the setting of CAVB should be performed. The use of fluorinated steroids as preventive treatment in at-risk pregnancies is not recommended. Furthermore, therapy with β-mimetic drugs to increase the fetal heart rate in complete heart block has been suggested, but the long-term benefits of such treatment have not been clearly established.

FETAL TACHYARRHYTHMIAS

Fetal tachycardia is defined by a sustained fetal ventricular heart rate of greater than 180 bpm. Sustained fetal tachycardia can potentially cause significant morbidity and mortality and requires immediate referral for further evaluation and management. Identifying the accurate diagnosis ensures the proper choice of medical therapy. The association of congenital heart malformations with fetal tachycardia is rare and has been reported in the range of 1% to 5% of cases (34). Echocardiographic measurement techniques that may help in the differential diagnosis of fetal tachycardia include the atrial and ventricular tachycardia and variability rates and the atrioventricular (AV) and ventriculoatrial (VA) time intervals.

Sinus Tachycardia

Sinus tachycardia is characterized by equal atrial and ventricular rates in the range of 180 to 200 bpm, 1:1 AV conduction, normal AV interval duration, and variability in the heart rate. Etiologies include maternal fever, infections, maternal drug ingestion such as β-mimetics, and fetal distress. Management of sinus tachycardia includes identifying and treating the underlying cause when possible.

Supraventricular Tachycardia

Supraventricular tachycardia (SVT) is the most common cause of fetal tachycardia and accounts for about 66% to 90% of all cases (35). In SVT, the tachycardia range is typically around 220 to 240 bpm, there is 1:1 ratio of atrioventricular conduction, and the fetal heart rate is monotonous with lack of atrial or ventricular rate variability (Fig. 25-14). SVT is most commonly present due to an accessory pathway between the atrium and the ventricle, which allows retrograde re-entry of VA conduction. A circuit is thus formed that allows for normal antegrade AV conduction through the AV node and a retrograde fast re-entry from the ventricles to the atria (VA) through the accessory pathway. Given that the re-entry VA pathway is commonly shorter than the normal AV conduction, SVTs are typically associated with a short VA interval or a VA/AV ratio of less than 1. This mechanism accounts for 90% of fetal SVTs (36), and at birth 10% of those are found to have Wolff-Parkinson-White syndrome. Other forms of SVTs include a long VA interval, those in whom the V and A wave are superimposed, and atrial re-entrant tachycardia (37). SVTs with a long VA interval include sinus tachycardia, ectopic atrial tachycardia, and permanent junctional reciprocating tachycardia. The A wave is superimposed to the V wave in junctional ectopic tachycardia. Unlike the typical fetal SVT with fast VA re-entry, SVTs with long VA interval are rare, refractory to treatment, and may be associated with congenital abnormalities such as rhabdomyomas (38,39).

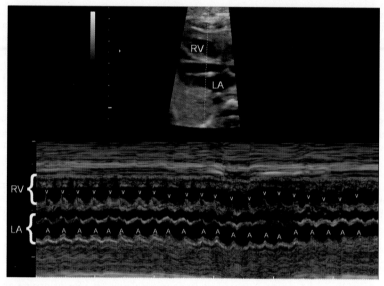

Figure 25-14. M-mode recording of a fetus with supraventricular tachycardia. The M-mode cursor line intersects the right ventricle (RV) and left atrium (LA). The atrial contractions are marked with A and the ventricular contractions are marked with V. Note the presence of atrial and ventricular tachycardia with a 1:1 ratio of atrioventricular conduction and monotonous heart rate with lack of atrial or ventricular rate variability.

Atrial Flutter

Atrial flutter in the fetus is defined by a rapid regular atrial rate of 300 to 600 bpm, accompanied by variable degrees of AV conduction block, resulting in a slower ventricular rate, typically around 220 to 240 bpm (Fig. 25-15). The atrioventricular conduction block is 2:1 in 80% of cases and 3:1 in the remainder (40). Atrial flutter is another form of SVT involving accessory circuits within the atria that results in atrial re-entrant tachycardia. Atrial flutter accounts for about 10% to 30% of all fetal tachyarrhythmias (35) and tends to occur later in gestation. Atrial flutter is associated with chromosomal abnormalities and structural heart or other defects in up to 30% of cases (41). The incidence of fetal hydrops in atrial flutter is similar to that in rapid re-entrant SVT and is in the order of 35% to 40% (40).

Ventricular Tachycardia

Ventricular tachycardia is rare and presents with ventricular rates of more than 180 bpm in the setting of AV dissociation. Atrial rates are typically normal. Underlying etiology includes fetal myocarditis or long QT syndrome (42,43). Diagnosis of ventricular tachycardia can be challenging and is based on the demonstration of a fast and regular ventricular rhythm with no temporal relationship to the atrial rhythm. The atrial rhythm is typically slower than the ventricular rhythm. On rare occasions retrograde atrial activation occurs and 1:1 atrial-to-ventricular rate is seen. In this setting, tissue Doppler imaging and fetal magnetocardiograms may be helpful in the diagnosis.

Atrial Fibrillation

Atrial fibrillation is a rare form of fetal tachycardia that involves a rapid and irregular atrial rate with a blocked AV conduction. The ventricular rate is thus rapid and irregular with variability. Often atrial fibrillation cannot be reliably differentiated from atrial flutter in the fetus.

 MANAGEMENT OPTIONS FOR FETAL TACHYARRHYTHMIAS

When fetal tachyarrhythmia is diagnosed at a time in gestation when fetal lung maturity can be established, delivery is the preferred method of treatment. Furthermore, when fetal

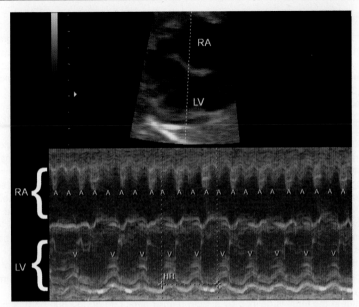

Figure 25-15. M-mode recording of a fetus with atrial flutter. The M-mode cursor line intersects the right atrium (RA) and left ventricle (LV). The atrial contractions are marked with A and the ventricular contractions with V. Note the presence of atrial and ventricular tachycardia with a 2:1 ratio of atrioventricular conduction.

tachyarrhythmia is intermittent with no evidence of fetal hemodynamic compromise, careful and frequent follow-up without medical treatment is recommended. Sustained fetal tachyarrhythmia may result in hemodynamic compromise due to impaired diastolic filling, venous congestion, and reduced cardiac output. In this setting, drug therapy with antiarrhythmic medications is warranted. Initiation of drug therapy is best performed in an inpatient setting in order to closely monitor serum levels and maternal response to the medications.

Digoxin is still considered by many as the first-line drug of choice in treating fetal tachyarrhythmia. Digoxin serum levels in the fetus are 70% to 100% that of maternal serum levels in nonhydropic fetuses (44). Serum levels of digoxin in hydropic fetuses are unreliable and typically do not achieve therapeutic levels despite near-toxic maternal levels (45). Conversion rates in hydropic fetuses with SVT or atrial flutter treated with digoxin are in the range of 6% to 7% (40). Furthermore, digoxin therapy is not effective in SVT with long VA interval such as ectopic atrial tachycardia and permanent junctional reciprocating tachycardia (39). Nevertheless, digoxin appears to be effective in treating SVT with short VA interval and atrial flutter in nonhydropic fetuses (about 90% of fetal tachyarrhythmias), with reported conversion rates in the range of 40% to 60% (40).

Oral sotalol, a beta-blocking agent, is used as the first line of treatment for tachyarrhythmias in some centers (28). Oral sotalol is recommended as the drug of choice for SVT with long VA interval and for hydropic fetuses either alone or in combination with digoxin. Fetal serum levels of sotalol are identical to maternal levels and placental transfer is almost complete. Close maternal monitoring of the QT interval is recommended with initiation of treatment.

Flecainide, amiodarone, and other antiarrhythmic medications are typically reserved as second-line treatment in cases that are unresponsive to digoxin and/or sotalol. Flecainide has shown success when used in cases where digoxin monotherapy failed to correct cardiac tachyarrhythmias (46) and also as first-line treatment in some centers. In severely hydropic fetuses that failed conventional treatment, direct fetal therapy into the umbilical vein or intramuscularly have been reported (47,48). Repeated injections are typically required for effective therapy.

■ KEY POINTS: FETAL ARRHYTHMIAS

■ Irregular fetal cardiac rhythm is the leading cause for referrals to fetal echocardiography centers for rhythm disturbances and the vast majority of those are benign atrial ectopic beats.

■ Premature atrial contractions are associated with congenital heart disease in up to 1–2% of cases and can progress to sustained tachycardia in utero or in the first 3 to 4 weeks of life in up to 2–3% of cases.

■ Fetal bradycardia is defined by a sustained fetal heart rate of less than 100 bpm.

■ Causes of fetal bradycardia include sinus bradycardia, blocked atrial bigeminy/trigeminy or high degree atrioventricular block.

■ Up to 40% of congenital atrioventricular heart block cases occur in fetuses with congenital cardiac malformations with the remaining 60% occurring in association with maternal connective tissue diseases.

■ Fetal tachycardia is defined by a sustained fetal ventricular heart rate of greater than 180 bpm.

■ Sinus tachycardia is characterized by equal atrial and ventricular rates in the range of 180–200 bpm, 1 to1 atrioventricular conduction, normal atrioventricular interval duration and variability in the heart rate.

■ Supraventricular tachycardia (SVT) is the most common cause of fetal tachycardia and accounts for about 66–90% of all cases.

■ In SVT, the tachycardia range is typically around 220–240 bpm, there is 1:1 ratio of atrioventricular conduction and the fetal heart rate is monotonous with lack of atrial or ventricular rate variability.

■ Atrial flutter in the fetus is defined by a rapid regular atrial rate of 300–600 bpm, accompanied by variable degrees of atrioventricular conduction block, resulting in a slower ventricular rate, typically around 220–240 bpm.

■ Ventricular tachycardia is rare and presents with ventricular rates of more than 180 bpm in the setting of atrioventricular dissociation.

■ Atrial fibrillation is a rare form of fetal tachycardia that involves a rapid and irregular atrial rate with a blocked atrioventricular conduction.

■ Digoxin is still considered by many as the first-line drug of choice in treating fetal tachyarrhythmia in nonhydropic fetuses.

References

1. Southall DP, Richards J, Hardwick RA, et al. Prospective study of fetal heart rate and rhythm patterns. *Arch Dis Child* 1980;55:506–511.
2. Reed KL. Fetal arrhythmias: etiology, diagnosis, pathophysiology, and treatment. *Semin Perinatol* 1989;13:294–304.
3. Dancea A, Fouron JC, Miro J, et al. Correlation between electrocardiographic and ultrasonographic time-interval measurements in fetal lamb heart. *Pediatr Res* 2000;47:324–328.
4. Fouron JC, Fournier A, Proulx F, et al. Management of fetal tachyarrhythmia based on superior vena cava/aorta Doppler flow recordings. *Heart* 2003;89:1211–1216.
5. Carvalho JS, Perfumo F, Ciardelli V, et al. Evaluation of fetal arrhythmias from simultaneous pulsed wave Doppler in pulmonary artery and vein. *Heart* 2007;93:1448–1453.
6. Friedman DM, Kim MY, Copel JA, et al. Utility of cardiac monitoring in fetuses at risk for congenital heart block. The PR Interval and Dexamethasone Evaluation (PRIDE) prospective study. *Circulation* 2008;117:485–493.
7. Rein AJ, O'Donnell C, Geva T et al. Use of tissue velocity imaging in the diagnosis of fetal cardiac arrhythmias. *Circulation* 2002;106:1827–1833.
8. Nii M, Shimizu M, Roman KS, et al. Doppler tissue imaging in the assessment of atrioventricular conduction time: validation of a novel technique and comparison with electrophysiologic and pulsed wave Doppler-derived equivalents in an animal model. *J Am Soc Echocardiogr* 2006;19:314–321.
9. Tutschek B, Zimmermann T, Buck T, et al. Fetal tissue Doppler echocardiography: detection rates of cardiac structures and quantitative assessment of the fetal heart. *Ultrasound Obstet Gynecol* 2003;21:26–32.
10. Zhao H, Cuneo BF, Strasburger JF, et al. Electrophysiological characteristics of fetal atrioventricular block. *J Am Coll Cardiol* 2008;51:77–84.
11. Hornberger LK, Collins K. New insights into fetal atrioventricular block using fetal magenetocardiography. *J Am Coll Cardiol* 2008;51:85–86.
12. Seki Y, Kandori A, Kumagai Y, et al. Unshielded fetal magnetocardiography system using two-dimensional gradiometers. *Rev Sci Instruments* 2008;79:036106.
13. Simpson JM, Yates RW, Sharland GK. Irregular heart rate in the fetus—not always benign. *Cardiol Young* 1996;6:28–31.
14. Simpson LL. Fetal supraventricular tachycardias: diagnosis and management. *Semin Perinatol* 2000;24:360–372.

15. Vergani P, Mariani E, Ciriello E, et al. Fetal arrhythmias: natural history and management. *Ultrasound Med Biol* 2005;31:1–6.
16. Fish F, Benson DJ. Disorders of cardiac rhythm and conduction. In: Allen HD, Gutgesell H, Clark EB, et al., eds. *Heart disease in infants, children, and adolescents,* 6th ed. Philadelphia: Lippincott William & Wilkins, 2001;482–533.
17. Larmay HJ, Strasburger JF. Differential diagnosis and management of the fetus and newborn with an irregular or abnormal heart rate. *Pediatr Clin North Am* 2004;51:1033–1050.
18. Hofbeck M, Ulmer H, Beinder E, et al. Prenatal findings in patients with prolonged QT interval in the neonatal period. *Heart* 1997;77:198–204.
19. Beinder E, Grancay T, Menendez T, et al. Fetal sinus bradycardia and the long QT syndrome. *Am J Obstet Gynecol* 2001;185:743–747.
20. Michaelsson M, Engle MA. Congenital complete heart block: an international study of the natural history. *Cardiovasc Clin* 1972;4:85–101.
21. Siren MK, Julkunen H, Kaaja R. The increasing incidence of isolated congenital heart block in Finland. *J Rheumatol* 1998;25:1862–1864.
22. Brucato A, Frassi M, Franceschini F, et al. Risk of congenital complete heart block in newborns of mothers with anti-Ro/SSA antibodies detected by counterimmunoelectrophoresis: a prospective study of 100 women. *Arthritis Rheum* 2001;44:1832–1835.
23. Costedoat-Chalumeau N, Amoura Z, Lupoglazoff JM, et al. Outcome of pregnancies in patients with anti-SSA/Ro antibodies: a study of 165 pregnancies, with special focus on electrocardiographic variations in the children and comparison with a control group. *Arthritis Rheum* 2004;50:3187–3194.
24. Moak JP, Barron KS, Hougen TJ, et al. Congenital heart block: development of late-onset cardiomyopathy, a previously underappreciated sequela. *J Am Coll Cardiol* 2001;37:238–242.
25. Villain E, Marijon E, Georgin S. Is isolated congenital heart block with maternal antibodies a distinct and more severe form of the disease in childhood? *Heart Rhythm* 2005;2(1S):S45.
26. Buyon JP, Hiebert R, Copel J, et al. Autoimmune-associated congenital heart block: demographics, mortality, morbidity and recurrence rates obtained from a national neonatal lupus registry. *J Am Coll Cardiol* 1998;31:1658–1666.
27. Nii M, Hamilton RM, Fenwick L, et al. Assessment of fetal atrioventricular time intervals by tissue Doppler and pulse Doppler echocardiography: normal values and correlation with fetal electrocardiography. *Heart* 2006;92:1831–1837.
28. Jaeggi ET, Nii M. Fetal brady- and tachyarrhythmias: new and accepted diagnostic and treatment methods. *Semin Fetal Neonatal Med* 2005;10:504–514.
29. Sonesson SE, Salomonsson S, Jacobsson LA, et al. Signs of first degree heart block occur in one-third of fetuses of pregnant women with anti-SSA/Ro 52 kd antibodies. *Arthritis Rheum* 2004;50:1253–1261.
30. Friedman DM, Kim MY, Copel JA, et al. Utility of cardiac monitoring in fetuses at risk for congenital heart block: the PR interval and Dexamethasone Evaluation (PRIDE) prospective study. *Circulation* 2008;117:485–493.
31. Jaeggi ET, Fouron JC, Silverman ED, et al. Transplacental fetal treatment improves the outcome of prenatally diagnosed complete atrioventricular block without structural heart disease. *Circulation* 2004;110:1542–1548.
32. Buyon JP, Clancy RM. Maternal autoantibodies and congenital heart block: mediators, markers and therapeutic approach. *Semin Arthritis Rheum* 2003;33:140–154.
33. Kutzler MA, Ruane EK, Coksaygan T, et al. Effects of three courses of maternally administered dexamethasone at 0.7, 0.75 and 0.8 of gestation on prenatal and postnatal growth in sheep. *Pediatrics* 2004;113:313–319.
34. Simpson J, Silverman NH. Diagnosis of cardiac arrhythmias during fetal life. In: Yagel S, Silverman NH, Gembruch U, eds. *Fetal cardiology.* London: Martin Dunitz, 2003;333–344.
35. Van Engelen AD, Weitjens O, Brenner JI, et al. Management outcome and follow up of fetal tachycardia. *J Am Coll Cardiol* 1994;24:1371–1375.
36. Kleinman CS, Nehgme RA. Cardiac arrhythmias in the human fetus. *Pediatr Cardiol* 2004;25:234–251.
37. Fouron JC. Fetal arrhythmias: the Sainte-Justine hospital experience. *Prenat Diagn* 2004;24:1068–1080.
38. Jaeggi E, Fouron JC, Fournier A, et al. Ventriculo-atrial time interval measured on M mode echocardiography: a determining element in diagnosis, treatment, and prognosis of fetal supraventricular tachycardia. *Heart* 1998;79:582–587.
39. Strasburger JF. Prenatal diagnosis of fetal arrhythmias. *Clin Perinatol* 2005;32:891–912.
40. Krapp M, Kohl T, Simpson JM, et al. Review of diagnosis, treatment and outcome of fetal atrial flutter compared with supraventricular tachycardia. *Heart* 2003;89:913–917.
41. Larmay HJ, Strasburger JF. Differential diagnosis and management of the fetus and newborn with an irregular or abnormal heart rate. *Pediatr Clin North Am* 2004;51:1033–1050.
42. Cuneo BF, Ovadia M, Strasburger JF, et al. Prenatal diagnosis and in utero treatment of torsades de pointes associated with congenital long QT syndrome. *Am J Cardiol* 2003;91:1395–1398.
43. Zhao H, Strasburger JF, Cuneo BF, et al. Fetal cardiac repolarization abnormalities. *Am J Cardiol* 2006;98:491–496.
44. Api O, Carvalho J. Fetal dysrhythmias. *Best Pract Res Clin Obstet Gynaecol* 2008;22(1):31–48.
45. Frohn-Mulder IM, Stewart PA, Witsenburg M, et al. The efficacy of flecainide versus digoxin in the management of fetal supraventricular tachycardia. *Prenat Diagn* 1995;15:1297–1302.
46. Krapp M, Baschat AA, Gembruch U, et al. Flecainide in the intrauterine treatment of fetal supraventricular tachycardia. *Ultrasound Obstet Gynecol* 2002;19:158–164.
47. Leiria TL, Lima GG, Dillenburg RF, et al. Fetal tachyarrhythmia with 1:1 atrioventricular conduction. Adenosine infusion in the umbilical vein as a diagnostic test. *Arq Bras Cardiol* 2000;75:65–68.
48. Mangione R, Guyon F, Vergnaud A, et al. Successful treatment of refractory supraventricular tachycardia by repeat intravascular injection of amiodarone in a fetus with hydrops. *Eur J Obstet Gynecol Reprod Biol* 1999;86:105–107.

Page numbers followed by "f" denote figures; "t," tables